Ultrasound in Clinical Diagnosis

Ultrasound in Clinical Diagnosis
From pioneering developments in Lund to global application in medicine

Edited by

Bo Eklöf, MD, PhD
Clinical Professor Emeritus of Surgery, University of Hawaii, USA
Lund University, Sweden

Kjell Lindström, PhD, MDhc
Professor Emeritus, Department of Electrical Measurements,
Lund Institute of Technology, Lund University, Sweden

Stig Persson, MD, PhD
Associate Professor of Cardiology, Lund University, Sweden

OXFORD
UNIVERSITY PRESS

OXFORD
UNIVERSITY PRESS

Great Clarendon Street, Oxford OX2 6DP

Oxford University Press is a department of the University of Oxford.
It furthers the University's objective of excellence in research, scholarship,
and education by publishing worldwide in

Oxford New York

Auckland Cape Town Dar es Salaam Hong Kong Karachi
Kuala Lumpur Madrid Melbourne Mexico City Nairobi
New Delhi Shanghai Taipei Toronto

With offices in

Argentina Austria Brazil Chile Czech Republic France Greece
Guatemala Hungary Italy Japan Poland Portugal Singapore
South Korea Switzerland Thailand Turkey Ukraine Vietnam

Oxford is a registered trade mark of Oxford University Press
in the UK and in certain other countries

Published in the United States
by Oxford University Press Inc., New York

© Oxford University Press, 2012

The moral rights of the authors have been asserted
Database right Oxford University Press (maker)

First published 2012

All rights reserved. No part of this publication may be reproduced,
stored in a retrieval system, or transmitted, in any form or by any means,
without the prior permission in writing of Oxford University Press,
or as expressly permitted by law, or under terms agreed with the appropriate
reprographics rights organization. Enquiries concerning reproduction
outside the scope of the above should be sent to the Rights Department,
Oxford University Press, at the address above

You must not circulate this book in any other binding or cover
and you must impose the same condition on any acquirer

British Library Cataloguing in Publication Data
Data available

Library of Congress Cataloging in Publication Data
Data available

Typeset in Minion by Cenveo, Bangalore, India
Printed and bound by
CPI Group (UK) Ltd, Croydon, CR0 4YY

ISBN 978–0–19–960207–0

10 9 8 7 6 5 4 3 2

Whilst every effort has been made to ensure that the contents of this book are as complete, accurate and
up-to-date as possible at the date of writing, Oxford University Press is not able to give any guarantee or
assurance that such is the case. Readers are urged to take appropriately qualified medical advice in all cases.
The information in this book is intended to be useful to the general reader, but should not be used as a
means of self-diagnosis or for the prescription of medication.

Foreword

Now that more than one-quarter of all clinical imaging procedures uses ultrasound and the number of ultrasonic scans which are performed each year exceeds all of those done by X-ray computed tomography, magnetic resonance, and radionuclide scanning combined, it is all too easy to forget the origins of this hugely important medical technology. Sixty years ago, however, the use of ultrasound as an investigative tool was little more than a laboratory curiosity. Moreover, the part played by the pioneers is all too easily forgotten and, indeed, it may mistakenly be thought to have been trivial by today's researchers and practitioners, with their well-funded and better-equipped laboratories, their vastly more sophisticated hospitals, and their ignorance of the brilliance and tenacity of the early enthusiasts and the scepticism which they endured amongst their contemporaries.

This fascinating book serves more than one purpose. Perhaps most importantly, it is an historical record of the pioneering developments in clinical ultrasonic diagnosis which took place in Lund, beginning with what we now recognize as one of the greatest medical innovations of the twentieth century. This was the conception and realization, by Inge Edler and Hellmuth Hertz, of the technique called 'echocardiography'—so familiar in modern medical practice that 'echo' has become its simple epithet. It was followed by Lars Leksell's invention of 'echo-encephalography' and his demonstration of its clinical utility. Few will know that this had initially been unfruitful, but that Leksell had subsequently been inspired to carry on by Edler and Hertz.

Medical technologies are often characterized by having short lifetimes of popularity. This was certainly the case for echo-encephalography. It was never widely adopted, because what little reliability it had depended on the skill of the operators: it quickly fell into complete disuse with the arrival of computed tomography. Not so for echocardiography: its clinical utilization is now universal and the range of its contemporary capabilities would surely stagger those who conceived and used the primitive devices of 60 years ago.

Besides its historical content, this book also includes scholarly reviews of the state-of-the-art in adult and paediatric cardiology, obstetrics and gynaecology, vascular disease in several countries, and, primarily from a technical perspective, radiology, as well as an overview contrast study. The general field of echocardiography is discussed in breadth and in depth. In all of these disparate subjects, one thing is clear. This is that innovation may be driven by the needs of clinicians—that is, by 'clinical pull'—or by the inventiveness of scientists and engineers—that is, by 'technology push'—but that progress is most relevant, rapid, and efficient when clinicians and technologists work as one. Nowhere is this more manifest than in the partnership of Edler and Hertz in the history of the emergence of echocardiography in Lund.

Such was the inertia with which the medical community embraced the benefits of innovative technologies—indeed, that inertia has hardly yet diminished—that it was not until the 1960s that the significance of echocardiography began to dawn on the world beyond Lund. In 1966, I myself was privileged to have been amongst the first of those who visited there to learn what could be done and to return home intent on its emulation. The memory of the courtesy with which Professor Edler received a colleague so ignorant and junior as myself remains fresh with me. Later, I was privileged to have Professor Hertz not only as a colleague but also as a friend and my own association with Kjell Lindström has a warmth which I cherish to the present day.

When Ian Donald, Regius Professor of Midwifery at the University of Glasgow, and his colleagues the clinician James MacVicar and the engineer Tom Brown published their seminal work on the investigation of abdominal masses by ultrasound in 1958, it was in Lund and not in the United Kingdom that their ideas were first taken seriously. There, Bertil Sundén, who at the time was working under the supervision of Alf Sjövall, had already begun to experiment with ultrasound, having been greatly influenced by Leksell. He visited Donald and this led to a most productive collaboration between their two centres. Thus, the potential of ultrasound to transform the practice of their specialty was demonstrated not only in Glasgow but also in Lund to the sceptical and conservative community of obstetricians and gynaecologists worldwide. Eventually in 1973, Donald was appointed a Commander of the Order of the British Empire by Her Majesty the Queen, which, being one step below a Knighthood, now seems to many people to have been too small a recognition of his immense contributions. Sadly, Tom Brown, upon whose engineering brilliance Donald understood that his own success depended, received almost no public acclaim at all.

The 1950s was a period of greatly accelerating progress in medicine, driven by the application of science and engineering. Freed from the shackles of World War II, the dividend of peace included technologies which found many new uses in medicine. In cardiology, Andre Cournand, Werner Forssmann, and Dickinson Richards were the recipients of the Nobel Prize in Physiology and Medicine in 1956: their citation was 'for their discoveries concerning heart catheterization and pathological changes in the circulatory system'. Edler and Hertz had to wait longer for the recognition of the profound implications of their demonstration of the ultrasonic examination of the heart in 1953: it was not until 1977 that they received the equivalent of the Nobel Prize, the Albert Lasker Clinical Medical Research Award. Edler's citation was 'for pioneering the clinical application of ultrasound in the medical diagnosis of abnormalities of the heart—probably the most important non-invasive tool for cardiac diagnosis since the electrocardiograph machine' and that of Hertz was 'for pioneering the development of ultrasound technology in medicine'. From our present-day perspective, neither echocardiography nor cardiac catheterization can be said to be the more important: whether used separately or together, they are both absolutely and completely indispensable in the practice of contemporary cardiology. The same indispensability applies to ultrasound in obstetrics and gynaecology, and in vascular studies, in the development of which those in Lund have played so prominent a role.

The co-editors of this book, Bo Eklöf, Kjell Lindström, and Stig Persson, have placed on record the pioneering developments in ultrasonic clinical diagnosis which occurred in Lund and the applications which sprang from them and which now have global impact. They and all the contributors to this book deserve our sincere thanks and hearty congratulations.

Peter N.T. Wells CBE FRS
Distinguished Research Professor
Cardiff University, United Kingdom

Preface

Inge Edler, cardiologist, and Hellmuth Hertz, physicist, in Lund on 29 October 1953, performed the first successful ultrasoundcardiogram (UCG), later renamed echocardiogram. A few weeks later, on 16 December, the neurosurgeon Lars Leksell diagnosed an intracranial bleeding in a 16-month-old boy using the same equipment, and echoencephalography was born. The Lundensian obstetrician Bertil Sundén was in 1962 able to take the first ultrasound picture of twins in pregnancy. These three world premieres at the Lund University were the foundation for the tremendous development of diagnostic ultrasound. Inge Edler (1911–2001), Hellmuth Hertz (1920–1990), and Lars Leksell (1907–1986) are all deceased, but Bertil Sundén (b. 1923) is still going strong.

Before it is too late, the history in Lund will be told, and with this history as background we will engage the leading ultrasound experts of today to bring us up to date with the use of ultrasound in its ever-increasing importance for diagnosis in many areas of medicine. Two of the editors have followed this history: Stig Persson was the successor of Inge Edler at the Lund University Hospital and Kjell Lindström the successor of Hellmuth Hertz at the Lund Institute of Technology. Our idea for this book was to have Swedish experts to describe the development in Sweden, followed by international authorities to describe the global development and state-of-the-art in the use of ultrasound in diagnosis in several disciplines of medicine. You can follow this development in cardiology, obstetrics/gynaecology, vascular disease, radiology, ophthalmology and otorhinolaryngology. In neurology/neurosurgery different diagnostic modalities have taken over. Finally, the industrial development of refined technologies has been important.

Edler and Hertz were several times nominated for the Nobel Prize in Medicine, but the prize has still not been awarded to the field of medical ultrasound. However, the American Lasker Awards often presage future recognition by the Nobel committee, so they have become popularly known as 'America's Nobels'. To date, 80 Lasker laureates have later received the Nobel Prize.

The Albert Lasker Clinical Medical Research Award for 1977 was jointly given to Dr Inge Edler and Professor Hellmuth Hertz, both Lund, Sweden, with the following Award descriptions:

Inge Edler

For pioneering the clinical application of ultrasound in the medical diagnosis of abnormalities of the heart—probably the most important non-invasive tool for cardiac diagnosis since the electrocardiograph machine.

Hellmuth Hertz

For pioneering the development of ultrasound technology in medicine.

As indicated by the title of this book the text will mainly deal with the clinical diagnostic ultrasound (Edler) and not to any larger extent with the necessary underlying ultrasound physics and technology (Hertz).

However, Hertz and his students at Lund University continued to develop new ultrasound methods and technologies for use in different medical applications. For this work a few classical ultrasound textbooks played the most important role, giving us a thorough knowledge as well as inspiration. These books were Ludwig Bergmann's *Der Ultraschall und Seine Anwendung in Wissenschaft und Technik*, 1954, and Peter N.T. Wells' *Physical Principles of Ultrasonic Diagnosis*, 1969, and *Biomedical Ultrasonics*, 1977.

Examples of such ultrasound applications are the first two-dimensional real-time pictures of the moving heart (1967), intracardiac blood flow measurements using continuous wave ultrasound Doppler (1969), fetal breathing measurements, high-intensity focused ultrasound, measurement methods for ultrasound beam characterization, ultrasound tracking methods for real-time blood vessel measurements, technology for blood perfusion measurements, ultrasound vector Doppler tomography, CMUTs (capacitive micromachined ultrasonic transducers), use of ultrasound contrast, and more recently, applications of high-frequency ultrasound in microfluidics and ultrasound communication with dolphins.

New technology can often result in various spin-offs. Such an interesting development came out of the clinical need for a continuous recording of ultrasound M-mode curves or two-dimensional ultrasound pictures. Existing ultraviolet-recorders or photographic film needed subsequent development, which was time-consuming. However, Hertz was aware of a unique electrocardiogram-recorder, developed in Lund by Dr Rune Elmqvist (also the inventor of the implantable cardiac pacemaker in 1958), the Mingograph ink-jet recorder. By inventing an electrical method to intensity-modulate the recorder's ink jet, Hertz was in the mid 1960s able to print out continuous M-mode curves or even colour pictures of a stunning quality.

It is today possible to buy rather cheap ink jet recorders for your personal computer. But if you switch over the ink for chemical solutions, drugs, or even small cells, and use the ink jet recorder as a real micro-sampler (volume size nanolitre to picolitre) and control these samples by ultrasound microfluidics, you might end up with a perfect tool for tomorrows 'lab-on-a-chip'.

Some of this work will be described in more detail elsewhere as one of the authors in this book, the former Vice Chancellor of Lund University, Håkan Westling, is currently working on a separate biography of the life of C. Hellmuth Hertz.

This book would not have been possible without the significant collaboration of eminent Swedish and international experts who contributed their time, efforts, and talents to this publication. We would like to thank Peter Wells for his well-written Foreword. The Royal Physiographic Society in Lund has played a major role in the development. The original paper by Edler and Hertz, 'The Use of Ultrasonic Reflectoscope for the Continuous Recording of the Movements of Heart Valves' was published in their proceedings in 1954, and Edler and Hertz were later awarded their highest distinction. The secretary of the Society, Rolf Elofsson, has been involved in this project from the start and the Society has financially sponsored this publication. Special thanks go to the team at Oxford University Press, Nicola Wilson, Jenny Wright, Victoria Mortimer and Vimal Stephen whose professional and friendly guidance hopefully will result in a book that will be valuable and interesting to read for those who are interested in the development of ultrasound diagnosis in medicine.

Bo Eklöf, Kjell Lindström, and Stig Persson
Helsingborg, Malmö, and Lund, Sweden
15 January 2011

Contents

Contributors *xv*
Abbreviations *xvii*

1. Ultrasound in Lund—three world premieres *1*
   Håkan Westling
2. The development of echocardiography in Sweden *8*
   Stig Persson, Jan Eskilsson, and Nils-Rune Lundström
3. Ultrasound in cardiology—state of the art *21*
   Fausto J. Pinto
4. Ultrasound in paediatric cardiology—state of the art *33*
   Luc L. Mertens
5. The development of echoencephalography in Sweden *43*
   Leif G. Salford
6. The development of ultrasound in obstetrics and gynaecology in Sweden *50*
   Karel Maršál and Bertil Sundén
7. A history of ultrasound in obstetrics and gynaecology *63*
   Stuart Campbell
8. Eugene Strandness and the development of Doppler ultrasound in vascular disease *81*
   David S. Sumner and Kirk W. Beach
9. The development of ultrasound in vascular disease in Sweden *95*
   Tomas Jogestrand and Olav Thulesius
10. Ultrasound in vascular disease—state of the art *106*
    Kimon Bekelis and Nicos Labropoulos
11. The development of ultrasound in radiology in Sweden *121*
    Torbjörn Andersson
12. The early development of diagnostic ultrasound in Denmark *129*
    Jørgen Jørgensen
13. Ultrasound in radiology—state of the art *137*
    David O. Cosgrove
14. Use of contrast in ultrasound *153*
    Tomas Jansson and Anders Nilsson
15. The development of ultrasound in ophthalmology *161*
    Karl C. Ossoinig

16 The development of ultrasound in otorhinolaryngology *172*
Pernilla Sahlstrand Johnson and Magnus Jannert

17 The industrial development of ultrasound—a Swedish perspective *178*
Gunnar Arveheim

Appendix: 'The Use of Ultrasonic Reflectoscope for the Continuous Recording of the Movements of Heart Walls.'—The original paper by Edler and Hertz (1954) *189*

Index *209*

Contributors

Torbjörn Andersson, MD, PhD
Professor of Radiology, Örebro
University, Sweden

Gunnar Arveheim
Director,
Sigtuna, Sweden

Kirk W. Beach, PhD, MD
Emeritus Research Professor, Vascular
Surgery, University of Washington,
Seattle, WA, USA

Kimon Bekelis, MD
Resident, Department of Neurosurgery,
Dartmouth-Hitchcock Medical Center,
Lebanon, NH, USA

Stuart Campbell, MD, PhD
Professor Emeritus,
St George's Hospital Medical School,
University of London, UK

**David O. Cosgrove, BMBCh,
MA, FRCR, FRCP**
Professor Emeritus, Imaging Sciences
Department, Imperial College,
London, UK

Jan Eskilsson, MD, PhD
Associate Professor,
Lund University, Sweden

Magnus Jannert, MD, PhD
Associate Professor,
Lund University, Sweden

Tomas Jansson, PhD
Associate Professor, Department
of Measurement Technology and
Industrial Electrical Engineering,
Faculty of Engineering, LTH,
Lund University, Sweden

Tomas Jogestrand, MD, PhD
Professor, Department of Clinical
Physiology, Karolinska University
Hospital, Huddinge, Sweden

Jørgen Jørgensen, MD, PhD
Associate Professor,
Aarhus University Hospital,
Denmark

**Nicos Labropoulos, BSc(Med),
PhD, DIC, RVT**
Professor of Surgery and Radiology,
Stony Brook University, Stony Brook,
NY, USA

Nils-Rune Lundström, MD, PhD
Professor Emeritus,
Lund University, Sweden

Karel Maršál, MD, PhD
Professor of Obstetrics and Gynecology,
Lund University, Sweden

Luc L. Mertens, MD, PhD
Associate Professor of Paediatrics,
The Labatt Family Heart Center,
University of Toronto, Canada

Anders Nilsson, MD, PhD
Associate Professor, Department of
Radiology, Uppsala University, Sweden

Karl C. Ossoinig, MD
Professor Emeritus of Ophthalmology,
University of Iowa, Iowa City, IA, USA

Stig Persson
Associate Professor of Cardiology,
Lund University, Sweden

Fausto J. Pinto, MD
Professor of Cardiology,
Lisbon Cardiovascular Institute,
University of Lisboa, Portugal

Pernilla Sahlstrand Johnson, MD
Consultant, Department of
Oto-Rhino-Laryngology,
Skåne University Hospital,
Malmö, Lund University, Sweden

Leif G. Salford, MD, PhD
Professor of Neurosurgery, Lund
University, Sweden

David S. Sumner, MD
Distinguished Professor Emeritus,
Department of Surgery, Division of
Vascular Surgery, Southern Illinois
University School of Medicine,
Springfield, Illinois, USA

Bertil Sundén, MD, PhD
Associate Professor,
Lund University, Sweden

Olav Thulesius, MD, PhD
Professor Emeritus,
Linköping University,
Linköping, Sweden

Håkan Westling, MD, PhD
Professor Emeritus and
former Vice Chancellor,
Lund University, Sweden

Abbreviations

2-D	two-dimensional	HIFU	high-intensity focused ultrasound
3-D	three-dimensional	HLHS	hypoplastic left heart syndrome
ABD	automatic border detection	ICP	intracranial pressure
AFI	automated functional imaging	IUGR	intrauterine growth-restricted
AME	air–mucosa echo	IVUS	intravascular ultrasound
ARS	acute rhinosinusitis	LA	left atrial/atrium
BPD	biparietal diameter	LV	left ventricular/ventricle
BWE	back-wall echo	MCE	myocardial contrast echocardiography
CAD	coronary artery disease	MRI	magnetic resonance imaging
CDI	colour Doppler imaging	MV	mitral valve
CEUS	contrast-enhanced ultrasound	NO	nitric oxide
CIMT	carotid intima–media thickness	PACS	picture archiving and communication system
CMR	cardiovascular magnetic resonance		
CRS	chronic rhinosinusitis	PET	positron emission tomography
CT	computed tomography	PI	pulsatility index
CW	continuous wave	ROI	region of interest
DSE	dobutamine stress echocardiography	RV	right ventricular/ventricle
DU	Duplex ultrasound	SAE	stimulated acoustic emission
DVT	deep vein thrombosis	SPECT	single-photon emission computed tomography
EAE	European Association of Echocardiography		
		TGC	time gain compensation
ECG	electrocardiogram	TOE	transoesophageal echocardiogram
EF	ejection fraction	UBM	ultrasonic biomicroscopy
FMD	flow-mediated dilatation		

Chapter 1

Ultrasound in Lund—three world premieres*

Håkan Westling

In the historical section of the monograph *Ultrasound in Medical Diagnosis*, published in 1976, one can read that a substantial part of the early development of the ultrasound-echo method took place in the little university town of Lund in Sweden. It is not without pride that the Lundensians Inge Edler and Hellmuth Hertz comment upon this in a later review article. They also describe what happened in Lund in the 1950s which they thought contributed in a decisive way to diagnostics in cardiology, neurosurgery, and obstetrics and gynaecology. Apart from the cardiologist Edler and the physicist Hertz the pioneers were the neurosurgeon Lars Leksell and the obstetrician Bertil Sundén. Hertz and his pupils were to a high degree responsible for the technical development and the application in all three specialities.

Examination of the heart—first done on 29 October 1953

During the late 1940s and the early 1950s surgery of the heart was started in Lund. The first common lesion to be corrected in adults was mitral stenosis. The valve was opened by forced dilatation. Results were often good but there was a diagnostic problem. In some patients the symptoms were not due simply to a small valve opening. There was also a leakage of blood 'backwards', mitral insufficiency. This condition of course could not be improved by such a primitive operation. Instead, the procedure might make the condition worse. There was thus a great need for improved diagnostics before operation.

This was when the young internist Inge Edler entered the scene. Born in 1911 he had started his career in internal medicine in Malmö but in 1950 he moved to Lund where he became responsible for the preoperative heart evaluations. He immediately focused his interest on the possibilities of making a quantitative diagnosis of mitral stenosis and to determine the existence of mitral insufficiency. Edler's nurse was married to a physicist, Jan Cederlund. Hence it was natural for Edler to ask Cederlund if the radar technique developed during World War II could be used for examination of the heart. Cederlund forwarded the question to his friend Hellmuth Hertz, also a physicist. He said no, but rang up Cederlund after a couple of days and asked for the name of the doctor. Hertz had

---

* This chapter has been partly reproduced from Nilsson J and Westling H (2004). Ultrasound in Lund—three world premieres. *Clinical Physiology and Functional Imaging*, **24**:137–40, with permission.

figured out that it might be possible to use ultrasound. In this way the fruitful collaboration between Edler and Hertz started.

Hellmuth Hertz was born in Berlin in 1920. His father Gustav was a physicist and had received the Nobel Prize for physics in 1926, together with the American James Franck. The uncle of Gustav was Heinrich Hertz; his name was used for the unit of frequency, e.g. in radio waves. Thus the young Hellmuth had an important heritage in physics. During World War II he was taken prisoner by the Americans in North Africa and was transferred to the United States. After the war Hellmuth did not want to return to Germany, neither did he want to stay in the United States. Through studies of mathematics he made contact with his father's friend James Franck in Chicago. Franck contacted another Nobel laureate, Niels Bohr in Copenhagen, who in his turn talked to Professor Torsten Gustafson in Lund. He was a physicist who was good at recognizing talent and arranged for a 1-year scholarship for Hellmuth. This was in 1947. After that Hellmuth Hertz worked as a junior assistant in physics, under Professor Sten von Friesen.

It was not by chance that Hertz suggested that ultrasound should be tried out in diagnostics. As part of his training in physics he had just plodded his way through the 'bible of ultrasound', *Der Ultraschall* by Ludwig Bergmann. After establishing contact with Edler, Hertz immediately went to Kockum's shipbuilding yard in nearby Malmö. He knew that there was ultrasound equipment used to test welding-seams in ships. A sound impulse of high frequency (ultrasound) was sent through the material. If there were irregularities inside, echoes were formed and reflected back to the outside where they could be detected.

Hertz put the ultrasound probe upon his chest and immediately saw an echo that moved in pace with the heart! He was allowed to borrow the machine to Lund over a weekend in May 1953. To their fascination Edler and Hertz could observe echoes from their own hearts as well as from patients. But the machine was not suitable in its present form—to be able to record the movements of the echoes it needed to be modified and supplied with a film camera.

Soon after this Hellmuth Hertz got married and travelled on a honeymoon to Germany. There he left his wife Birgit for a couple of hours to visit Mr Gellinek, one of the directors at Siemens-Reiniger in Erlangen. Hertz's father had worked there 18 years before. Gellinek quickly grasped the importance of the heart observations and Hertz was allowed to borrow an ultrasound machine for 1 year. A couple of months later this machine arrived in Lund—and never left the town.

The 33-year-old assistant at the Department of Physics and the 42-year-old cardiologist started a scientific collaboration that was to last for more than 30 years (Fig. 1.1). Somewhat surprisingly, they were quite different types of personality. Hertz was impulsive and insisted upon the immediate trial of new ideas. Edler, on the other hand, was quiet and more reflective, in fact more practically than scientifically oriented. Maybe the difference in personalities was the reason why they relatively seldom published together. In the cardiological literature Edler most often appeared alone, even if the article contained some physics. The opposite held for Hertz, who only put his name on articles where his own contribution was the dominant one.

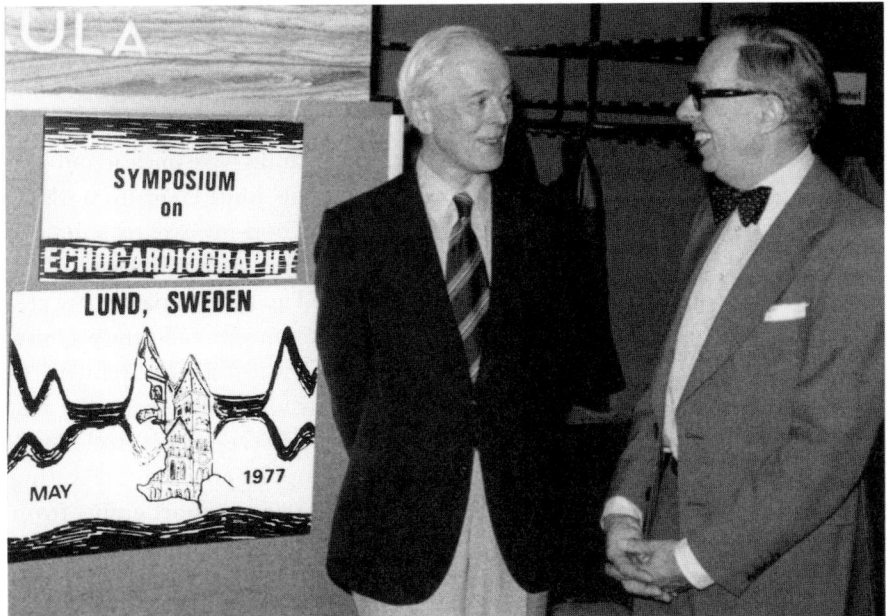

Fig. 1.1 Inge Edler and Hellmuth Hertz welcoming participants to an international symposium on echocardiography in Lund in 1977.
© Håkan Westling, Jan Nilsson, and Per Wollmer, Lund University. Used with permission.

Anyway, in the autumn of 1953 the new Siemens machine could be tested. It had been supplied with an addition that recorded the movement of the heart echoes. The film camera had been built in the workshop of the physics department. On 29 October 1953 the first moving pictures were recorded from the heart. The first echoes came from the hind wall of the left ventricle and from another structure, initially thought to be the wall of the left atrium. An article was published in the *Proceedings of the Royal Physiographical Society in Lund* in 1954—a cardiological classic.

Later on, Edler and his cardiological co-workers, mainly Arne Gustafson, could establish that the most important echo, the second one mentioned above, did not come from the atrial wall but from the anterior leaflet of the mitral valve. The crucial experiments were made in the kitchen of an un-used ward for internal medicine. Calf hearts were used for model experiments. Heart and valve movements were obtained by a pump. Simultaneous filming of the ultrasound echo and the moving mitral valve showed that they 'belonged together'. Further confirmation was obtained in humans using ingenious autopsy experiments.

Recording the movements of the anterior mitral valve became a cornerstone in the preoperative evaluation of candidates for mitral valve surgery. The valvular movements were quite different in stenosis and insufficiency—Edler's vision had come true. The ultrasound method also became useful for detecting blood clots or tumours in the left atrium and for demonstrating the presence of fluid in the pericardial sac.

The subsequent development of echocardiography was dramatic. Soon it was possible to obtain two-dimensional pictures and to visualize in detail the movement patterns of valves and heart walls. Apart from Lund the greater part of this development took place outside Sweden. Swedish cardiologists and thoracic surgeons were used to more sophisticated invasive techniques and thought that the echocardiographic pictures were unclear and difficult to interpret. An exception was the paediatric cardiologist Nils-Rune Lundström who came to Lund and immediately realized the value of an entirely non-invasive technique when investigating small children. And in due time the method was generally accepted also in Sweden. At a recent poll among colleagues, Inge Edler (see Fig. 1.2) was named the greatest cardiologist in Sweden during the 20th century, in competition with full-time professors.

Hellmuth Hertz also had a great career. As professor of 'electrical measurements' at the new Institute of Technology in Lund he obtained a basis for developing many areas of applied physics. Together with talented junior co-workers he created new techniques for two-dimensional echocardiography and for using the Doppler effect for measuring the rate of blood flow. Unfortunately, Hertz did not receive any support grants from the Swedish Board of Technical Development. The advisors to the Board felt that the method

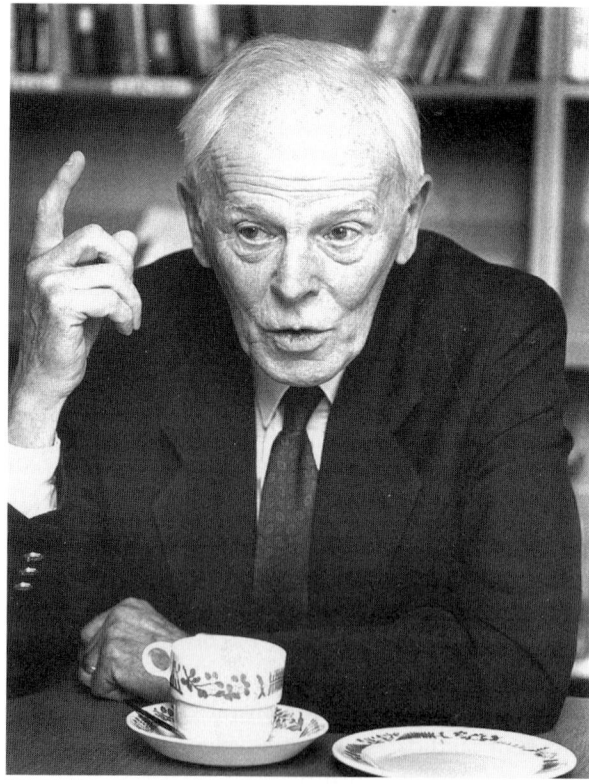

Fig. 1.2 Inge Edler insisting upon something.
© Håkan Westling, Jan Nilsson, and Per Wollmer, Lund University. Used with permission.

lacked medical and commercial interest. This refusal was a long-lasting disappointment for Hertz. Thereafter his developmental work was instead concentrated on the so-called ink-jet writer which was exploited industrially outside of Sweden.

Edler and Hertz were of course nominated for the Nobel Prize several times but they had to be satisfied with the prestigious Lasker Award. The motivation for the prize was rather impressive: 'For pioneering the clinical application of ultrasound in the medical diagnosis of abnormalities in the heart—probably the most important non-invasive tool for cardiac diagnosis since the electrocardiography machine.'

Examination of the brain—first done on 16 December 1953

Attempts to use ultrasound in the field of neurosurgery were made early. The transmission of sound through the brain was studied—but echoes were not recorded. In Lund, the neurosurgeon Lars Leksell started to register echoes soon after Edler and Hertz. He used their equipment and also obtained advice which is gratefully acknowledged in his first paper of 1955.

To his surprise, Leksell found that it was possible to register ultrasound echoes from the interior of the brain whereas previous investigators had found that the skull bones absorbed too much of the sound (Fig. 1.3). That Leksell was successful was probably due

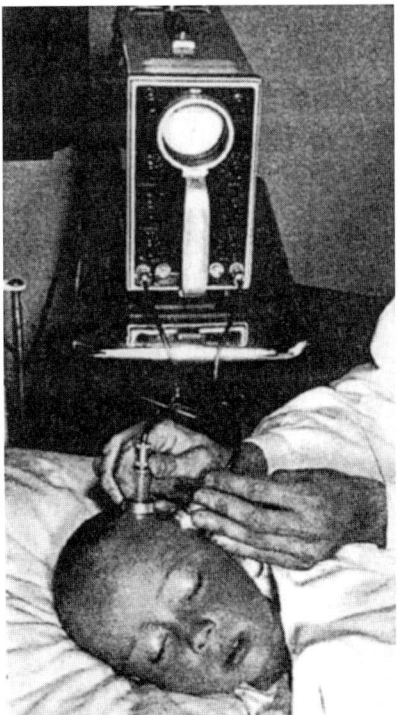

Fig. 1.3 Lars Leksell recording an echoencephalogram on 16 December 1953.
© Håkan Westling, Jan Nilsson, and Per Wollmer, Lund University. Used with permission.

to the fact that he examined children with thin skull bones. The interesting echo came from the midline and it was assumed that it came from the epiphysis. In some illustrative cases Leksell showed that the midline echo was displaced to one side if the patient had an intracranial bleeding on the other side. The first patient was a 16-month-old boy who was examined on 16 December 1953, just 7 weeks after the first heart patient examined by Edler and Hertz.

In his elegant memoirs, Leksell describes vividly another patient in which ultrasound was of decisive clinical importance. Leksell's main interest at that time was extradural haematomas. This patient, a girl of 6 years, was admitted to the hospital deeply unconscious and an intracranial haematoma was suspected. An ultrasound examination showed a displaced midline echo. A hole was burred in the temporal bone on the suspected side—there was no sign of bleeding. Firmly believing that the 'ultrasound was right', Leksell widened the hole and found a large haematoma over the frontal lobe. The blood was sucked out and the patient woke up. Leksell concluded that the diagnosis would have been missed without the help of ultrasound.

The work of Leksell was carried on by Stig Jeppsson who wrote a doctoral thesis on the subject. Echoencephalography was for a long time a handy routine method for the examination of patients with suspected intracranial bleeding. In due time it was replaced by CAT (computer-assisted tomography).

Ultrasound in obstetrics and gynaecology

One day, Professor Alf Sjövall, head of the Department of Obstetrics and Gynaecology, returned from the doctors' luncheon room and reported to his colleagues a conversation with Lars Leksell, the neurosurgeon. Sjövall had been convinced that ultrasound would be useful also in obstetrics and gynaecology. The young resident Bertil Sundén was given the task to explore this. In May 1958 he peformed some trials with Leksell's equipment, without any obvious success. Soon after that, in June, Ian Donald in Glasgow published a new method for ultrasound examination of the abdominal cavity. Alf Sjövall immediately sent Bertil Sundén to Scotland and during some memorable weeks he was introduced into the new technique. Sundén obtained a grant from the Swedish Medical Research Council to buy the new Scottish wonder. It weighed almost 700kg and it took some real effort to install it on the top floor of the clinic building.

Sundén now started to work intensely with the new machine. First, he could show convincingly that examinations with the current technique had no harmful effects, at least not in rats. Both fertility and offspring were quite unaffected. Then Sundén made a survey of the use of ultrasound in his speciality. Obstetrical problems were the most near-lying. Examination with x-rays was potentially harmful to the fetus. Ultrasound examination proved to give valuable information for the diagnosis of early pregnancy, the position of the fetus, twin pregnancy, and some malformations. Sundén was able to take the first ultrasound pictures of twins (Fig. 1.4); this was in 1962. Soon ultrasound examination became a routine practice.

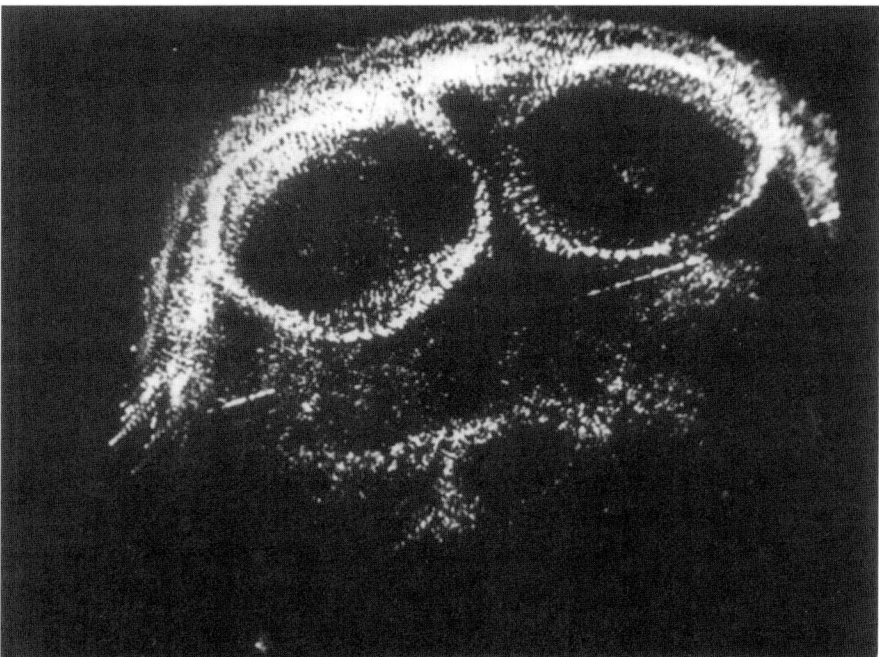

Fig. 1.4 The first echo picture of twins, taken by Bertil Sundén in 1962.
© Håkan Westling, Jan Nilsson, and Per Wollmer, Lund University. Used with permission.

Why Lund?

It may be asked why this powerful development of ultrasound in three widely different medical specialities took place in the Medical Faculty of Lund. It was (of course) not the result of some sort of planning. On the contrary, the development is characterized more by random meetings between persons. But it was not any type of person. One recalls the statement from a biography on Louis Pasteur: 'In the fields of observation, chance favours only the mind that is prepared.' It has also been noted that the University Hospital in Lund was rather small and that most of the doctors took their luncheon in a special room. This is a nowadays overlooked and underestimated link in the communication between different specialists in the care of patients as well as in research.

But in a historical perspective one must still conclude that there were two main factors in the development. First, the present of chiefs that gave talented young workers considerable freedom to follow new leads, and second—but not least—the existence of biomedically-oriented physicists, with Hellmuth Hertz in the lead. With his knowledge, enthusiasm, and generosity he provided invaluable help not only theoretically but also in practicalities—it may be mentioned that the first ultrasound machine of Bertil Sundén had electrical shielding made by used tobacco tins.

Chapter 2

The development of echocardiography in Sweden

Stig Persson, Jan Eskilsson, and Nils-Rune Lundström

The start and the first period of development

Stig Persson

Medical history is filled with innovations contributing to the continuous development of medical science, but some achievements may be thought of as real feats. One event which really deserves such a designation should be the introduction of ultrasound in medical diagnosis. This is a real example of creative thinking that cut across scientific borders and which required a lot of careful and time-consuming work with equipment of initially very primitive standards.

As described by Håkan Westling in the first chapter of this book, it all started in the late 1940s when the young Swedish cardiologist Inge Edler started to take an interest in techniques used during World War II. The account of the very first course of events differ, however, in small details from what I learnt when Edler himself gave me his version. His general aim was to investigate if it would be possible to turn any of the horrors of the war to something positive in the service of mankind. It is true that his first idea was intended for radar and that he got in contact with the physicist Hellmuth Hertz to get advice. When Hertz had judged the idea as unrealistic—the wavelength of radar would not permit a resolution necessary for the visualization of human organs—Edler became interested in the hunt for submarines in the North Sea, where ultrasound was used for detection and as a tool for directing the torpedoes against the right target. Again, he got in touch with Hertz who had recently studied the basics of ultrasound and who immediately realized that it would be a good idea to test it in medical diagnosis. The description of the testing of an ultrasound reflectoscope from Kockum's shipyard in Malmö, Sweden, in May 1953 and another one from Siemens-Reiniger-Werke in West Germany during the autumn of the same year coincides with Westling's report. It is really fascinating to see how human creativity may convert technical equipment originally meant for industrial, non-destructive detection of flaws in materials to the use for diagnosis of defects in the human body.

Inge Edler was born in 1911, studied medicine at Lund University, Sweden, and was first employed at Malmö General Hospital in 1944 where he became responsible for the heart catheterization laboratory in 1948. In 1950 he moved to Lund University Hospital as director of its cardiovascular laboratory. After a short break between 1960 and 1963, when he worked as head of the Department of Internal Medicine at the hospital of Ängelholm, he returned to Lund as appointed head of the Department of Cardiology where he stayed until his retirement in 1977. As Hellmuth Hertz was also employed at Lund University, the fruitful collaboration between the two suggests that Lund may be designated 'the birthplace of echocardiography'.

As Edler himself humbly points out in his overview 'The history of cardiac ultrasound' in 1985 (1), he and Hertz were not the first ones to use ultrasound in medical diagnosis—in 1942 Dussik reported attempts with ultrasound as a diagnostic tool (2) with neurological disease as the target. During the following decade a number of attempts were made to use ultrasound in different specialities, including cardiology by Kiedel (3), but the results were not successful enough to encourage its clinical application. It was not until Edler and Hertz started their investigations with the borrowed reflectoscope that the development started to take a practical clinical direction (Fig. 2.1). However, the possibilities to continue the scientific development and the clinical implications of echocardiography were, in the beginning, both limited and primitive. Much of the initial work was performed on calf hearts mounted in simple glass reservoirs and took place in a kitchen of a closed ward at the hospital. To produce heart movements another glass reservoir connected to the heart chambers was brought up and down by climbing a ladder. Assisting in these preliminary studies were some of Edler's younger co-workers, Arne Gustafson,

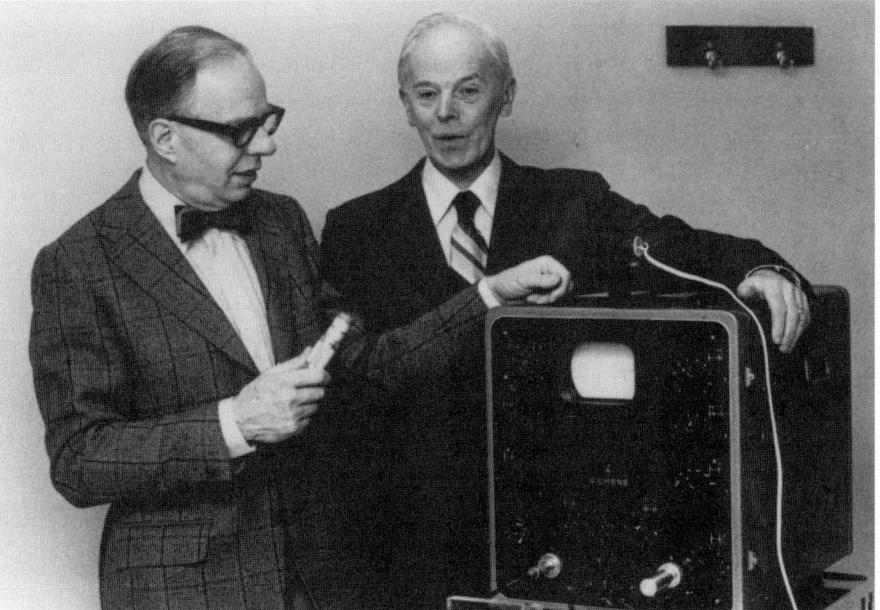

Fig. 2.1 Inge Edler (to the right) and Hellmuth Hertz with the ultrasound reflectoscope used for the recordings of the first echocardiograms.
Reproduced from Holmer N-G, Lindström K, Lundström NR, et al. Ekokardiografins tidiga historioa. *Läkartidningen*, 2002; **99**(12):1360–2, with permission.

Tord Karlefors, and Bo Christensson, of whom Gustafson in particular devoted himself to echocardiography in his later career. These experimental studies were accompanied by investigations on corpses at the pathological institution and by anatomical and physiological studies as well as investigations of the influence of ultrasound on human tissues. Hertz contributed with, besides irreplaceable competent advice, the construction of a device for the printout of the movements of the echo-producing structures in the heart. He placed a cine camera in front of the oscilloscope screen. As the film was wound forward at a constant speed the A-mode echo signals appeared as curves corresponding to the movements of the echo-giving structures. Thus the M-mode technique was introduced into clinical application. This technique was used with the Siemens apparatus in 1953, and the first ultrasound cardiogram was recorded in 29 October 1953 (Fig. 2.2).

During the 1950s Edler literally lived with ultrasound besides his full-time work as a clinical cardiologist and thus his family also played a great part in the course of events. His wife Karin, herself an ophthalmologist, gave him her full support. Their four children—Lars, Eva, Anders, and Agneta—have told how he often brought the ultrasound reflectoscope home during weekends and to the summer house during holidays. He could be seen with the apparatus even on Christmas Eves before joining the family for dinner. The family used to help him by providing coffee and meals when he worked late at the clinic and by

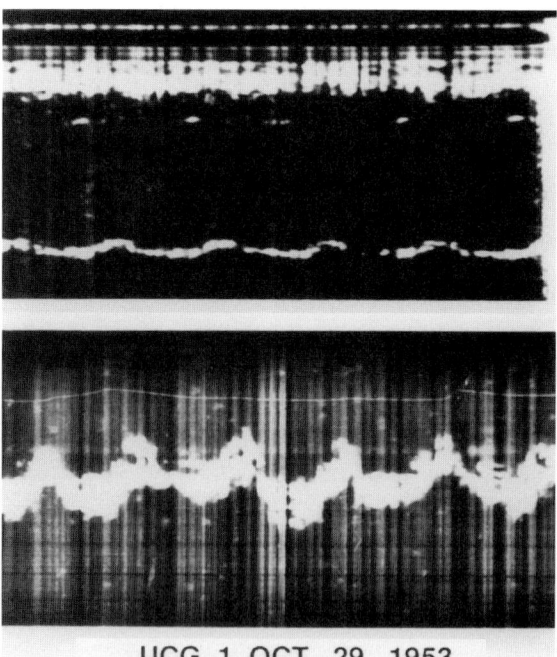

Fig. 2.2 The first recorded echocardiogram from 29 October 1953. Upper panel shows echo from the anterior chest wall (at the top) and the posterior wall of the left ventricle. Lower panel shows the movements of the posterior left ventricular wall at a larger scale.
Reproduced from Holmer N-G, Lindström K, Lundström NR, et al. Ekokardiografins tidiga historioa. *Läkartidningen*, 2002; **99**(12):1360–2, with permission.

also buying and bringing calf hearts to the home. The family also served as 'guinea pigs', and Anders has described how he was forced to swallow a special ultrasound transducer in the middle of the 1950s. However, this attempt failed and, as we know, it took a long time before transoesophageal echo was introduced in the clinical routine.

In this way the developmental work proceeded in spite of simple circumstances and primitive equipment. For example, the transducers with quartz crystals used in the beginning had a sensibility probably 100 times less than those in use today. It is obvious, though, that Edler and Hertz really believed in their work on ultrasound and the first paper on echocardiography was published in the *Proceedings of the Royal Physiographic Society in Lund* (*Kungliga Fysiografiska Sällskapets i Lund Förhandlingar*) in May 1954 (4). During the following years Edler and Hertz worked on improving the technique and finding extended fields of application in examining the heart. Although most of the scientific work was devoted to the movements of the mitral valve, the first clinical application was to diagnose and follow-up pericardial effusion in 1955. The diagnosis of a tumour, a myxoma, in the left atrium in 1956 was described by Edler himself as a climax of the first 3-year investigation. A number of papers were published in scientific journals, at the beginning mostly Scandinavian. At the 3rd European Congress of Cardiology in Rome in 1960, Edler and co-workers presented a movie showing the movements of the aortic and mitral valves, which may still be seen at the Museum of Medical History in Lund. In 1961 Edler presented his summarized findings in his thesis, 'Ultrasoundcardiography' (5), in which he describes the use of ultrasound as a diagnostic aid and its effects on biological tissues, the ultrasound reflections of mitral and aortic valve movements as studied experimentally, and of atrioventricular valve motility in the living human. His co-worker Arne Gustafson concentrated his scientific interest around the mitral valve. His thesis 'Ultrasoundcardiography in mitral stenosis' (6), which was presented in 1966, accounts for relationships between echocardiography and clinical and haemodynamic as well as surgical findings.

Although echocardiography rapidly became a tool in the routine examination of heart patients in Lund, there were difficulties in spreading the message and to get colleagues at other departments in Scandinavia interested in picking up the method. However, during the 1960s there was a growing interest in diagnostic ultrasound in other parts of the world, in particular in the United States and the Netherlands. During these years, Edler and Hertz made numerous trips over the Atlantic and to Europe to visit interested cardiologists and, in particular, factories dealing with the development of ultrasound techniques for medical use.

Parallel to this, Hertz and co-workers were engaged in creating two-dimensional cross-sectional images of the heart with ultrasound. The first instrument was a mechanically oscillating transducer producing a sector scan which was built in Lund in 1960. The technique was successively improved and with the aid of mechanical mirror systems Hertz and co-workers made it possible to present the first two-dimensional images of the heart in real-time. This was done at the Department of Technology at Lund University in 1967 (Fig. 2.3). Although the enthusiasm for the rapid development of ultrasound diagnosis of the heart was great in Lund, it was not so among economic contributors to scientific work

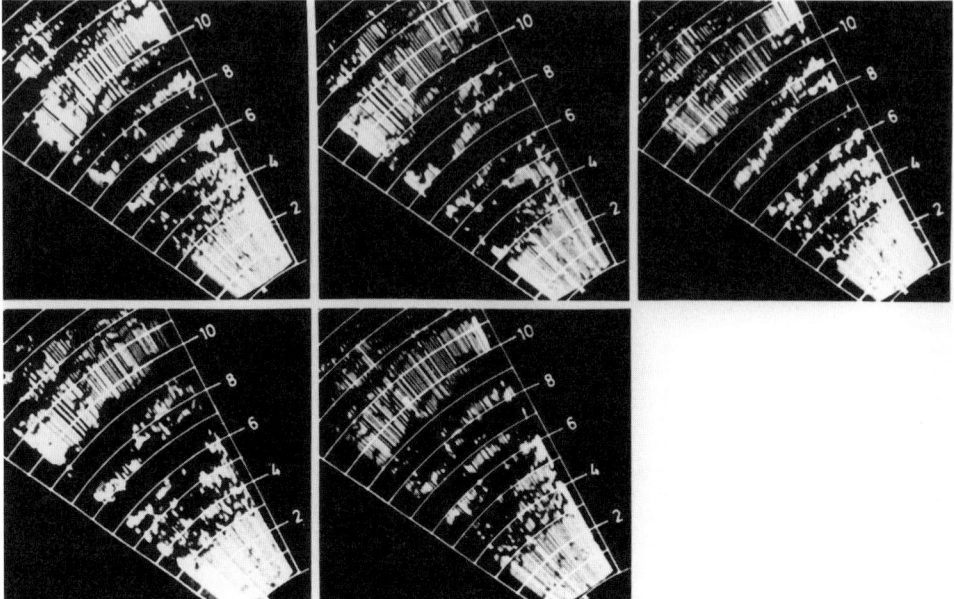

Fig. 2.3 The first imaging of the movements of the heart using the two-dimensional cross-sectional technique developed by Hertz and co-workers in Lund 1967.
Reproduced from Holmer N-G, Lindström K, Lundström NR, et al. Ekokardiografins tidiga historioa. *Läkartidningen*, 2002; **99**(12):1360–2, with permission.

in Sweden. Thus the Swedish Board of Technical Development regarded the project as lacking medical and commercial potential and refused Hertz and his group any support grant. This was, of course, a great disappointment for Hertz, and it explains why the initiative and the continued development of two-dimensional echo moved from Lund to other countries. This decision of the Board should probably be regarded as one of its great historical mistakes.

At the beginning of the 1960s attempts were made in Lund to register intracardial blood flow with the aid of Doppler equipment. In this context, the principal work was done by Edler and one of Hertz's young co-workers, Kjell Lindström, co-editor of this book. Lindström tells that Edler's skill as a clinical cardiologist with an excellent capability to listen to heart sounds was a great advantage in this context. After a great deal of development work the equipment could be tested on isolated heart preparations and later on patients. At the first World Congress on Ultrasound Diagnosis in Vienna in 1969 they were able to present the first 40 clinical intracardial Doppler measurements evaluating leakage in the aortic and mitral valves, besides their experiments on heart preparations.

The pioneering work on ultrasound diagnosis during the 1950s and 1960s should definitely be ascribed to the collaboration between Inge Edler and Hellmuth Hertz. In recognition, they shared the Albert Lasker prize, one of the most prominent of medical awards, in 1977. In the cardiological world, however, the clinician Edler is the one who

> **Box 2.1 A list of Inge Edler's international distinctions**
>
> | | |
> |---|---|
> | 1971 | Honorary member of the American Ultrasound Association. |
> | 1974 | Honorary member of the German Ultrasound Association. |
> | 1977 | Albert Lasker Prize together with Helmut Hertz. |
> | 1978 | Honorary member of the Swedish Ultrasound Association. |
> | 1979 | Honorary member of the Yugoslavian Ultrasound Association. |
> | 1983 | Rotterdam Echocardiography Award. |
> | 1984 | 'Award for scientific work of extraordinary significance' from the Royal Physiographic Society in Lund. |
> | 1987 | Honorary member of the Swedish Society of Cardiology. |
> | 1988 | 'History of Medical Ultrasound Pioneer Award' from the American Institute of Ultrasound in Medicine, the World Federation of Ultrasound in Medicine and Biology, and the Medical Sciences Division of the National Museum of American History, Smithsonian Institution. |
> | 1988 | Münchener and Aachener Preis für Technik und Angewandte Naturwissenschaft [Aachen and Munich Prize for Technology and Applied Science]. |
> | 1991 | Eric K. Fernström's Great Nordic Prize. |
> | 1991 | Honorary member of the American College of Cardiology. |
> | 2000 | Chosen as 'The Swedish Cardiologist of the Twentieth Century' by the members of the Swedish Society of Cardiology. |

has received most attention in the international arena. He has been designated as 'the father of echocardiography' on numerous occasions and has been awarded honorary memberships and distinctions from numerous international associations as shown in Box 2.1. In 2000 he was chosen by the members of the Swedish Cardiological Society as 'The Swedish Cardiologist of the Twentieth Century'.

The continued development of adult echocardiography in Sweden

Jan Eskilsson

During the early 1960s the main clinical application of echocardiography was for evaluating mitral valve disease. The early results by Edler in Sweden and Effert in West Germany were confirmed by Joyner, Reid, and Bond in the United States. Their report from 1963 (7) marks in practice the introduction of echocardiography in the United States and as from then the continued development moved successively from Sweden and, in particular, to the United States. One of the great pioneers there was Harvey Feigenbaum in Indianapolis. In 1965 he and his co-workers presented an improved technique for diagnosing and evaluating pericardial effusion and in the late 1960s they also described methods for measuring left ventricular wall thickness, left ventricular internal dimensions, and stroke volumes. It is obvious that the possibility of studying left ventricular function to a great extent stimulated the growing interest for echocardiography internationally.

During most of the 1960s the interest in echocardiography was generally very small in Sweden outside Lund. However, Ingemar Wallentin in Gothenburg showed an increasing interest and at the end of the decade he introduced the technique in Gothenburg. As a clinical physiologist he combined in his clinical work the use of M-mode echo with other non-invasive cardiac investigations like apexcardiogram and external pulse wave recordings. In Stockholm, a reluctance towards echocardiography remained for several years. One exception was the cardiologist Kaj Lindvall who started to perform M-mode studies of the left ventricular regional function in patients with myocardial infarction in the 1970s.

At this time a new technique was emerging—two-dimensional echocardiography, 2-D echo, which rather rapidly replaced M-mode as the standard echocardiographic technique. M-mode echo could still be used with success in special patient populations, e.g. in the long-term follow-up of patients who had undergone commissurotomy for mitral stenosis, as was for a long period carried out in Lund (8). As pointed out in the previous section, Hellmuth Hertz and co-workers in Lund built an instrument for real-time 2-D imaging of the heart in 1960. They used a mechanically oscillating transducer and a special ultrasonic mirror system which were applied via a water bath contact. With this equipment they could produce a sector scan where, however, only 7 frames/s could be recorded. The technique was successively improved and later on Hertz and his young co-worker Kjell Lindström were able to produce 16 frames/s by using rotating mirror systems. Thus they were able to record the first 2-D images of the heart in real-time in 1967 (see Fig. 2.3). As already mentioned in the first part of this chapter the continued development of 2-D echo then moved from Lund to other countries, mainly due to the fact that the project did not receive any support grants from the Swedish Board of Technical Development.

In 1971, Bom in Rotterdam presented the first real-time 2-D system for practical clinical use. With his equipment a linear scan of the heart was obtained, but the large transducer needed for this was a major obstacle. For instance, not only the intercostals space but also the adjacent ribs were covered by the transducer which to a large extent complicated the interpretation of the images. With the introduction of the mechanical sector scanner by Griffith and Henry Bethesda in 1973, and of the phased array system by Thurstone and von Ramm in Durham in 1976, 2-D echo gradually became established as the golden standard within echocardiography.

During the 1970s and 1980s the annual symposia on echocardiography in Rotterdam played an important role as a meeting point for people interested in ultrasound. Among active participants from Sweden, the clinical physiologist Bengt Wranne from Linköping should be mentioned. In May 1977 a very special meeting took place in Lund. It was arranged as a mark of honour to Inge Edler at his retirement from the appointment as head of the Department of Cardiology at the University of Lund. This symposium (9) focused a great deal on 2-D echo and it is easy to conclude that it contributed to an increased interest in 2-D echo among Swedish cardiologists. From the early 1980s onwards, 2-D echo was established as a routine examination in most of the hospitals in the country. For many years, however, there was a disagreement between physicians representing clinical physiology and clinical cardiology on which department should be responsible for the echocardiographic examinations. This was, in fact, an unfortunate situation which, if anything, had a negative influence on the further development of echocardiography in Sweden.

During the 1960s Edler and Kjell Lindström performed some pioneer work on Doppler cardiography in Lund parallel to the development work on 2-D echo. The Doppler technique was ready for clinical use at about the same time as 2-D echo, but the latter was easier to accept for the cardiological community. Therefore, in Sweden as well as in other countries, Doppler cardiography came into clinical use several years after the introduction of 2-D echo. It should be pointed out that an important role in the transformation of the Doppler technique into a useful clinical tool was played by the Norwegian cardiologist Liv Hatle in Trondheim, who made numerous trips to her colleagues in Lund during this first period of development.

Echocardiographic registration of the mitral valve ring was first described by Edler in 1965, but a more detailed ultrasound study of the movements of the mitral ring was published in 1967 by Feigenbaum's group in the United States (10). Although this study was mainly concerned with the normal ring echo, a smaller amplitude was observed in patients with dilated hearts and significant haemodynamic abnormalities. It may now be stated that it took the echocardiographic community more than 20 years to realize the importance of this finding for the study of left ventricular function, as the vital role of the movement of the heart along its long axis for the ventricular pump function was not highlighted by the Swede Stig Lundbäck until 1986 (11). The echo recording of left atrioventricular plane displacement has now gained recognition as a valuable tool for the assessment of left ventricular systolic function, mainly thanks to Swedish studies by, among others, Christer Höglund, Mahbubul Alam, Birger Wandt, and Ronnie Willenheimer.

Transoesophageal echo (TOE) was introduced in Sweden in the late 1980s. One of the pioneers in this field was Johan Landelius in Uppsala and from the early 1990s TOE was established as a routine investigation, when needed, in universities as well as in regional hospitals. As an example of its use in scientific work, Anders Roijer and co-workers in Lund may be mentioned, who investigated patients with ischaemic stroke in order to find a possible cardiogenic origin.

During the last decade much interest has been focused upon tissue Doppler and contrast echocardiography in Sweden as well as elsewhere. For example, Reidar Winter in Malmö used contrast-enhanced transthoracic Doppler echocardiography for measurements of coronary flow reserve, and Lars-Åke Brodin in Stockholm has made innovative and significant contributions within the field of tissue Doppler. Another interesting application of clinical echocardiography has been developed in northern Sweden, which is partly characterized by remote and sparsely populated areas with long distances between hospitals and echolabs. Here Kurt Boman and co-workers in Skellefteå have constructed a system in which a centrally-situated operator can handle an echo transducer far away with the aid of a robot, thus making echocardiographic diagnosis possible without an educated echocardiographer present at the bed-side.

The development of paediatric echocardiography in Sweden
Nils-Rune Lundström

A unit for paediatric cardiology did not exist in Lund during the first 10 years of the development of ultrasound for cardiac use by Edler and Hertz. When I started paediatric cardiology in Lund in 1963, physical diagnosis and heart catheterization were the important diagnostic tools. I, of course, heard about the work of Inge Edler but it seemed to be of interest mainly in the diagnosis of mitral stenosis, a lesion rarely seen in childhood. After a few years such a patient did, however, appear and I contacted Inge Edler. He examined the patient and demonstrated the usefulness of this diagnostic tool. This was, of course, interesting but the usefulness in paediatric cardiology with its wide variation in malformations of the heart was still not obvious. Shortly thereafter I met a young patient with severe symptoms indicating pulmonary venous congestion, possibly a mitral stenosis. I contacted Inge Edler again and we made an ultrasound examination of the patient together. We found a normal echo from the mitral valve but behind that an abnormal echo with a clear movement in atrial systole (Fig. 2.4). These findings indicated an abnormal structure in the left atrium. Further investigation with heart catheterization and angiocardiography revealed an obstructing membrane in the left atrium, a cor triatriatum. The patient was successfully operated on with removal of the membrane. A new echocardiographic examination revealed that the abnormal echo had disappeared. This episode convinced me of a possible value of ultrasound, even in paediatric cardiology. These initial experiences of ultrasound in paediatric cardiology were followed by a period when Inge Edler showed me how to use his equipment and examine patients and he also gave me opportunity to borrow his equipment until we could obtain our own. I, of course, then examined patients with various diagnoses, but equally important was to examine a large number of normal infants and children to establish normal ultrasound values for various intracardiac dimensions.

My first presentation of the use of ultrasound in paediatric cardiology was made at the 1st World Congress on Ultrasonic Diagnostics in Medicine in Vienna 1969 (12). Characteristic abnormal ultrasound findings were then presented for several cardiac malformations such as Ebstein's anomaly of the tricuspid valve, congenital mitral stenosis, cor triatriatum, hypoplastic left heart syndrome, and membranous subaortic stenosis. At this time I could find only one published article concerning ultrasound diagnosis in congenital heart disease, and this was a preliminary observation on one patient with a membranous subaortic stenosis.

The meeting in Vienna demonstrated the broad early experience of the use of ultrasound as a diagnostic tool in Lund. Presentations were of course given by Edler and Hertz but also by Arne Gustafsson in cardiology, Kjell Lindström concerning cardiac Doppler, Bertil Sundén in obstetrics, and by myself in paediatric cardiology.

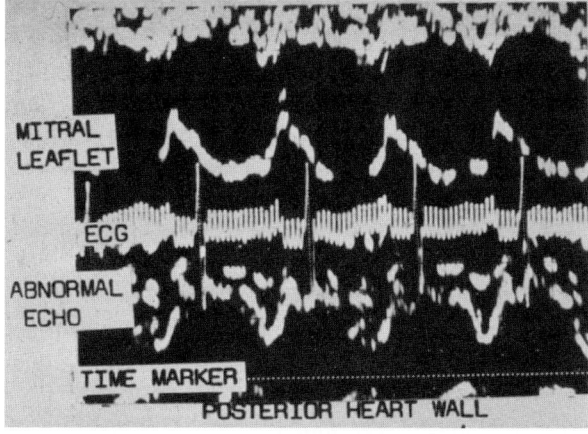
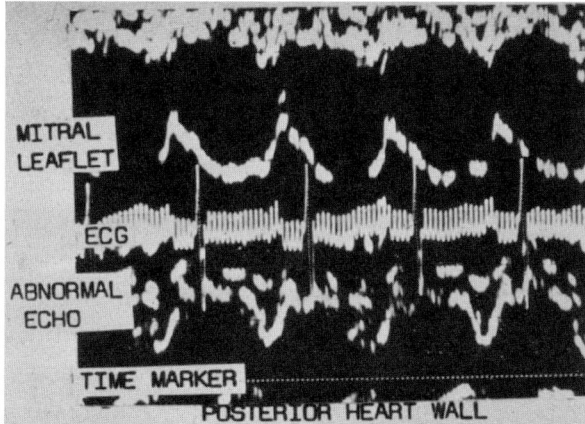

Fig. 2.4 M-mode echocardiography of an infant registered in 1968. The movement of the mitral leaflet is normal but behind that an abnormal echo is seen, later proven to originate from a membrane in the left atrium.
Reproduced from Lundström N-R. Ultrasound cardiographic studies of the mitral valve region in young infants with mitral atresia, mitral stenosis, hypoplasia of the left ventricle and cor triatriatum. *Circulation* 1972; **45**:324–34, with permission from Wolters Kluwer Health.

During the following years we published a series of articles in *Acta Paediatrica Scandinavica* about the clinical applications of echocardiography in infants and children. These articles included normal values of various intracardiac measurements in infants and children of various age and size as well as validation of the relevance of these measurements by comparison with measurement made on angiocardiography. During the same period I also published three articles in *Circulation* about the diagnosis of specific cardiac malformations by echocardiography (13, 14.). One of these articles can illustrate the problem of validating new findings in a small paediatric cardiology unit such as ours. This study was about the diagnosis of Ebstein's malformation of the tricuspid valve, a relatively rare malformation. I examined all patients with this diagnosis seen in our unit with M-mode echocardiography and found consistent abnormal findings (Fig. 2.5). There is, however, variation in the extent of this malformation and a larger patient material would be an advantage. More patients were available at two other paediatric cardiology units in the country but they were situated far away. I therefore took the ultrasound equipment in my car and travelled 600–700km to the two other hospitals and could thereby get a more adequate number of patients included in the study. The abnormal findings were still consistent in all patients.

During the early part of the 1970s the use of M-mode echocardiography in paediatric cardiology was spread to several centres in the United States and Europe. Some years later it was possible for me to bring the experience of several American and European paediatric echocardiographers together and publish a book on echocardiography in congenital heart disease (15).

As described earlier, M-mode echocardiography was of clinical importance in paediatric cardiology but there were limitations. With complex malformations it is important to demonstrate the connection and spatial relationship between different structures in the heart and this is more easily done by two-dimensional echocardiography than with the M-mode technique. The M-mode registrations are also more difficult to understand by those not familiar with the technique. This technique was therefore spread to only a few paediatric cardiologists in Sweden.

The development of two-dimensional echocardiography in the 1970s spread interest for ultrasound as a diagnostic tool in paediatric cardiology. The early two-dimensional pictures were rather crude but the technical development was rapid and it soon became

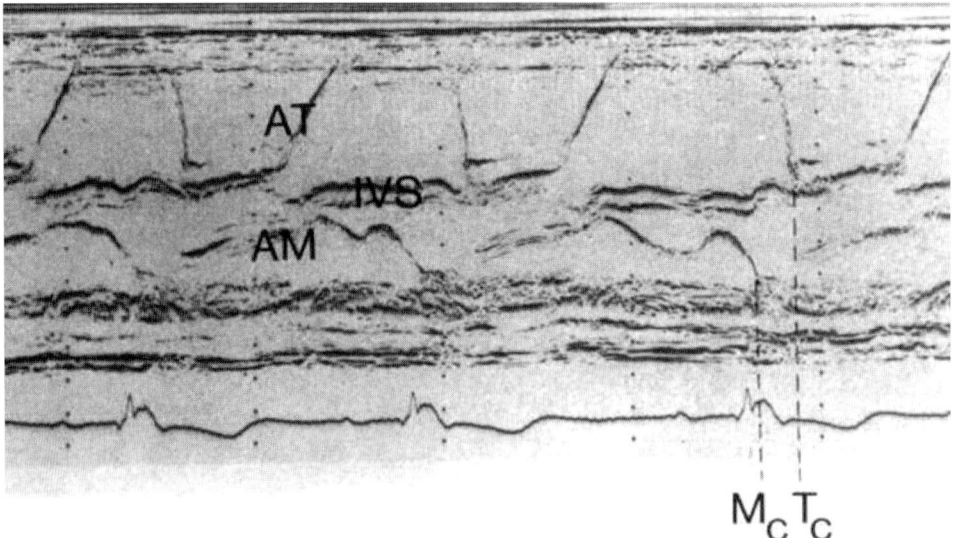

Fig. 2.5 M-mode echocardiogram of a patient with Ebstein's malformation of the tricuspid valve. Echoes from the anterior tricuspid (AT) and anterior mitral (AM) leaflets are seen and between them echoes from the interventricular septum (IVS). The most typical abnormal finding is the late closure of the tricuspid valve (Tc) compared to the mitral valve closure (Mc).

possible to make a detailed ultrasound diagnosis of even complex malformations of the heart.

The introduction of Doppler echocardiography in the late 1970s added another important diagnostic tool—particularly useful in combination with two-dimensional echocardiography.

In 1979 we could bring a group of experienced European and American paediatric echocardiographers and a paediatric cardiac pathologist together in Lund. As a result of this meeting, a book showing the usefulness of ultrasound in the diagnosis of heart malformations and in particular complex malformations was published in 1980 (16).

During the following decades the technical development of the ultrasound technique has been enormous. New applications such as transoesophageal echocardiography and colour-Doppler have been introduced as well as quite new techniques such as three-dimensional echocardiography. All these techniques have been found to be of great value in paediatric cardiology.

Echocardiography has over the last decades been firmly established as the most important diagnostic method in paediatric cardiology. The method is indispensable at the first examination of a patient but is also useful at follow-up examinations. The ultrasound technique has also made it possible to diagnose heart malformations in the fetus. Echocardiography is now routinely used during surgery to control the result of the surgical procedure. The introduction of this non-invasive method has also markedly reduced the need for heart catheterization in infants and children, with its inherent risks and discomfort for the patients.

References

1. Edler I. The history of cardiac ultrasound. In: Giuliani ER (ed) *Two-dimensional real-time ultrasonic imaging of the heart.* Boston/Dordrecht/Lancaster: Martinus Nijhoff Publishing; 1985, pp. 1–16.
2. Dussik K. Über die Möglichkeit hochfrequente mechanische Schwingungen als diagnostisches Hilfsmittel zu verwenden. *Z Neurol* 1942; **174**:153–68.
3. Keidel WD. Über eine Methode zur registrierung der Volumänderungen des Herzens am Menschen. *Z Kreislaufforsch* 1950; **39**:257–71.
4. Edler I, Hertz CH. The use of the ultrasonic reflectoscope for the continuous recording of the movements of heart walls. *Kungl Fysiogr Sällsk i Lund förhandl* 1954; **24**(5):40–58. [Reproduced in *Clin Physiol Funct Imaging* (2004) 24:118–36.]
5. Edler I. Ultrasoundcardiography. *Acta Med Scand* 1961; **170**(Suppl. 370):5–124.
6. Gustafson A. Ultrasound cardiography in mitral stenosis. *Acta Med Scand* 1966; **180**(Suppl. 461): 5–123.
7. Joyner CR, Reid JM, Bond JP. Reflected ultrasound in the assessment of mitral valve disease. *Circulation* 1963; **27**:503–11.
8. Eskilsson J. Mitral stenosis after closed commissurotomy. A clinical and echocardiographic long-term follow-up study. *Acta Med Scand* 1982; **211**(Suppl. 664):7–116.
9. Gustafson A, Persson S (eds). Proceedings of symposium on echocardiography. Lund, Sweden May 13–14, 1977. *Acta Med Scand* 1979; **205**(Suppl. 627):7–327.
10. Zaky A, Grabhorn L, Feigenbaum H. Movement of the mitral ring: a study in ultrasoundcardiography. *Cardiovasc Res* 1967; **1**:121–31.
11. Lundbäck S. Cardiac pumping and the function of the ventricular septum. *Acta Physiol Scand* 1986; **550**(suppl):1–101.

12. Lundström N-R. Reflected ultrasound in the diagnosis of congenital heart disease. Proceedings of the 1st World Congress on Ultrasound in Medicine, Vienna. *Verlag der Wiener Medizinischer Akademie* 1969; **3**:395–405.
13. Lundström N-R. Ultrasoundcardiographic studies of the mitral valve region in young infants with mitral atresia, mitral stenosis, hypoplasia of the left ventricle and cor triatriatum. *Circulation* 1972; **45**:324–34.
14. Lundström N-R. Echocardiography in the diagnosis of Ebstein's anomaly of the tricuspid valve. *Circulation* 1973; **47**:597–605.
15. Lundström N-R (ed). *Echocardiography in Congenital Heart Disease.* Amsterdam: Elsevier/North Holland Biomedical Press; 1978.
16. Lundström N-R (ed). *Pediatric Echocardiography–Cross Sectional, M-mode and Doppler.* Amsterdam: Elsevier/North Holland Biomedical Press; 1980.

Chapter 3

Ultrasound in cardiology—state of the art

Fausto J. Pinto

Introduction

Echocardiography represents the most widely used diagnostic tool in cardiology. From its beginnings, in 1953, when Professor Inge Edler first used it in Lund, Sweden, there always was a clinical question underlying its use and development (1). This might be one of the main reasons why echocardiography has always been one of the most popular diagnostic methods to be used clinically and several authors have named it as the fastest growing technique in cardiology. (2). In fact, there are a variety of areas where echocardiography has proven to be fundamental not only for clinical orientation but also for significantly increasing the understanding of the underlying pathophysiology of the disease process. The other important aspect is the fact that, at the same time, significant technological developments have occurred that have made it possible to develop adequate transducers able to accompany the clinical questions. Some of the main features and contributions of echocardiography in different clinical conditions can be summarized as follows.

Heart failure

Heart failure remains one of the main killers in the developed world with its prevalence increasing worldwide mainly as the result of coronary artery disease (CAD), responsible for almost two-thirds of cases of left ventricular (LV) dysfunction. (3, 4) Echocardiography has played a major role in the understanding of the different mechanisms involved in the development of the different types of heart failure (5–7). In addition, it has helped to monitor and develop new therapeutic targets and strategies in heart failure.

Assessment of left ventricular function

LV function represents the most important prognostic indicator in patients with heart disease regardless of their aetiology (8). Echocardiography has been the main diagnostic tool to assess how much systolic and diastolic function are involved in the mechanism of heart failure in a particular patient (9, 10).

Systolic function

Regarding systolic function, echocardiography can provide different measurements that contribute to a more objective assessment of function, including: global and regional function, degree of ventricular remodelling, contractile reserve, presence of ischaemia and/or viability, particularly in patients post-acute coronary syndromes or post-myocardial revascularization, and the concomitant presence of valvular heart disease, which may significantly impact on the assessment of LV function (particularly the presence of significant volume overload, such as in mitral and/or aortic regurgitation). The use of different modalities such as M-mode, two-dimensional echo, and Doppler flow assessment can provide an array of anatomical and functional information that is very useful in the assessment of patients with heart failure (Figs. 3.1 and 3.2). There are several measurements that can be performed, including internal diameters, areas, volumes, ejection fraction (EF), cardiac output, LV mass, dP/dt (from the mitral regurgitation jet). EF has been widely used as a surrogate of systolic function. More recently, the identification of heart failure with preserved EF has raised some questions on the accuracy of EF in the assessment of cardiac function. The possibility of studying other parameters showed that in most of these patients with heart failure and preserved EF there is, for instance, an impairment of longitudinal function as assessed either by measuring annular motion or by using tissue Doppler

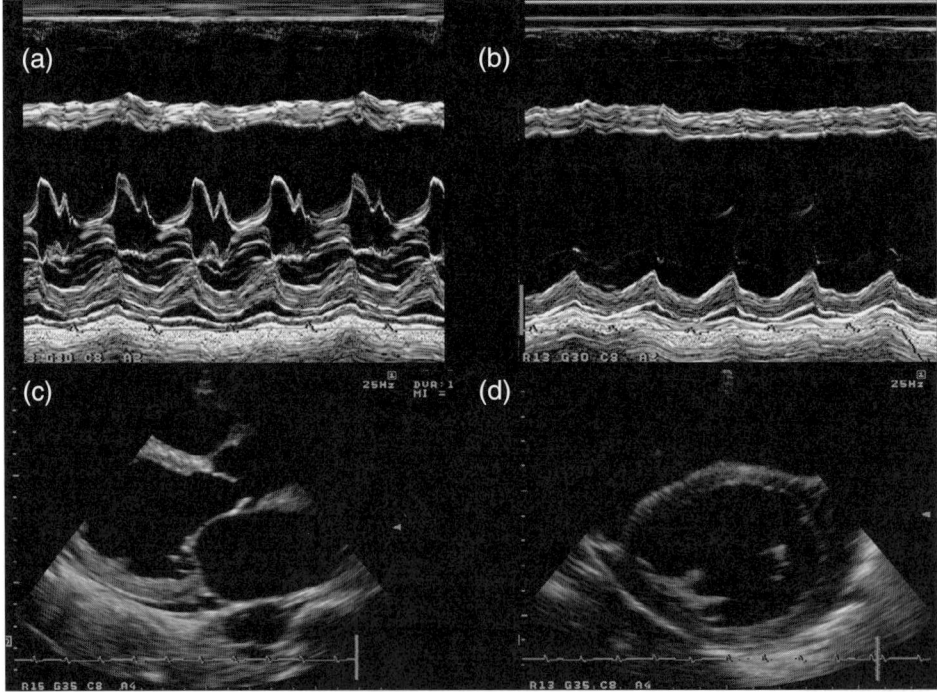

Fig. 3.1 M-mode (a,b) and two-dimensional (c,d) images of a patient with dilated cardiomyopathy, showing an enlarged left ventricle with impaired contractility.

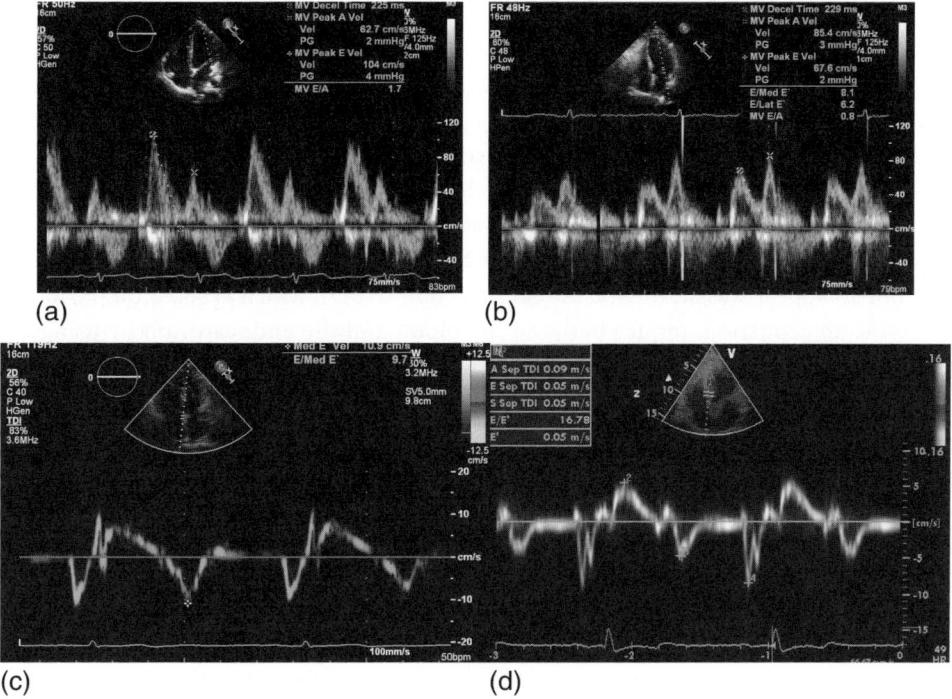

Fig. 3.2 Doppler flow tracings of a normal individual (a) and a patient with impaired relaxation (e<a) (b). Doppler myocardial imaging obtained at the septal part of the mitral ring in a normal individual (c) and a patient with impaired e' velocities (d). (This figure is reproduced in colour in the colour plate section.)

velocities or speckle tracking methodologies (11, 12). This has been shown also to have some prognostic implications (13).

Diastolic function

Echocardiography also provides the ability to study the diastolic phase of the cardiac cycle, supplying substantial information (14–16). Diastolic dysfunction can be defined as the presence of an abnormal filling of the LV together with increased filling pressures. The main causes for diastolic dysfunction are ischaemic heart disease, hypertensive heart disease, cardiomyopathies, systemic diseases—such as amyloidosis, haemochromatosis or Fabry's disease, among others—and valvular heart disease. The introduction of Doppler flow assessment in clinical practice helped to improve our ability of studying and understanding LV filling. The mitral valve (MV) inflow, together with the pulmonary venous flow and the size of the left atrium (LA) provide important information with real clinical applications. The most useful parameters to observe and measure in the mitral inflow are: deceleration time of early inflow (e-wave), duration of the atrial (*a*) wave in the mitral and pulmonary venous flow, and *e/a* ratio. A Valsalva manoeuvre should be routinely performed to differentiate the pseudonormalization patterns from the normal. If there is an *e/a* ratio superior to 2, with a deceleration time inferior to 150ms it means there is restrictive physiology with high filling pressures. In addition, LA size can also provide some information, since an enlarged LA indicates chronic increased chamber pressure.

The use of tissue Doppler added a new dimension to the understanding of diastolic function or, to be more precise, of the filling phase of the cardiac cycle. The main advantage regards the direct measurement of myocardial function, by sampling directly the myocardium with less limitations than blood-flow velocities analysis.

The need to overcome some of these limitations led to the development of new technological refinements and methodologies, which have appeared over the last few years. The first one to appear was automatic border detection (ABD), which is based on the ability to define an acoustic interface between the blood and the endocardium by using the integrated backscatter information from the blood pool and tissues. This method has the advantage of representing the cardiac cycle over time mimicking the volume curves, but it is very much operator dependent as well as image-quality dependent. Some data have been published on its use to assess diastolic function and also to improve border detection, such as in the continuous estimation of cardiac output for haemodynamic monitoring of patients in the operating room and intensive care settings. With further development, this method may measure cardiac output in selected patient care settings (17). This technique may also be regarded as complementary to Doppler echocardiography. The combined use of the methods may improve the diagnosis of LV relaxation abnormalities (18). The waveform of LV area obtained by the ABD technique identifies the phases of the cardiac cycle and correlates with Doppler values of LV diastolic function. Therefore, this new method of ABD has potential uses in the assessment of LV diastolic function (19).

Another method for improving endocardial definition is colour kinesis. In this situation, the heart motion is followed throughout the cardiac cycle and is represented with different colours, according to the amount of motion. One of its developments is called ASMA (automatic segmental motion assessment) and it allows assessment of regional LV function, including the display of a histogram bar graphic. Again, one of the major limitations with this method regards its dependence on image quality and border definition.

One of the main technical refinements over the last few years has been the introduction of second harmonic imaging into the ultrasound systems. With this method an ultrasound beam is sent at a certain frequency and received at doubled frequency. This allows a dramatic improvement of the image quality without losing penetration and it improves significantly the ability to detect endocardial borders (20). The use of second harmonic imaging also allowed the development of contrast ultrasound, since it improved the ability to detect the ultrasound bubbles in the blood pool, as well as in the myocardium. The use of contrast echo to improve endocardial border definition, particularly in some instances, such as during stress echocardiography, is supported by several studies (21).

The use of Doppler to assess myocardial velocities was first introduced in the 1980s, but only in the 1990s did it achieve widespread use. It is based on the ability to sample myocardium and obtain myocardial velocities at a specific site (Fig. 3.2). The rationale behind its use is based on the fact that myocardial velocities are less dependent than blood pool velocities, therefore representing more precisely the different events that occur throughout the cardiac cycle. Some important applications of this method have been differentiating a pseudo normal from a normal pattern, constriction versus restriction, in patients with hypertrophic cardiomyopathy, and more recently in cardiac resynchronization, where it has been used for selection, monitoring, and follow-up of these patients (22–24). Another important application has been on the study of so-called subclinical diseases, such as cardiomyopathies (hypertrophic, Friedrich ataxia, Duchene, etc.), diabetes, ageing, drugs, and athlete's heart. Despite all these applications, the use of pure tissue velocities still has some limitations, with angle dependency and load dependence being the more significant. This was the rational to develop a method that could be more accurate and better assess the sequence of events that occur at a very fast rate in the myocardium, for which the human eye has no capacity to differentiate (our eye can differentiate up to 80ms and some phenomena occur much faster). In recent years the use of strain and strain rate has been adopted as a new modality. With this method we are actually assessing myocardial deformation. Strain is basically the amount of deformation of a certain segment of myocardium, while strain rate is the rate at which this deformation occurs throughout the cardiac cycle. This seems to be a more direct and accurate surrogate of regional LV function (13). Further developments allowed the ability to quantify the amount of myocardial deformation (strain) at the different segments and obtain a bull's eye view of the heart similar to what we've been used to seeing in nuclear cardiology (Fig. 3.3). This is called automated functional imaging (AFI).

Valvular heart disease
Non-invasive haemodynamics

Echocardiography plays an important role in the assessment of valvular heart disease for several reasons: assessment of valve morphology and function, therefore helping to

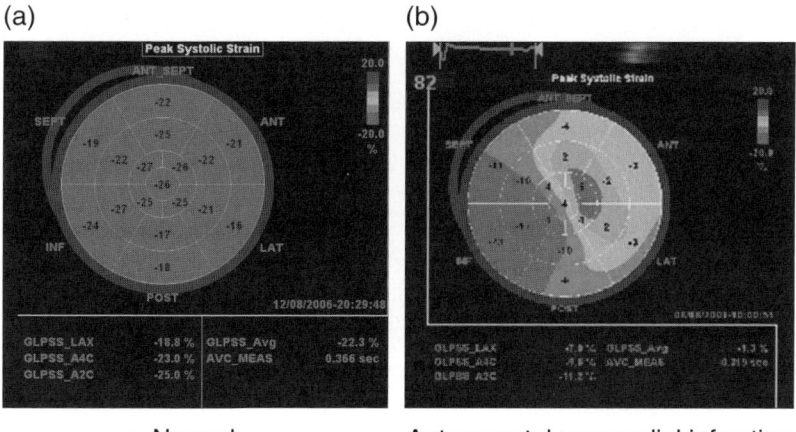

Fig. 3.3 Automatic functional imaging (AFI) with a bull's eye display of a normal individual (a) and a patient who suffered an anteroseptal infarction, with the corresponding segmental abnormalities (b). (This figure is reproduced in colour in the colour plate section.)

determine the mechanism of valve disease, impact of valve disease in chamber function, LV function, LA function, etc. but one of the most relevant contributions has been the ability to non-invasively assess cardiac haemodynamics. The work of Liv Hatle and co-workers in the 1970s and 1980s using Doppler flow assessment to determine non-invasively the cardiac haemodynamics has changed the whole concept of haemodynamic assessment in the living patient (25–27). One of the areas where its application has been more useful is in the assessment of valvular heart disease severity. In fact, with the use of Doppler determinations it is possible to obtain variables such as gradients across valves (using the Bernoulli equation), valve areas (continuity equation), regurgitant volumes, determine pulmonary artery pressure, etc.

The use of transoesophageal echocardiography (TOE) has improved the assessment of valve disease, in particular, mitral valve disease. More recently the development of three-dimensional technology adapted to TOE probes expanded the use of this method not only for diagnostic purposes but also in the operating room to guide surgical treatment (Fig. 3.4). It has also been used in the catheterization laboratory to guide interventional procedures, such as percutaneous closure of atrial septal defects, percutaneous valve implantations, closure of perivalvular leaks, occlusion of LA appendage, etc. (28, 29)

Coronary artery disease

The use of echocardiography in patients with known or suspected coronary artery disease can be quite extensive, including assessment of baseline cardiac function; detection of changes in wall motion contractility either at rest or induced by exercise or pharmacologically, suggesting myocardial ischemia; detection of myocardial viability, helping to identify the subgroup of patients that will benefit from myocardial revascularization;

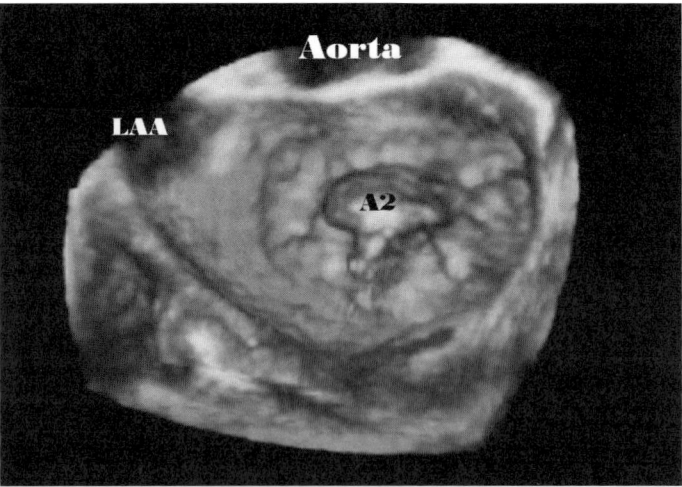

Fig. 3.4 Transoesophageal three-dimensional echocardiogram of a patient with a mitral valve prolapse involving the middle scallop of the anterior leaflet (A2). (This figure is reproduced in colour in the colour plate section.)

detection of acute complications in the setting of acute myocardial infarction, e.g. cardiac rupture, ventricular septal defect, acute mitral regurgitation, etc. (30).

Diagnosing myocardial ischaemia and viability

In patients with known or suspected coronary artery disease the main question to ask is if there is induced myocardial ischaemia. The use of stress echocardiography has been an important development to use as a clinical tool that can be easily applied, even at bedside if necessary, to rule out or confirm myocardial ischaemia. With a very high sensitivity and specificity, similar to the competing modalities, as scintigraphy, it has the main advantage of being radiation free and also provides other relevant information at the same time, such as morphology and function of cardiac valves and chambers (31).

In addition, the inclusion of the novel ultrasound modalities, such as Doppler myocardial imaging has further improved the accuracy of using echocardiography for assessing myocardial ischaemia. For instance, it has been shown that during coronary occlusion there is a significant decrease in absolute strain, as well as a displacement of peak strain to end systole or even early diastole, in what is called post-systolic thickening (32). This has also been shown as a marker of myocardial viability. More recently, the added value of strain in stress echo using dobutamine, increasing its sensitivity and specificity, has been shown by a few groups (33).

Chronic left ventricular dysfunction

In assessing patients with chronic LV dysfunction there are two important questions to investigate: 1) how to distinguish ischaemic from non-ischaemic cardiomyopathy and 2) how to identify the candidates that will benefit most from revascularization.

The importance of myocardial viability has been shown in several studies where the patients who showed significant viability and were revascularized had a much better prognosis (34, 35). However, it also shows that revascularization in the absence of viability can be highly deleterious. This highlights the need for proper investigation of these patients. A number of non-invasive imaging procedures have been developed to evaluate myocardial viability and to identify markers of functional recovery, including dobutamine stress echocardiography (DSE), myocardial contrast echocardiography (MCE), single-photon emission computed tomography (SPECT), positron emission tomography (PET), and cardiovascular magnetic resonance (CMR) imaging. All of them have shown similar sensitivity and specificity (36). The use of stress echo has been shown to predict survival (37). It is also important to understand that the worse the LV function is in the presence of viability, the better are the results of revascularization (38). In addition there is a direct correlation between the degree of myocardial viability and functional recovery. Only when more than four segments show myocardial viability is a significant improvement in functional recovery observed. This is very important since it means that both presence and significant extension of viability have to occur to predict functional recovery. More recently the same authors also showed that once the patients with significant viability are identified and the sooner they are revascularized the better for the outcome and prognosis (39).

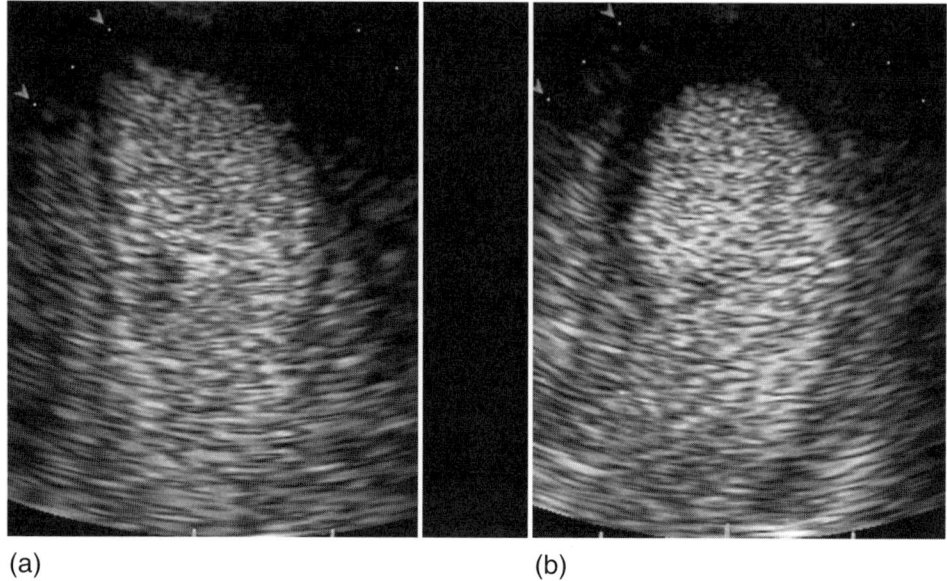

(a) (b)

Fig. 3.5 Myocardial perfusion imaging using contrast echocardiography showing a perfusion defect in the distal septum and apex in a patient with a tight left anterior descending lesion. (a) Two- and (b) four-chamber views denote different projections of the image. (This figure is reproduced in colour in the colour plate section.)

MCE is a technique that uses microbubbles during echocardiography. These microbubbles remain exclusively within the intravascular space, and their presence within any myocardial territory denotes the status of microvascular perfusion within that region. It has been used to diagnose myocardial ischaemia and myocardial viability (40, 41) (Fig. 3.5). It has also been shown that the extent and severity of contrast perfusion defects after acute myocardial infarction predict mortality and combined mortality/reinfarction independent of clinical factors, electrocardiogram (ECG) parameters, cardiac biomarkers, and resting LV EF (42).

Subclinical disease

The early diagnosis of disease represents a major goal in medicine. Early detection means earlier ability to intervene. Echocardiography has been shown to be able to detect early changes in some disease processes that may help to change the natural history of some conditions. Among these some have had more visibility:

1. Patients undergoing **chemotherapy** with cardiac toxic agents. Echocardiography, particularly by using tissue Doppler, has been shown to be more sensitive for the detection of early impairment of systolic function than the crude measurement of EF (43).
2. Some **infiltrative diseases**, such as Fabry's disease or amyloidosis, may benefit from early diagnosis and subsequently an earlier intervention can be started. In Fabry's

disease, for example, it has been shown that early intervention will delay and even prevent myocardial involvement or promote its regression (44).

3. In **obesity,** the use of new parameters such as torsion has shown that apparently healthy individuals with obesity already show abnormalities that can be detected by ultrasound (45).

4. **Diabetes**—the use of echocardiography in diabetic patients can detect early changes in myocardial function that can be attributed to early diabetic cardiomyopathy (46).

5. **Aging**—the aging process implies a set of physiological changes in heart function and structure that can be detected by ultrasound assessment. For instance, the changes that occur in diastolic function, with an increasingly more rigid LV with aging can be detected and differentiated from true diastolic dysfunction. The mild fibrotic changes that can be observed with aging can also be followed-up. It is very important to distinguish the normal aging changes from truly pathological conditions (47).

6. **Athlete's heart**—one of the more difficult differential diagnoses is the one between athlete's heart and cardiomyopathy in certain athletes. This is of utmost relevance since the presence of underlying heart disease in an athlete can be deleterious and even fatal. On the other hand, to label an athlete with a cardiac condition can halt a potential career. Echocardiography has also been shown to be helpful in these circumstances. For example, the presence of higher tissue velocities in the athlete's heart, particularly when challenged either by exercise or DSE, is one of the ways to make the differential diagnosis (48).

Conclusions

It is clear that echocardiography has become the most used diagnostic method in cardiology. Its major impact has been on improving the understanding of many disease processes as well as helping in medical diagnosis, therefore impacting directly on patient care. New technological refinements will further expand the use of echo, such as Doppler myocardial imaging, contrast echocardiography, particularly myocardial perfusion assessment, and three-dimensional echo. The future is open to novelty and to the wit of the newcomers.

References

1. Edler I, Hertz CH. The use of ultrasonic reflectoscope for the continuous recording of the movements of heart walls. 1954. *Clin Physiol Funct Imaging* 2004; 24:118–36.
2. Braunwald E. Shattuck lecture – Cardiovascular medicine at the turn of the millennium: triumphs, concerns and opportunities. *N Eng J Med* 1997; **337:**1360–9.
3. Alderman EL, Fisher LD, Litwin P, Kaiser GC, Myers WO, Maynard C, et al. Results of coronary artery surgery in patients with poor left ventricular function (CASS). *Circulation* 1983; **68**(4):785–95.
4. Krishnamani R, El Zaru M, DeNofrio D. Contemporary medical, surgical, and device therapies for end-stage heart failure. *Curr Treat Options Cardiovasc Med* 2003; 5(6):487–99.
5. Carerj S, La Carrubba S, Antonini-Canterin F, Di Salvo G, Erlicher, Liguori E, et al. The incremental prognostic value of echocardiography in asymptomatic stage A heart failure. *J Am Soc Echocardiography* 2010; 23:1025–34.

6. Colonna P, Pinto FJ, Sorino M, Bovenzi F, D'Agostino, De Luca I. The emerging role of echocardiography in the screening of patients at risk of heart failure. *Am J Cardiol* 2005; **96**(12 Suppl. 1):42–51.
7. Marwick TH, Raman CV, Carrió I, Bax JJ. Recent developments in heart failure imaging. *JACC Cardiovasc Imaging* 2010; **3**:429–39.
8. Mosterd A, Hoes AW. Clinical epidemiology of heart failure. *Heart* 2007; **93**:1137–46.
9. Pinto FJ. Echocardiography in left ventricular dysfunction. *Ital Heart J* 2004; Suppl. **6**:41S–47S.
10. Grothues F, Braun-Dullaeus R. Serial assessment of ventricular morphology and function. *Heart Fail Clin* 2009; **24**:410–14.
11. Leong DP, De Pasquale CG, Selvanayagam JB. Heart failure with normal ejection fraction: the complementary roles of echocardiography and CMR imaging. *JACC Cardiovasc Imaging* 2010; **3**:409–20.
12. Triantafyllou KA, Karabinos E, Kalkandi H, Kranidis AI, Babalis D. Clinical implications of the echocardiographic assessment of left ventricular long axis function. *Clin Res Cardiol* 2009; **98**:521–32.
13. Stanton T, Leano R, Marwick TH. Prediction of all cause mortality from global longitudinal speckle tracking: comparison with ejection fraction and wall motion scoring. *Circ Cardiovasc Imaging* 2009; **2**:356–64.
14. Gibson D, Francis D. Clinical assessment of left ventricular diastolic function. *Heart* 2003; **89**:231–8.
15. Paulus WJ, Tschope C, Sanderson JE, Rusconi C, Flachskampf FA, Rademakers FE, *et al*. How to diagnose diastolic heart failure: a consensus statement on the diagnosis of heart failure with normal left ventricular ejection fraction by the Heart Failure and Echocardiography Associations of the European Society of Cardiology. *Eur Heart J* 2007; **28**:2539–50.
16. Oh JK, Hatle L, Tajik AJ, Little WC. Diastolic heart failure can be diagnosed by comprehensive two-dimensional and Doppler echocardiography. *J Am Coll Cardiol* 2006; **47**:500–6.
17. Pinto FJ, Siegel LC, Chenzbraun A, Schnittger I. On-line estimation of cardiac output with a new automated edge detection system using transesophageal echocardiography: a preliminary comparison with thermodilution. *J Cardiothorac Vasc Anesth J* 1994; **8**:625–30.
18. Chenzbraun A, Pinto FJ, Milton S, Schnittger I, Popp RL. Comparison of acoustic quantification and Doppler echocardiography in assessment of left ventricular diastolic parameters. *Br Heart J* 1993; **70**:448–56.
19. Chenzbraun A, Pinto FJ, Popylisen S, Schnittger I, Popp RL. Filling patterns in left ventricular hypertrophy: a combined acoustic quantification and Doppler study. *J Am Coll Cardiol* 1994; **23**:1179–85.
20. Van Camp G, Franken P, Schoors D, Hagers Y, Koole M, Demoor D, *et al*. Impact of second harmonic imaging on the determination of the global and regional left ventricular function by 2D echocardiography. *Eur J Echocardiogr* 2000; **1**:122–9.
21. Agati L, Tonti G, Galiuto L, Di Bello V, Funaro S, Madonna MP, *et al*. Quantification methods in contrast echocardiography. *Eur J Echocardiogr* 2005; Suppl. **2**:S14–S20.
22. Hatle L, Sutherland G. Regional myocardial function – a new approach. *Eur Heart J* 2000; **21**: 1337–57.
23. Bijnens BH, Cikes M, Claus P, Sutherland GR. Velocity and deformation imaging for the assessment of myocardial dysfunction. *Eur J Echocardiogr* 2009; **10**:216–26.
24. Abraham T, Kass D, Tonti G, Tomassoni GF, Abraham WT, Bax JJ, *et al*. Imaging cardiac resynchronisation therapy. *JACC Cardiovasc Imaging* 2009; **2**:486–97.
25. Hatle L. Non-invasive measurements of intracardiac blood flow velocities with Doppler ultrasound. *Acta Med Scand* 1987; **221**:133–6.
26. Hatle L. Doppler echocardiographic evaluation of mitral stenosis. *Cardiol Clin* 1990; **8**:233–47.
27. Baumgartner H, Hung J, Bermejo J, Chambers JB, Evangelista A, Griffin BP, *et al*. EAE/ASE Echocardiographic assessment of valve stenosis: EAE/ASE recommendations for clinical practice. *Eur J Echocardiogr* 2009; **10**:479.

28. Cobanu A, Bennett S, Azam M, Clark A, Vinereanu D. Incremental value of three-dimensional transoesophageal echocardiography for guiding double percutaneous MitraClip® implantation in a 'no option' patient. *Eur J Echocardiogr* 2010; **12**(2):E11.
29. Saric M, Perk G, Purgess JR, Kronzon I. Imaging atrial septal defects by real-time three dimensional transesophageal echocardiography: step by step approach. *J Am Soc Echocardiogr* 2010; **23**:1128–35.
30. Nihoyannopoulos P, Pinto FJ. Ischemic heart disease. In: Badano L, Fox K, Sicari R, Zamorano JL (eds) *The EAE Textbook of Echocardiography*. Oxford: Oxford University Press; 2011, chapter 12.
31. Sicari R, Nihoyannopoulos P, Evangelista A, Kasprzak J, Lancellotti P, Poldermans D, et al. Stress echocardiography expert consensus statement: European Association of Echocardiography (EAE) (a registered branch of the ESC). *Eur J Echocardiogr* 2008; **9**:415–37.
32. Kukulski T, Jamal F, Herbots L, D'hooge J, Bijnens B, Hatle L, et al. Identification of acutely ischemic myocardium using ultrasonic strain measurements: A clinical study in patients undergoing coronary angioplasty. *J Am Coll Cardiol* 2003; **41**:810–19.
33. Voigt JU, Nixdorff U, Bogdan R, Exner B, Schmiedehausen K, Platsch G, et al. Comparison of deformation imaging and velocity imaging for detecting regional inducible ischaemia during dobutamine stress echocardiography. *Eur Heart J* 2004; **25**:1517–25.
34. Baker DW, Jones R, Hodges J, Massie BM, Konstam MA, Rose EA. Management of heart failure. III. The role of revascularization in the treatment of patients with moderate or severe left ventricular systolic dysfunction. *JAMA* 1994; **272**(19):1528–34.
35. Holmes DR, Jr, Detre KM, Williams DO, Kent KM, King SB, III, Yeh W, et al. Long-term outcome of patients with depressed left ventricular function undergoing percutaneous transluminal coronary angioplasty. The NHLBI PTCA Registry. *Circulation* 1993; **87**(1):21–9.
36. Rizzello V, Poldermans D, Bax JJ. Assessment of myocardial viability in chronic ischemic heart disease: current status. *Q J Nucl Med Mol Imaging* 2005; **49**(1):81–96.
37. Beanlands RS, Hendry PJ, Masters RG, deKemp RA, Woodend K, Ruddy TD. Delay in revascularization is associated with increased mortality rate in patients with severe left ventricular dysfunction and viable myocardium on fluorine 18-fluorodeoxyglucose positron emission tomography imaging. *Circulation* 1998; **98**(19 Suppl.):II51–56.
38. Senior R, Lahiri A. Dobutamine echocardiography predicts functional outcome after revascularisation in patients with dysfunctional myocardium irrespective of the perfusion pattern on resting thallium-201 imaging. *Heart* 1999; **82**(6):668–73.
39. Bax JJ, Schinkel AF, Boersma E, Rizzelo V, Elhendy A, Maat A, et al. Early versus delayed revascularization in patients with ischemic cardiomyopathy and substantial viability: impact on outcome. *Circulation* 2003; **108**(Suppl 1):II39–42.
40. Wei K, Jayaweera AR, Firoozan S, Linka A, Skyba DM, Kaul S. Basis for detection of stenosis using venous administration of microbubbles during myocardial contrast echocardiography: bolus or continuous infusion? *J Am Coll Cardiol* 1998; **32**(1):252–60.
41. Janardhanan R, Moon JC, Pennell DJ, Senior R. Myocardial contrast echocardiography accurately reflects transmurality of myocardial necrosis and predicts contractile reserve after acute myocardial infarction. *Am Heart J* 2005; **149**(2):355–62.
42. Dwivedi G, Janardhananan R, Hayat SA, Swinburn JM, Senior R. Prognostic value of myocardial viability detected by myocardial contrast echocardiography early after acute myocardial infarction. *J Am Coll Cardiol* 2007; **50**(4):327–34.
43. Ho E, Brown A, Barrett P, Morgan RB, King G, Kennedy MJ, et al. Subclinical anthracycline-and trastuzumab-induced cardiotoxicity in the long term follow up of asymptomatic breast cancer survivors: a speckle tracking echocardiographic study. *Heart* 2010; **96**:701–7.
44. Cikes M, Sutherland GR, Anderson LJ, Bijnens BH. The role of echocardiographic deformation imaging in hypertrophic myopathies. *Nat Rev Cardiol* 2010; **7**:384–96.

45. Kosmala W, O'Moore-Sullivan TM, Plaksej R, Kulliczkowska-Plaksej J, Przewlocka-Kosmala M, Marwick TH. Subclinical impairment of left ventricular function in young obese women: contribution of polycystic ovary disease and insulin resistance. *J Clin Endocrinol Metab* 2008; **93**:3748–54.
46. Jellis CL, Stanton T, Leano R, Martin J, Marwick TH. Usefulness of at rest and exercise hemodynamics to detect subclinical myocardial disease in type 2 diabetes mellitus. *Am J Cardiol* 2010; **107**(4):615–21.
47. Cheng S, Xanthakis V, Sullivan LM, Lieb W, Massaro J, Aragam J, *et al.* Correlates of echocardiographic indices of cardiac remodeling over the adult life course: longitudinal observations from the Framingham Heart Study. *Circulation* 2010; **122**:570–8.
48. Vinereanu D, Florescu N, Sculthorpe N, Tweddel AC, Stephens MR, Fraser AG. Left ventricular long axis diastolic function is augmented in the hearts of endurance-trained compared with strength-trained athletes. *Clinical Science* 2002; **103**:249–57.

Chapter 4

Ultrasound in paediatric cardiology— state of the art

Luc L. Mertens

Introduction

The development of ultrasound technology to visualize cardiac structures, based on the pioneering work by Edler and Hertz at the University of Lund in Sweden, has literally created a revolution in the field of paediatric cardiology. Before the era of cardiac catheterization and echocardiography the diagnosis of congenital heart disease was mainly based on combining physical findings, cardiac auscultation, electrocardiogram (ECG), and chest X-ray. This was largely based on the work by Helen B. Taussig at John Hopkins in the 1930s who established the field of clinical paediatric cardiology by integrating pathology knowledge with clinical findings. Diagnosis at that time was based on clinical skills and was more an art than science. The introduction of paediatric cardiac surgery in the 1950s was made possible due to the simultaneous development of cardiac catheterization and angiography which allowed an accurate description of the different cardiac lesions and the associated haemodynamics prior to surgery. For a long period catheterization was the diagnostic gold standard and all surgical patients underwent an invasive cardiac evaluation. In the 1970s, echocardiography was developed as a clinical tool and due to its non-invasive nature, was introduced quickly in paediatric cardiology. As anatomical diagnosis is challenging by M-mode echocardiography, it was really the development of two-dimensional (2-D) echocardiography in the late 1970s and early 1980s that deeply influenced the field. For the first time the congenital defects could be imaged non-invasively and the 2-D images were extensively validated by comparing them with pathological and surgical findings. Adding pulsed, continuous, and colour Doppler data to the 2-D images resulted in a complete detailed description of congenital cardiac defects and their haemodynamic consequences. Further optimization of ultrasound technology specifically for paediatric imaging, such as the development of higher-frequency probes and increasing the standard grey-scale frame rates, further improved spatial and temporal resolution and overall image quality (see Fig. 4.1). Based on its excellent diagnostic accuracy and its non-invasive nature, echocardiography quickly became the primary non-invasive diagnostic technique for all children with heart disease. Currently every paediatric patient with suspected heart disease will undergo an echocardiographic examination as the first (and often only) diagnostic test. Specialized paediatric echocardiography laboratories were established within larger paediatric cardiology centres and these contributed

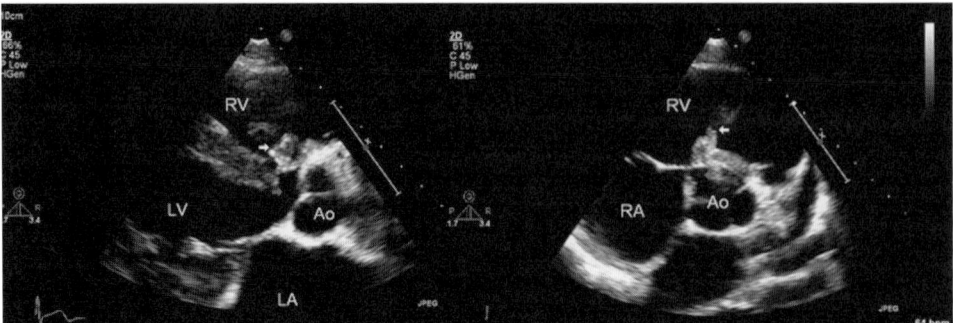

Fig. 4.1 Transthoracic imaging. Left: transthoracic parasternal long-axis view. Patient with small perimembranous ventricular septal defect (VSD; lower arrow) and a large vegetation (upper arrow) due to infective endocarditis. Right: parasternal short axis view. The ventricular septal defect (lower arrow) can be imaged in the perimembranous region of the interventricular septum, partially shrouded by tricuspid valve tissue. There is a large vegetation that extends from the VSD to the right ventricular outflow tract. (This figure is reproduced in colour in the colour plate section.)

significantly to the development and standardization of paediatric echocardiography. In the remainder of the chapter the application of different echocardiographic techniques to paediatric cardiology will be described in more detail.

Transthoracic echocardiography

Infants and children generally have excellent imaging windows for echocardiography allowing acquisition of high quality 2-D images. Apart from the standard adult imaging windows, additional views are used in paediatric echocardiography. This includes the use of subcostal (subxyphoid) and suprasternal views which are extremely useful for defining cardiac anatomy. Paediatric image orientation differs from standard adult imaging as most paediatric echocardiography laboratories image the heart in the anatomical orientation with the superior structures on top of the screen (with the apex down on an apical four-chamber view). This is related to the focus of paediatric echocardiography on anatomical imaging and viewing the anatomy as realistically as possible. Apart from static image cuts, acquisition of so-called dynamic 'sweeps' (from posterior to anterior and from right to left) provides a stack of 2-D cuts which are very useful for mentally reconstructing three-dimensional (3-D) anatomy. The American Society of Echocardiography published guidelines on the performance of a paediatric echocardiography describing the different views in detail (1). Also the measurements performed during paediatric echocardiograms have been standardized in recently published recommendations (2). A complete paediatric 2-D echocardiography includes:

1 Full description of cardiac anatomy using the segmental approach. This includes description of: cardiac position, cardiac situs, systemic and pulmonary venous return, atrioventricular connection, and ventriculoarterial connection. The presence of atrial and ventricular septal defects is described. The aortic arch laterality (left or right arch) and branching pattern are identified and extra-cardiac shunts, like a patent arterial

duct, are looked for. In every patient the coronary origins are described and identified by colour flow imaging (Fig. 4.2). The segmental approach provides a conceptual framework for describing even the most complex congenital lesions. It has become 'the language of paediatric cardiology' although specific dialects exist. Specific diagnostic codes were developed into the International Pediatric and Congenital Cardiac Code which offers a standard language for describing congenital heart defects (3).

2 Evaluation of haemodynamics and valve function. Valvar stenosis and regurgitation are described and quantified. Estimates of pressure gradients and intracardiac pressures can be made to describe the haemodynamic impact of certain lesions.

3 Evaluation of systolic and diastolic ventricular function. Due to the complex geometric and variable cardiac loading conditions (changes in preload and afterload), this can be very challenging.

Paediatric echocardiography is an operator-dependent technique that requires special skills and thus special training. Both European and North American training recommendations have been published by the professional associations (4, 5). The European Association of Echocardiography (EAE) currently provides accreditation in congenital echocardiography that involves both a theoretical as well as a practical component. Teaching courses and updated textbooks focused on paediatric and congenital echocardiography are available that can help in updating expertise (6, 7). In the hands of well-trained

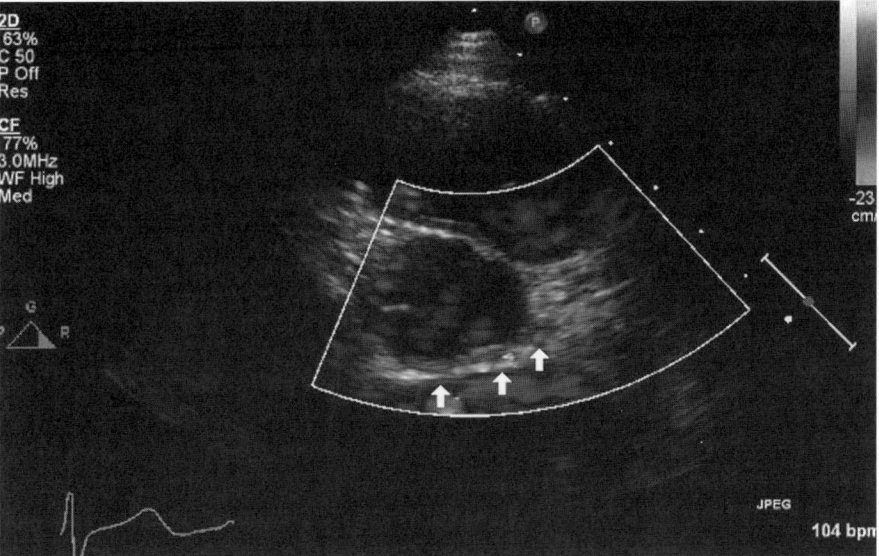

Fig. 4.2 Transthoracic imaging of abnormal coronary artery origin. Use of colour Doppler. Image obtained in 11-year old girl presenting with chest pain and ST-segment changes on ECG. An abnormal course of the left coronary artery (LCA) could be demonstrated by colour Doppler (arrows). The LCA originates from the right coronary sinus and runs posterior to the aorta to the left. The size of the LCA is small and on coronary angiography this segment was shown to be stenosed and hypoplastic. This demonstrates the high resolution of transthoracic echocardiography. (This figure is reproduced in colour in the colour plate section.)

echocardiographers and in the context of a protocolized and standardized echocardiographic laboratory with quality management strategies, the current technology allows a very accurate description of most paediatric congenital lesions. In Boston Children's Hospital only 87 diagnostic errors could be detected on more than 50 000 echocardiographic studies (8). This high diagnostic accuracy has resulted in that currently most patients are referred for cardiac surgery based on echocardiographic diagnosis only, while diagnostic cardiac catheterization has become more obsolete in the preoperative assessment. Additional imaging using cardiac magnetic resonance imaging or, more rarely, cardiac computed tomography may be required for specific indications, but are overall only rarely needed. In Toronto, before each surgical intervention, a complete transthoracic echocardiographic evaluation is performed using standardized imaging protocols that guarantee that all the required information is gathered. The echocardiographic data are presented in surgical conference where the completeness and accuracy information is evaluated. To further reduce the potential effect of human error, every preoperative study is reviewed by two experienced staff echocardiographers prior to surgery. If missing information is detected, either further transthoracic images or transoesophageal images during surgery may be obtained.

One of the challenges for quantification of paediatric echocardiography is the effect of somatic growth on the size of cardiac structures such as valves, volumes, ventricular walls, and vessels. Reporting absolute values has no meaning and correcting for weight and height of body surface area is based on the assumption of a well-defined (linear) relationship between the measurement and the allometric parameter. This has resulted in the development of the z-score method as the method of choice to adjust for the effect of age and body size on the measurement of cardiac structures (9). A z-score is the position of a certain measurement relative to the mean of a population expressed in standard deviations. The problem, however, is that no 'universal' z-scores have been developed and that the published data might not be applicable to every laboratory due to the potential effect of race and environment on the measurements. Nevertheless, currently most paediatric laboratories report their measurements of cardiac and vascular dimensions as z-score values allowing correcting for the effect of growth on the measurements.

Transoesophageal echocardiography

Since transthoracic imaging windows are generally excellent in children, it is not necessary to use transoesophageal echocardiography (TOE) for diagnostic purposes. Most diagnoses can reliably be established by transthoracic echocardiography. The only exception might be the diagnosis of endocarditis, especially in adolescents where TOE might have a higher diagnostic sensitivity, although no good paediatric data are available addressing this question. The development of smaller multiplane paediatric TOE probes allowed this technique to be used even in smaller children and infants. Recently a miniaturized probe was developed for multiplane imaging in the smallest infants. The main indications for use of TOE in children are perioperative assessment in the operating room and monitoring interventional procedures in the catheterization laboratory. The perioperative use of

TOE has become the standard of care in most paediatric cardiac surgery programmes as it has been shown to reduce the need for surgical reinterventions (10). Especially when coming off cardiopulmonary bypass, residual lesions and a suboptimal surgical result can be identified and, if necessary, it can be decided to go back on bypass (Fig. 4.3). Based on that routine practice, in Toronto currently 10% of all children go back on bypass to further optimize the surgical result (unpublished data). This relatively high number is partially based on our intentional strategy to try to be valve-sparing in tetralogy of Fallot repair which increased the incidence of residual right ventricular (RV) outflow tract obstruction. In our practice we only rarely perform pre-bypass TOE studies as all preoperative information is usually available from the preoperative imaging studies. The imaging windows in TOE are more limited compared to transthoracic imaging, especially to image the pulmonary artery branches. If insertion of the TOE probe is not possible (small size of the child, oesophageal surgery) or if not all of the required information can be obtained by TOE, epicardial imaging directly on the open heart is a good alternative and can provide excellent images. In our experience this has been useful in identifying pulmonary artery stenosis when TOE was not able to visualize the pulmonary arteries. Apart from use in the operating room, TOE plays an important role in the catheterization laboratory for monitoring different interventional procedures. In particular, closure on atrial septal defects and patent foramen ovale by placement of devices is generally performed

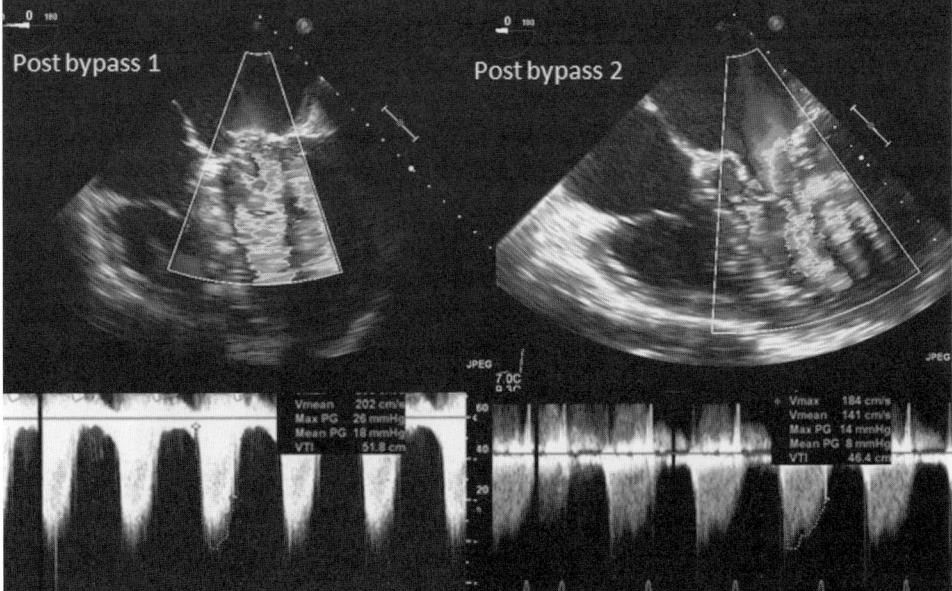

Fig. 4.3 Transoesophageal echocardiography (TOE). Use of perioperative TOE in a 13-year-old boy who underwent mitral valve repair for severe mitral regurgitation secondary to rheumatic fever. Left: after the first bypass TOE showed an immobile posterior leaflet with a narrow inflow jet and a mean gradient of 18mmHg. Right: after the second bypass the posterior leaflet mobility improved, the jet became wider, and the mean gradient was reduced to 8mmHg. (This figure is reproduced in colour in the colour plate section.)

under echocardiographic guidance and monitoring. Other procedures that can be monitored are device closure of ventricular septal defects, trans-septal puncture of the intra-atrial septum, closure of paravalvular leaks, and percutaneous implantation of aortic valves. Intracardiac ultrasound is a good alternative to TOE for atrial procedures but requires additional vascular access and is a relatively expensive technique as the intravascular probes are single-use. The recent development of a 3-D TOE probe for use in adults and in larger children (>20–25kg), allows real-time 3-D imaging in the operating room and in the interventional suite. In the operating room we mainly use 3-D TOE for the post-bypass assessment of valve surgery, especially the atrioventricular valve (Fig. 4.4). For interventional procedures the use of 3-D TOE could potentially be useful for better describing atrial septal defect morphology and size. Further data are required to demonstrate the additional value of 3-D imaging for these or other indications.

Fetal echocardiography

The development of fetal echocardiography in the late 1980s and 1990s was the logical next step in paediatric echocardiography. With the current technology a very detailed echocardiographic evaluation of the fetus heart can be performed from around 17–18 weeks' gestational age. All major congenital anomalies can be detected from around that age and if anomalies are detected the different treatment options can be discussed with the parents. Currently in different countries obstetrical ultrasound is used for screening

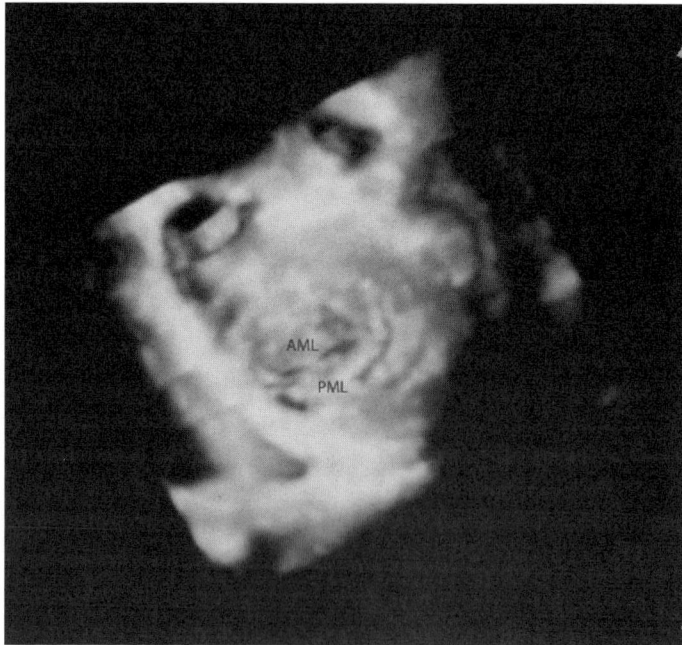

Fig. 4.4 3-D Transoesophageal echocardiography (TOE). In this 3-D picture the mitral valve imaged by 2-D in Fig. 4.3 the mitral valve is imaged from the atrial aspect. The leaflets could be imaged well by 3-D TOE. AML: anterior mitral leaflet; PML: posterior mitral leaflet. (This figure is reproduced in colour in the colour plate section.)

for fetal anomalies, including cardiac defects. Obstetrical ultrasonographers are specifically trained to detect cardiac malformations and if cardiac anomalies are suspected on a routine scan, the patients are referred to a specialized centre for a more detailed evaluation. Specifically-trained fetal echocardiographers can describe the cardiac defects in detail and provide counselling to the family regarding the diagnosis, therapeutic options, and expected outcome. This allows parents to make a well-informed decision about eventual termination of pregnancy in cases of lesions with poor prognosis and outcome. For the fetuses with congenital lesions where immediate postnatal haemodynamic instability can be expected or where an early postnatal intervention may be required, the delivery can be planned and organized to take place in a location where adequate neonatal cardiac care can be provided. Prenatal diagnosis with adequate planning of perinatal care has been shown to improve the outcomes for certain lesions such as transposition of the great arteries and hypoplastic left heart syndrome (HLHS, 11). Apart from the identification of structural defects, fetal echocardiography currently is also important for the detection and treatment of fetal arrhythmia. The most common rhythm disturbance that can be detected in fetal life is supraventricular tachycardia. This is usually detected at the time of an obstetrical ultrasound. If the tachycardia is very fast and incessant, this can result in cardiac dysfunction, development of fetal hydrops, and, ultimately, fetal demise. Maternal transplacental treatment of fetal tachycardia improves the outcome although some of the arrhythmia may be challenging to treat and may require usage of different drugs. Fetal intervention is a rapidly evolving field (12). Ultrasound-guided balloon dilatation of fetal critical aortic valve stenosis is performed in order to try to prevent the development of HLHS. The success of this therapy is still subject to debate and is still being investigated. Other procedures are being performed but the place of fetal intervention in the management of congenital heart disease is still controversial.

Three-dimensional echocardiography

During the last few years, 3-D echocardiography has gained more interest in paediatric cardiology since the development of a high-frequency paediatric transthoracic 3-D matrix probe that provides real-time 3-D imaging. For studying cardiac anatomy, it seems appealing to be able to visualize cardiac anatomy using 3-D images. For complex congenital heart disease this could be a great addition to conventional 2-D imaging, especially for defining spatial relationships. Directly showing 3-D anatomy instead of having to rely on mental reconstruction in the operator's mind can greatly enhance understanding of congenital lesions. Although significant improvements in 3-D imaging have been made, the technique is still not used in routine clinical practice in most laboratories. This is related to the lower spatial and temporal resolution of 3-D compared to 2-D and the lack of real good 3-D representation techniques. Further developments will be required before 3-D echocardiography will become fully integrated into clinical practice. Measurement of LV and RV volumes based on three-dimensional datasets is currently probably the most commonly indication to utilize 3-D echocardiography in our laboratory. Quantification of LV volumes using 3-D echocardiography is more reproducible than previous methods and also correlates well with volumes measured by cardiac magnetic resonance imaging. Also, RV volumes can be calculated using specific software applications but the methods used for the RV are still more cumbersome and require more extensive post-processing. It can, however, be expected that in the near future echocardiography will become the first-line technique for assessing RV volumes and ejection fraction (13).

Functional echocardiography

Apart from assessing anatomy, one of the main aims of an echocardiographic study is to assess cardiac function. For the evaluation of systolic ventricular function, congenital heart disease is challenging, related to the variability in anatomy and loading conditions affecting both measurement and interpretation of most functional parameters. Standard measurements used in adult echocardiography can be applied for the assessment of the structurally normal LV in children (mainly ejection fraction, fractional shortening) taking into consideration their intrinsic limitations (variability, effect of afterload). This becomes even more problematic when the LV is structurally abnormal. Also, for the

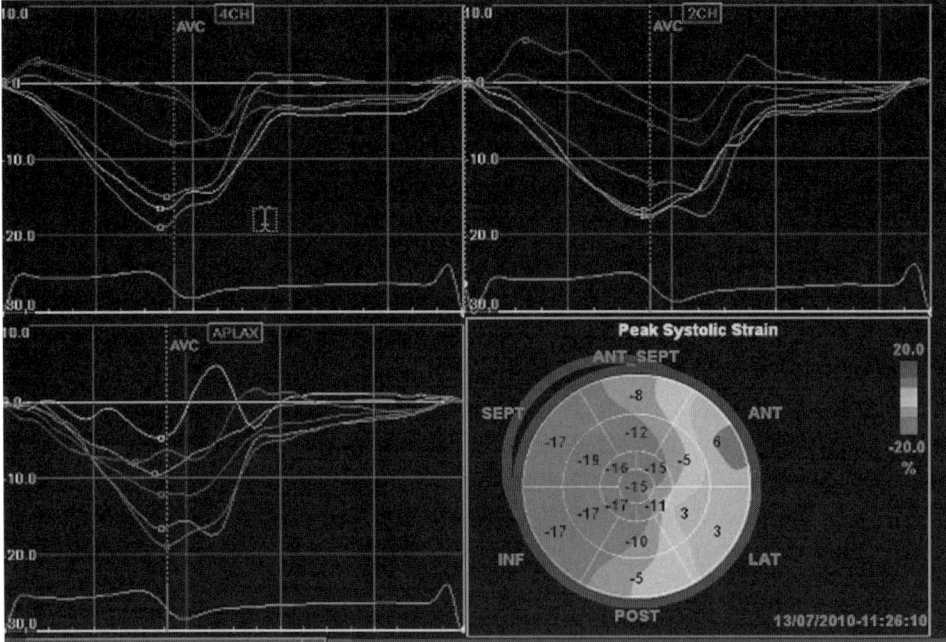

Fig. 4.5 Longitudinal strain measurement using automatic functional imaging. Images obtained in the girl presented in Fig. 4.2 with the abnormal origin of the left coronary artery from the right coronary artery with posterior looping. Longitudinal strain curves were obtained from apical four-chamber, three-chamber, and two-chamber views and were analysed using automatic functional imaging. Severely reduced peak systolic strain measurements were obtained in the anterolateral segments consistent with ischaemic changes in the left anterior descending coronary artery territory. The girl underwent coronary bypass surgery. This illustrates how current technology allows quantification of regional myocardial function. (This figure is reproduced in colour in the colour plate section.)

assessment of systolic function of the RV and the functionally univentricular heart, no good echocardiographic techniques are available and often subjective 'eyeballing' is used in routine clinical practice. During the last 15 years, new functional echocardiographic techniques have been introduced that are directly looking into the myocardium and thus are more geometry-independent. Tissue Doppler was the first technique developed and has been applied to patients with paediatric and congenital heart disease (14). As tissue Doppler velocities are influenced by cardiac translation and there is an effect of tethering on the measurements, cardiac deformation imaging was developed as better way to quantify regional myocardial function (Fig. 4.5). These seem promising techniques but introduction of this technology into routine clinical practice is slowed by the problem related to variability of the techniques, constant changes in technology, and lack of industry standards (15). Also for strain and strain rate measurements, normal data in the different age ranges are missing and there is no good understanding how the measurements can be used for clinical decision-making in congenital heart disease. It can be expected that standardization of strain analysis techniques will result in a more routine application in paediatric and congenital heart disease.

References

1. Lai WW, Geva T, Shirali GS, Frommelt PC, Humes RA, Brook MM, *et al.* Guidelines and standards for performance of a pediatric echocardiogram: a report from the Task Force of the Pediatric Council of the American Society of Echocardiography. *J Am Soc Echocardiogr* 2006; **19**(12):1413–30.
2. Lopez L, Colan SD, Frommelt PC, Ensing GJ, Kendall K, Younoszai AK, *et al.* Recommendations for quantification methods during the performance of a pediatric echocardiogram: a report from the Pediatric Measurements Writing Group of the American Society of Echocardiography Pediatric and Congenital Heart Disease Council. *J Am Soc Echocardiogr* 2010; **23**(5):465–95.
3. Franklin RC, Beland MJ, Krogmann ON. Mapping and coding of nomenclatures for paediatric and congenital heart disease. *Cardiol Young* 2006; **16**(2):105–6.
4. Mertens L, Helbing W, Sieverding L, Daniels O. Guidelines from the Association for European Paediatric Cardiology: standards for training in paediatric echocardiography. *Cardiol Young* 2005; **15**(4):441–2.
5. Sanders SP, Colan SD, Cordes TM, Donofrio MT, Ensing GJ, Geva T, *et al.* ACCF/AHA/AAP recommendations for training in pediatric cardiology. Task force 2: pediatric training guidelines for noninvasive cardiac imaging endorsed by the American Society of Echocardiography and the Society of Pediatric Echocardiography. *J Am Coll Cardiol* 2005; **46**(7):1384–8.
6. Eidem BW, Cetta F, O'Leary PW. *Echocardiography in Pediatric and Adult Congenital Heart Disease.* Philadelphia, PA: Lippincott, Wilkins and Williams; 2009.
7. Lai WW, Mertens L, Cohen M, Geva T. *Echocardiography in Pediatric and Congenital Heart Disease. From Fetus to Adult.* Oxford: Wiley-Blackwell; 2009.
8. Benavidez OJ, Gauvreau K, Jenkins KJ, Geva T. Diagnostic errors in pediatric echocardiography: development of taxonomy and identification of risk factors. *Circulation* 2008; **117**(23):2995–3001.
9. Sluysmans T, Colan SD. Theoretical and empirical derivation of cardiovascular allometric relationships in children. *J Appl Physiol* 2005; **99**(2):445–57.
10. Randolph GR, Hagler DJ, Connolly HM, Dearani JA, Puga FJ, Danielson GK, *et al.* Intraoperative transesophageal echocardiography during surgery for congenital heart defects. *J Thoracic Cardiovasc Surg* 2002; **124**(6):1176–82.

11. Bonnet D, Coltri A, Butera G, Fermont L, Le Bidois J, Kachaner J, *et al*. Detection of transposition of the great arteries in fetuses reduces neonatal morbidity and mortality. *Circulation* 1999; **99**(7):916–18.
12. McElhinney DB, Tworetzky W, Lock JE. Current status of fetal cardiac intervention. *Circulation* 2010; **121**(10):1256–63.
13. Mertens LL, Friedberg MK. Imaging the right ventricle-current state of the art. *Nat Rev Cardiol* 2010; 7:551–63.
14. Friedberg MK, Mertens L. Tissue velocities, strain, and strain rate for echocardiographic assessment of ventricular function in congenital heart disease. *Eur J Echocardiogr* 2010; **10**:585–93.
15. Koopman LP, Slorach C, Hui W, Manlhiot C, McCrindle BW, Friedberg MK, *et al*. Comparison between different speckle tracking and color tissue Doppler techniques to measure global and regional myocardial deformation in children. *J Am Soc Echocardiogr* 2010; 23(9):919–28.

Chapter 5

The development of echoencephalography in Sweden

Leif G. Salford

Although neurosurgery has a long history it was thanks to brave pioneering neurosurgeons such as Harvey Cushing in the United States—and in Sweden Herbert Olivecrona—that the speciality made huge progress during the first half of the 20th century. However, around 1950, the possibility to reveal pathological processes taking place inside the closed skull, was still very restricted. The only available rapid procedure was the neurological examination of the patient. X-ray of the skull is of restricted value, pneumo-encephalography was much too complicated and time-consuming for acute situations, and angiography was still in its infancy. Thus the neurosurgeon, receiving an acute patient with a suspected intracranial haematoma, had to make a qualified guess about where to start placing his trephine on the skull in order to save the life of the patient—often within minutes in the case of a bleeding between the skull bone and the dura. The mortality in those days was 40%, often because the diagnosis was made too late.

Thanks to an ingenious Swedish neurosurgeon, Lars Leksell, working at Lund University Hospital, a new approach to reveal the secrets inside the skull was introduced in clinical praxis—echoencephalography. Lars Leksell graduated from the Karolinska Institute (KI) and received his neurosurgical training in Herbert Olivecrona's department from 1935. He volunteered as a neurosurgeon in the Finnish Winter War in 1940 in Karelia. His team could operate on 24 head injuries per 24 hours and already by this point, Leksell showed his creative mind in constructing the double-action rongeur for more efficient removal of shell-splinters from the vicinity of the spinal cord. In 1941 he joined Professor Ragnar Granit (1967 Nobel laureate in Medicine) at the Institute of Neurophysiology where he presented his thesis on gamma nerve fibres in 1945. In 1946 he became the chief of the new neurosurgical unit in Lund and in 1958 he was appointed the first Professor of Neurosurgery at Lund University. In 1960 he succeeded Olivecrona as Professor and Chairman of the Neurosurgical Department at the Karolinska Institute/Hospital.

During his years in Lund, Leksell's originative mind designed the first stereotactic instrument to be based on the arc-centre principle 1949 and in 1951, in a collaboration with Börje Larsson, using the Uppsala University cyclotron, Leksell developed the concept of radiosurgery. They were the first to employ beams coming from several directions into a small area of the brain and treated the first patient 1958. This concept was further developed into the gamma knife, which aims gamma radiation to a target point in the patient's brain.

It is this untiringly working inventor who also realized the possibility for neurosurgery to utilize the pulse echo ultrasonic equipment. Widely used in metal testing, the technology of ultrasound was adapted for medicine during the 1940s. The Austrian brothers Karl and Friedrich Dussik built an apparatus in Austria to make images of the human brain and ventricles by transmission technique which they named 'hyperphonography' utilizing pulses of 0.1s at 1.2MHz produced by a quartz ultrasound generator. Their first ultrasound images were published in 1947 (1) and the work stimulated neurosurgeons and engineers at the Massachusetts Institute of Technology (MIT) in Boston to set up a project to 'detect intracranial pathology by ultrasound'. However, in the early 1950s, they showed that the images, which were registered by this technique from heads of humans, could also be received from empty skulls! Criticism was also raised that the degree of attenuation of the ultrasound beam on its passage through the skull was influenced by variations in the skull bone thickness, which might make the Dussik records questionable. These findings led to the statement by the United States Atomic Energy Commission, that ultrasound would not be useful in the diagnosis of brain pathologies as it would be impossible to detect intracranial processes through the intact skull. This dealt a severe blow to the development of the technique and the MIT project was terminated in 1954.

Leksell, however, by 1950 had borrowed an old Kelvin Hughes industrial flaw detector from his friend, Wylie McKissock, a neurosurgeon at the Atkinson Morley's hospital in London, in the hope of developing a method to rapidly and non-invasively locate intracranial haemorrhages in Lund. The apparatus had separate generating and receiving transducers, which made registrations from the head complicated and these first attempts were disappointing. Leksell temporarily gave up his tests and the instrument was returned.

Three years later, fate was very lucky for Leksell, as a collaboration had just started in the Lund University Hospital, between two young scientists, the cardiologist Inge Edler and the graduate student at the Department of Physics, Hellmuth Hertz, with the goal of proving that ultrasound could be used to monitor the heart—the start of what would become echocardiography. Leksell heard of the Edler–Hertz work and his interest in the technique was reawakened. He borrowed the apparatus during an emergency operation in 1954 and describes in his memoirs *Hjärnfragment* [*Brain Fragments*] from 1982 (2) how he successfully operated on a 6-year-old girl who was in a deep coma, after he had localized an extradural haematoma through the intact skull by revealing a dislocation of the midline echo towards the contralateral hemisphere. Leksell named the technique 'echo-encephalography' and started its development into a very useful tool in neurosurgery. He could not resist referring in his memoirs to the United States Atomic Energy Commission's statement, which coincided with his first operation 1954: 'it must be realized that there is no possibility of adapting this tool to detecting intracranial lesions . . . the distances involved would make the application foolish.' Leksell presented his observations at a meeting with the Swedish Society of Medicine in Stockholm in December 1954 and published his results in 1955/56 and 1958 (3, 4). He describes that by the use of a standard ultrasonic echo-apparatus (Krautkrämer Model USIP 9) operating at a frequency of 2Mc/s, the combined transmitter–receiver was applied to the shaved scalp using water or liquid paraffin as the coupling medium. The distance from the surface echo to the midline echo was measured by means of a calibrated scale on the oscilloscope screen as a one-dimensional trace, 'A-mode' (Fig. 5.1). The echo was photographed with a Polaroid camera.

Measurements of the distance from the scalp to the calcified pineal body, or the pineal recess, were made from lateral roentgenograms, using metal indicators on the skin and with appropriate correction for magnification. Leksell commented that 'lateral displacement of the calcified pineal body in the roentgenogram is a valuable diagnostic sign of an expanding intracranial lesion', but also that it was only about 15% of the cases that had sufficient calcification for identification. On the contrary, with improved ultrasonic equipment, the midline echo can be consistently identified almost as well in adults as in children, using a sound frequency of 2–4Mc/s. Leksell also reported his studies on cadaver brains, immersed in water, where the midline echo disappears after removing the pineal body from the brain. Thus he found that the pineal body is an important source of the midline echo—but he also emphasized that other structures, normally situated in the midline, may also give detectable echoes through the skull.

It was these first useful measurements of the midline echo that made Leksell famous in the echoencephalography field. The technique spread from Lund to neurosurgical and neurological use around the world and a lot of papers on the neurological use of ultrasound were published during the next 10 years. Leksell himself did not develop the use of echoencephalography in hydrocephalus, but he commented in his 1956 paper (3) that typical echoes can be obtained and that the ventricular walls may often be clearly identified. After 1958 Leksell did not publish further on echoencephalography

Stig Jeppsson, who had worked under Leksell and succeeded him as chief in Lund 1960, continued the work and defended his thesis 'Echoencephalography–the midline echo: an evaluation of its usefulness for diagnosing intracranial expansivities and an investigation into its sources' in 1961 (5). He showed that echoencephalography is quick, simple, and accurate as a routine examination as it is harmless and causes no inconvenience to the patient. Furthermore, it is infinitely repeatable, suited for checking clinical progress, rapid, and allows for immediate treatment. The examination is easily performed in small children, where angiography and pneumo-encephalography would require general anaesthesia. The dissertation also included a large patient material to evaluate limitations and accuracy of echoencephalography. Out of 579 examinations in patients with tumours,

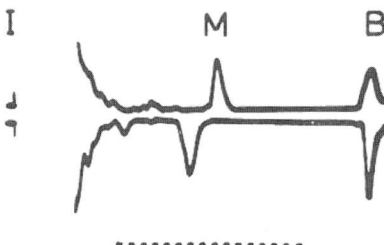

Fig. 5.1 Bilateral echoencephalogram from a patient with expansivity in the left temporal lobe. The upper trace is obtained from the left side of the head and the lower trace from the right. I: initial (surface) echo; M: midline echo.

trauma, or vascular lesions such as intracerebral haematomas and subarachnoidal haemorrhages, only 12 were wrong when compared to the findings at neuroradiological, surgical, pathological–anatomical, and clinical examinations. Jeppsson could conclude that the accuracy of the method was 98%!

In parallel with Jeppsson's work in Lund, Brita Lithander at the Paediatric Clinic, Karolinska Sjukhuset and the Neurological Clinic, Södersjukhuset in Stockholm had developed the use of the technique as suggested by Leksell in 1956. In her dissertation 1961, she demonstrated that useful echoes can be detected from the outer borders of the lateral ventricles in infants (6). This depends on their thin skull bones and can also be seen in adult patients with an increased intracranial pressure (ICP) leading to decreasing thickness of the skull bones. Lithander also found that echoes from the cerebral midline in children could be elicited over a much larger area on the lateral side of the skull than in adults and came to the conclusion that the midline echo is generated by the third ventricle, the transverse fissure, and the aqueduct—and not only by the pineal body. After her dissertation, Lithander left the field of echoencephalography 'because everything about echo-encephalography had then been discovered'—according to D.N. White, author of a thorough historical review on the early development of echoencephalography (7), who visited her in 1964.

From around 1962, Iréne Sjögren in the Department of Paediatric Neurology at Uppsala University continued the work on applying echoencephalography for the measurement of ventricular size in children. In her dissertation 1968 she presented a large study of about 1000 echoencephalographic examinations (8). She could conclude that the energy transferred during the examination is considerably below the level at which harmful effects may occur, even in small infants. The ventricles can be recorded by the technique, provided that the skull is less than 3mm. thick. She also concluded that the upper limit for the body of normal lateral ventricles is one-third of the diameter of the head. In her thesis, Dr Sjögren also developed a useful index for measuring the ventricular size in relation to the diameter of the skull with normal values less than 35% (Fig. 5.2). In a recent personal communication, she told me that the idea for the index came during a discussion between her and her physicist husband, when she stood in the kitchen, serving from a bowl with the size of a child's head.

Iréne Sjögren used her deep knowledge of echoencephalography in a somewhat unusual way! Together with her colleagues from Uppsala, Bo Vahlquist, Head of the Department of Paediatrics and Gunnar Engsner, a PhD student from the same department, she worked for the Scandinavian Institute of African Studies in Addis Ababa, Ethiopia during the years 1969–1973. Equipped with measuring tape to register head circumference, the research Siemens echoencephalograph (Kraut-Krämer System) from Uppsala, and a transillumination lamp, the group examined normal children and children with marasmus and kwashiorkor, and could show that especially the latter disease gave a large proportion of increased lateral ventricle indices and also enlarged space between brain and skull. This work led to a dissertation 1974 by Dr Engsner in Uppsala.

One of the opponents at Iréne Sjögren's dissertation was Kurt West, a neurosurgeon in Lund since 1962. He had taken care of the echo machine in Lund after Stig Jeppsson left

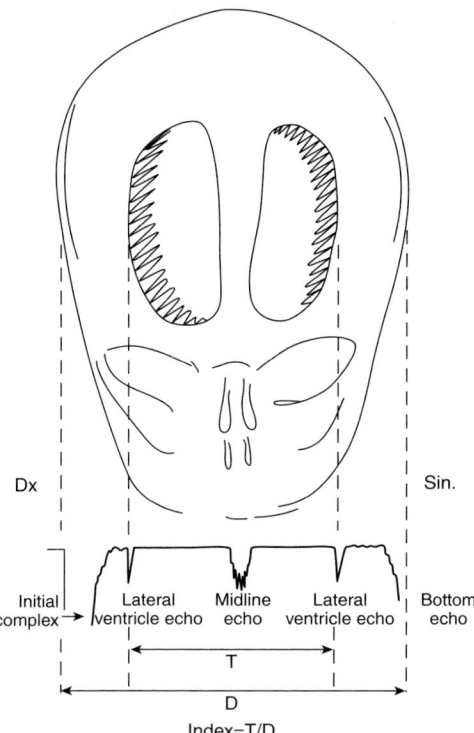

Fig. 5.2 Schematic picture of air-encephalogram compared to echoencephalogram and principles for index determination. Reproduced from Sjögren I. *Echoencephalography in paediatric practice with special regard to measurement of the ventricular size.* (Thesis.) Stockholm: P.A. Norstedt & Söner; 1968, with permission.

for Linköping to become the Chief of the Department of Neurosurgery there. West had, in parallel with Sjögren's work in Uppsala, started studies in Lund on communicating and non-communicating infantile hydrocephalus, utilizing the echoencephalograph. The patients were also investigated with pneumo-encephalography or ventriculography pre-operatively. West concluded that echoencephalography is of great value for the diagnosis, but felt that pneumo-encephalography and ventriculography were superior in the search for aetiological factors such as arachnoiditis, obstruction of the aqueduct, and papillomas of the choroid plexus. Kurt West also pioneered the use of ultrasound to measure residual urine in the bladder (9).

The author of this chapter joined the Department of Neurosurgery in Lund as locum physician in 1967 and became the department's first academic amanuensis on permanent staff in 1969. One of my first tasks was to be in charge of the echoencephalographic unit, once started by Leksell, and this continued until the early 1990s. During this period most provincial hospitals got their own equipment and trained staff to measure especially midline echoes, but also ventricular size. The technique was looked upon as a 'bedside' examination and continued in parallel with the great new technologies: from around 1973 computed tomography (CT) and from the 1980s magnetic resonance imaging (MRI). Several Swedish publications compared the echo technique with CT and found good correlations (10, 11). In Lund, we performed about 1800 echoencephalographic examinations per year during the 1970s, but then the number decreased and the last classical transcranial echoencephalography was performed in our department in 1992. Since then CT and MRI have totally taken over the diagnostic scene.

I also had the pleasure to work with diligent technicians during the great years of echoencephalography. Karl-Axel Kristiansson who joined us in the 1970s, made an interesting observation: in cases of increased ICP the midline echo and the echoes from the walls of the dilated third ventricle show a high-frequency fluttering of the peak of the echoes in combination with a high pulsating amplitude of the same echoes in most cases (Fig. 5.3). We thought that this finding might be used as a non-invasive device for measuring the ICP. During one year, 459 patients were included in a study. It was shown that 287 of them had ventricular dilatation. Forty-three of these patients were proven to have increased ICP by either an intraventricular pressure recording device, qualitative measurement of the ventricular ICP during the operation, or qualitative estimation of ICP through clinical signs such as papilloedema. All of them had their ventricular dilatation proven with CT examination. Of the 43 patients, 36 had fluttering echoes from the walls of the third ventricle and from the M-mode echo. We noted, with the help of echoencephalography, that during the development of a hydrocephalus, a dilatation of the third ventricle often precedes the dilatation of the lateral ventricles. This work was performed in collaboration with the physicists Nils Gunnar Holmer and Kjell Lindström of Lund University and the results were reported at the Swedish Society of Medicine in Stockholm in 1986.

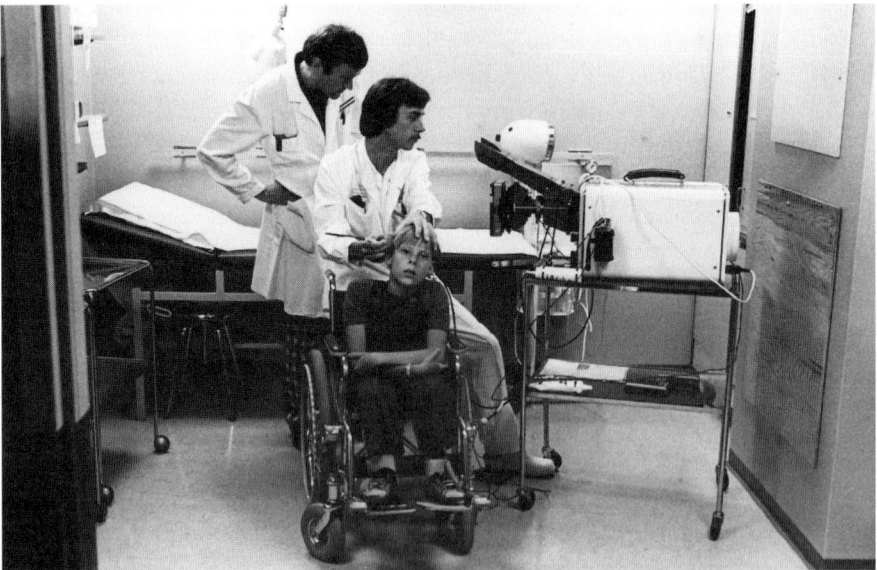

Fig. 5.3 Our echoencephalographist Karl-Axel Kristiansson demonstrates a fluttering echo to the author in 1981.

It may thus be concluded that the pioneering work of a series of Swedish neuroscientists in the 1950s and 1960s leading to a worldwide spread of the echoencephalographic diagnostic method has saved or improved hundreds of thousands of lives during the decades when it was the best solution for the clinician to acutely examine a skull trauma or to diagnose and follow the paediatric hydrocephalus patient.

References

1. Dussik KT, Dussik F, Wyt L. Auf dem Wege Zur Hyperphonograpie des Gehirnes. *Med Wochenschr* 1947; **97**:425–9.
2. Leksell L. *Hjärnfragment [Brain Fragments]*. Stockholm: P.A. Norstedt & Söners Förlag; 1982.
3. Leksell L. Echo-encephalography. I. Detection of intracranial complications following head injury. *Acta Chir Scand* 1956; **110**(4):301–15.
4. Leksell L. Echoencephalography. II. Midline echo from the pineal body as an index of pineal displacement. *Acta Chir Scand* 1958; **115**(4):255–9.
5. Jeppsson S. Echoencephalography–the midline echo: an evaluation of its usefulness for diagnosing intracranial expansivities and an investigation into its sources. *Acta Chir Scand* 1961; Suppl **272**: 1–151.
6. Lithander B. Clinical and experimental studies in echo-encephalography. *Acta Psychiatr Scand* 1961; **36**(Suppl. 159):1–53.
7. White DN. The early development of neurosonology: I: Echoencephalography in adults. *Ultrasound Med Biol* 1992; **18**(2):115–65.
8. Sjögren I. *Echoencephalography in paediatric practice with special regard to measurement of the ventricular size.* (Thesis.) Stockholm: P.A. Norstedt & Söner; 1968.
9. West K. Sonocystography. A method for measuring residual urine. *Scand J Urol Nephrol* 1967; **1**: 68–70.
10. Hanson J, Levander B, Liliequist B. Size of the intracerebral ventricles as measured with computer tomography, encephalography and echoventriculography. *Acta Radiol* 1975; **346**(Suppl.):98–106.
11. Knibestöl M, Brodtkorb E, Fagerlund M. Correlations between echo-encephalographic and computer tomographic measures of third and lateral ventricle size in children and adults. *Acta Neurol Scand* 1983; **68**(5):350–61.

Chapter 6

The development of ultrasound in obstetrics and gynaecology in Sweden

Karel Maršál and Bertil Sundén

In the field of obstetrics, the advent of diagnostic ultrasound was most welcome because of the obvious lack of a non-invasive method providing information on the fetus *in utero*. The subsequent very fast and widespread use of ultrasound in clinical obstetrics was vindication that the method fulfilled the expectations and that it literally 'opened a window into the uterus'. Ultrasound enabled direct examinations of fetal anatomy, measurements of fetal size and growth, and recording of intrauterine activities. Nowadays, 97% of all pregnant women in Sweden undergo at least one ultrasound examination during their pregnancy.

The pioneering work

The early positive results reported from the application of ultrasound in cardiology and neurosurgery at Lund University elicited interest to test the method on pregnant women at the Department of Obstetrics and Gynecology in Lund.

In 1957, Alf Sjövall, then professor in obstetrics and gynaecology, discussed over a lunch-table with neurosurgeon Lars Leksell his very first experience of diagnosing subdural hematoma using ultrasound (1). Professor Sjövall asked then Bertil Sundén, who worked at his department, to investigate early pregnancies with the Krautkrämer echoscope belonging to Leksell. The aim was to examine whether it would be possible to detect echoes from the fetus in early pregnancies and to differentiate it from myomatous enlargements of the uterus and from ovarian tumours.

The Krautkrämer echoscope offered only an A-mode display of ultrasound signals so no tangible results were obtained as the origin of the echoes could not be identified. At that time, it was unknown whether or not ultrasound might have any harmful effects on embryonic tissue and therefore these first investigations in early pregnancies were done on patients admitted for interruption of pregnancy.

After that Ian Donald published the first description of an echoscope generating a two-dimensional display in 1958 (2), Bertil Sundén went on a three-week visit to Professor Donald in Glasgow. There he met electronic engineer Tom G. Brown, employed by Smiths Industrial Division in Glasgow, who had built Donald's machine. During his stay in Glasgow Sundén performed several investigations on obstetric and gynaecological patients using Brown's equipment that was the only one of its type (3). The potential of this method was obvious and therefore, the Department of Obstetrics and Gynecology in Lund purchased an improved version of the apparatus built by Smiths Industrial Division. The machine was delivered to the Department of Obstetrics and Gynecology in Lund in the Autumn of 1961. It used pulsed ultrasound with pulse repetition frequency of 25 per second and worked at three frequencies, 1.5MHz, 2.5MHz, and 5MHz (Fig. 6.1).

A basic requirement of a method to be used in clinical practice is the absence of harmful effects. The ovaries and the fetus had been thought to be tissues potentially sensitive to ultrasound. With the apparatus used for clinical examinations Sundén performed a series of experiments on sexually mature albino rats—non-pregnant and pregnant—under the same conditions as used during clinical examinations. After insonation, a normal ovarian function and fertility of the exposed rats was preserved and the number and development of offspring were normal. There was no increase in the incidence of abortion, intrauterine death, premature birth, neonatal mortality, congenital deformities or abnormal postnatal development. The same applied to the second generation of animals.

The usefulness of ultrasound for obstetric and gynaecological diagnoses was studied by Sundén in more than 400 patients. In obstetric cases the ultrasound diagnoses were compared with the results of clinical examinations, the findings at spontaneous or induced abortions, X-ray findings and the findings at laparoscopy, cesarean section or at vaginal delivery. It was possible to record echoes from a fetus towards the end of the 8th week of pregnancy, which was earlier than possible with any other method. Typical images were obtained of fetuses at various gestational ages (Fig. 6.2) and presentations, and also the

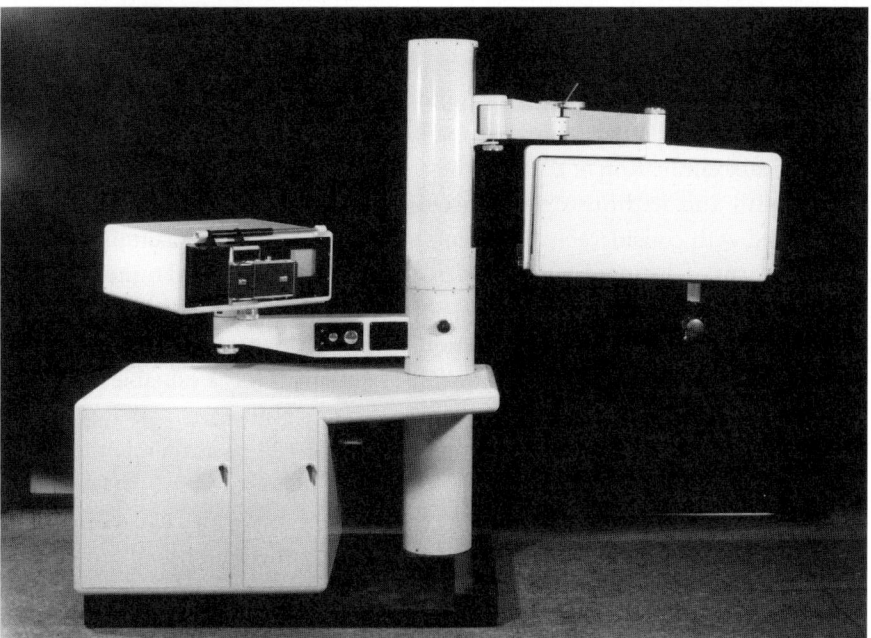

Fig. 6.1 Ultrasound scanner (Smiths Industrial Division, Glasgow, UK) used by Bertil Sundén for his studies in Lund in the early 1960s.

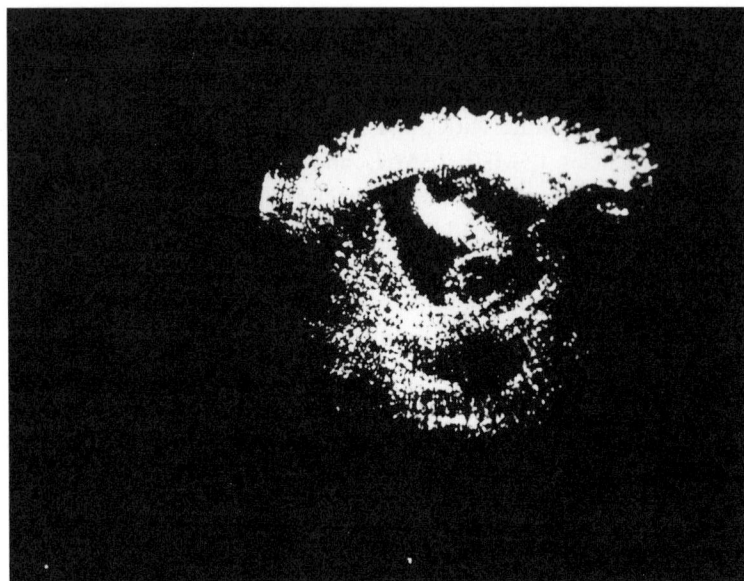

Fig. 6.2 Pregnancy at 13 postmenstrual weeks. Reproduced, with permission, from Sundén B (1964). On the diagnostic value of ultrasound in obstetrics and gynaecology. *Acta Obstet Gynecol Scand*, **43**(Suppl. 6):1–191, fig. 25. © John Wiley & Sons Ltd.

very first ultrasound picture in the world of a twin pregnancy (see Fig. 1.4, Chapter 1 this volume). The usefulness of the method was also demonstrated by the reports on typical ultrasound images of hydatidiform mole, hydramnios, hydrocephalus and acrania.

In gynaecology, Bertil Sundén investigated the ultrasound examination as a means of diagnosing pelvic tumors. The ultrasound diagnosis was compared with the clinical findings, the findings at laparoscopy or laparotomy, and with the results of macroscopic and histological examination of the specimens from surgery. Myomatous enlargement of the uterus with and without degenerative changes, and various ovarian tumours were examined with considerably diagnostic accuracy. Ultrasound examination proved reliable as a means of distinguishing between different gynaecological tumours of solid or cystic character (Fig. 6.3).

It was obvious that ultrasound examination in some cases provided information which could not be obtained by any other means while in others it was a valuable adjunct to the conventional methods of investigation.

The results of Sundén's studies were published in 1964 in an academic thesis entitled 'On the diagnostic value of ultrasound in obstetrics and gynaecology' (4) and they were presented at national and international congresses. In the following years visitors from all over the world came to Lund to study the method and Sundén published more papers on the diagnostic possibilities of ultrasound (5–7).

The academic thesis by Bertil Sundén is internationally recognized as 'the earliest and the most comprehensive publication in obstetric and gynaecological ultrasonography at that time'. Sundén successfully defended his thesis at a public dissertation at Lund

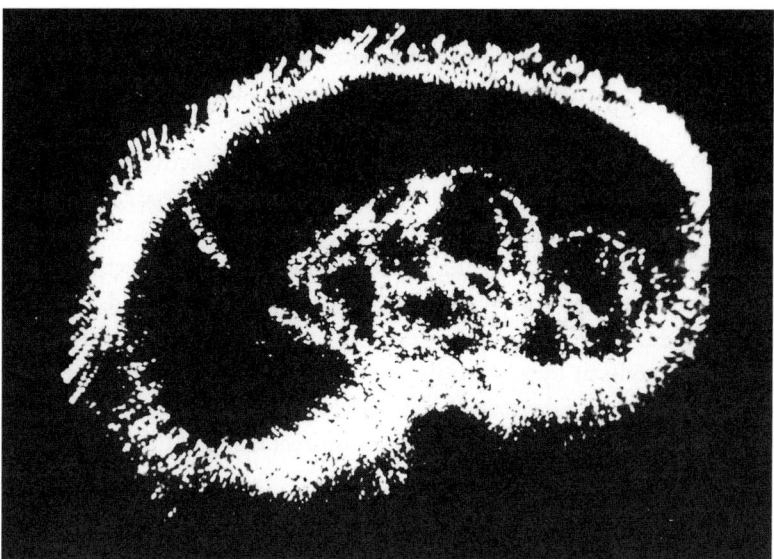

Fig. 6.3 Multilocular mucinous cystadenoma of the ovary. Reproduced, with permission, from Sundén B (1964). On the diagnostic value of ultrasound in obstetrics and gynaecology. *Acta Obstet Gynecol Scand*, **43**(Suppl. 6):1–191, fig. 83. © John Wiley & Sons Ltd.

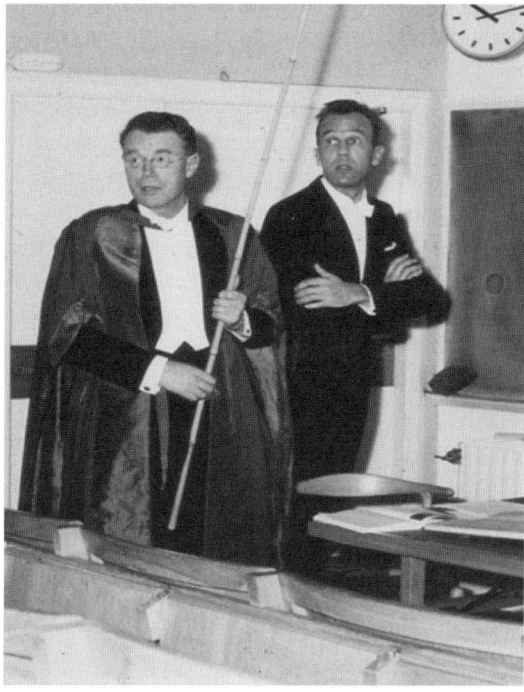

Fig. 6.4 Bertil Sundén defending his thesis 'On the diagnostic value of ultrasound in obstetrics and gynaecology' at Lund University in 1964. The opponent Professor Ian Donald to the left.

University in 1964. The first opponent appointed by the Faculty of Medicine was Professor Ian Donald (Fig. 6.4) and the second opponent was Professor Hellmuth Hertz. Later, Donald described his experience from the dissertation in Lund in an entertaining way and he praised Sundén for his work and defence of the thesis (8).

In the early 1970s, Professor Stig Kullander initiated a very active research programme in obstetric and gynaecological ultrasound at the University Department of Obstetrics and Gynecology at the Malmö General Hospital, one of the two university hospitals affiliated with Lund University. During the following years, various clinical applications of ultrasound in obstetrics and gynaecology were investigated and, in collaboration with the Department of Biomedical Engineering in Malmö and with the Department of Electrical Measurements at Lund Institute of Technology several new methods based on ultrasound techniques were developed, e.g. the semi-automatic method for recording of fetal breathing movements (9) and the method for recording of the aortic pulse waves in the fetus (10).

The continued development
Routine use of obstetric ultrasound

Forty years ago, many twin pregnancies remained undetected until delivery. The compound B-mode ultrasound technique enabled visualization of fetuses *in utero* and reliable diagnosis of multiple pregnancies. In 1973, Stig Kullander, Lars Grennert, and Per-Håkan Persson introduced in Malmö a routine ultrasound examination of all pregnant women at 28 gestational weeks with the aim to diagnose twin pregnancies in order to improve their perinatal outcome. To our knowledge, this was the first general ultrasound screening of a pregnant population in the world (11). Three years later, the Malmö department changed the time of examinations and offered all pregnant women two routine examinations—one at 19 gestational weeks for estimation of gestational age and one at 33 weeks for control of the intrauterine growth, in both cases using the ultrasound measurement of fetal biparietal diameter (11). This two-stage screening design was later introduced by Manfred Hansmann and Jochen Hackelör in the former Federal Republic of Germany and called 'the Malmö model'.

The potentials of ultrasound measurements of fetal size and weight for estimation of gestational age and fetal growth were systematically investigated by Persson, Grennert, Eik-Nes, Laurin, and others in Malmö. In mid-1980s, reference values for various fetal parameters and fetal weight were established and they still are the most widely used standards in Sweden (12). In 1990s, the Swedish Board of Health and Welfare accepted the intrauterine growth curve based on ultrasonically estimated fetal weights collected in a longitudinal multicentre study as the standard growth curve for evaluation of both fetal weights and birth weights (13). It was probably for the first time in the history of obstetric ultrasound that a growth curve based on normal fetal weights rather than on birth weights was recognized as the official standard.

After the pioneering work at Lund University, obstetric ultrasound spread fast to most Swedish obstetric units in late 1970s and early 1980s. Anders Selbing at the Department of Obstetrics and Gynecology at Linköping University demonstrated the advantage of pregnancy dating by ultrasound in the first trimester (14). However, that method was not adopted by other ultrasound units in Sweden, mainly because at that time the resolution of the ultrasound machines did not allow closer evaluation of fetal anatomy. In the 1980s, Waldenström et al. (15) in Uppsala and Falun performed one of the very few randomized trials evaluating the routine use of ultrasound in the early second trimester. They confirmed that routine dating of low-risk pregnancies at 13–19 postmenstrual weeks leads to a significant decrease in inductions of labour overall and due to prolonged pregnancy.

During the early days of obstetric ultrasound some of the major fetal malformations like anencephaly could already be detected (4). With improved resolution of modern ultrasound systems, it became possible to examine fetal anatomy in detail and to detect even very small fetal defects, e.g. cleft lip. The antenatal diagnosis of fetal malformations can in a minority of cases allow intrauterine treatment and in other cases timely planning of perinatal management and optimal postnatal treatment. An early antenatal diagnosis of severe developmental defects offers to the parents the option of termination of pregnancy. The ultrasound diagnosis of congenital defects is associated with sometimes difficult ethical and psychological considerations and problems. The psychological effects of fetal diagnosis based on ultrasound were thoroughly studied by Connie Jörgensen and colleagues in Lund. The results of their studies showed that the positive effects of prenatal diagnosis dominate and that the majority of pregnant women and their partners wish the ultrasound examination of the fetus to be performed (16).

The Swedish specialists in obstetric ultrasound contributed to the evaluation of modern fetal diagnosis by a multicentre randomized trial of impressive size (close to 40 000 pregnancies) that compared two policies of screening for Down syndrome (17). Despite the convincing study results and the experience from abroad, the option of estimating the individual risk of trisomy in the late first trimester has not been generally adopted in Sweden. Possibly, this reflects the kind of 'minimalistic' approach of care providers who try to obtain as much information as possible from just one ultrasound examination routinely offered in pregnancy.

Studies of fetal physiological functions

Real-time ultrasound techniques enabled studies of fetal physiology in humans and development of new biophysical methods for fetal surveillance in high-risk pregnancies. In early 1970s, Gerhard Gennser and Karel Maršál in Malmö started to study fetal breathing movements, first using the one-dimensional A-mode ultrasound as described by the Oxford research group. In 1974, the Malmö group could, for the first time, demonstrate the rhythmic movements of fetal thorax and abdomen in moving two-dimensional images using the mechanical real-time scanner Vidoson (Siemens, Erlangen, Germany). This was then the final proof of the existence of fetal breathing movements. Together with Kjell Lindström of the Lund Institute of Technology, a device was developed for semi-automatic recording of fetal breathing movements as changes in the diameter

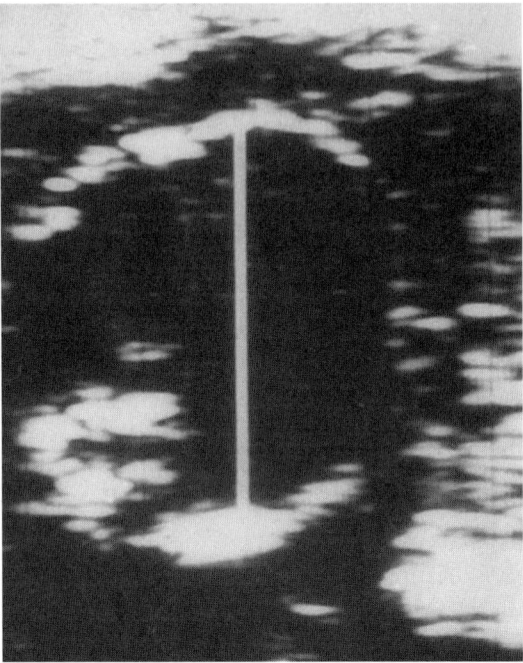

Fig. 6.5 Recording of fetal breathing movements. Image of fetal thorax in transverse section recorded with a mechanical real-time scanner Vidoson (Siemens, Erlangen, Germany).
The vertical white line indicates the chest diameter measured along the selected image line using a time-distance recorder (Diamove, Teltec AB, Lund, Sweden).

of fetal thorax detected by Vidoson (Fig. 6.5) (9). The method, called time–distance recording, was further technically improved and modified for recordings of the pulse waves of fetal aorta (Fig. 6.6) (10). The device (Diamove, Teltec AB, Lund, Sweden) was later applied for recordings of arterial pulsations and estimation of vascular wall stiffness in adults. The Malmö group also belonged to one of the few research groups studying fetal general and limb movements using real-time ultrasound (18).

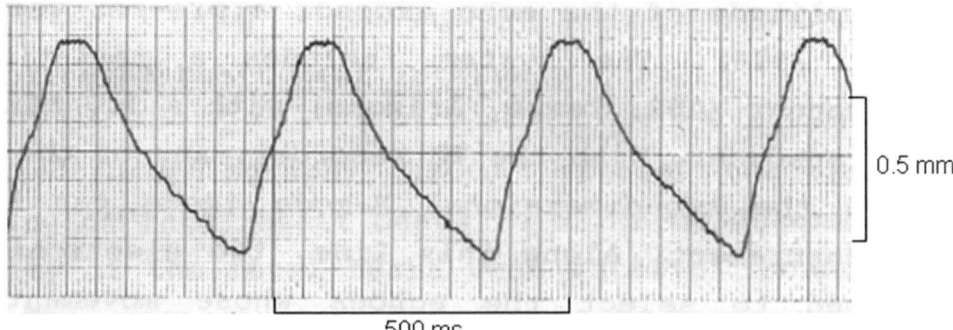

Fig. 6.6 Pulse wave of vessel diameter recorded from the fetal descending aorta at 35 gestational weeks using echo-tracking of vessel walls in the real-time image.

The new ultrasound methods enabled systematical investigations of various fetal functions. The physiological appearance of fetal breathing movements and the reference values of their incidence were established (19) and effects on fetal breathing of various external factors and maternal smoking (20) were demonstrated. It was shown that the characteristics of fetal aortic pulsations were changed in growth-restricted fetuses, possibly indicating an increased blood pressure (21).

Shortly after the first report in the literature on Doppler ultrasound recordings of blood velocity signals from the umbilical artery in 1978, a laboratory for studies of fetal and uteroplacental circulation was established by Karel Maršál in Malmö. Sturla Eik-Nes, who was the first to record the Doppler signals from fetal aorta (22), worked in 1978–1980 on his academic thesis in Malmö. From Trondheim, Norway, he brought with him the method combining a stand-alone pulsed Doppler device (Pedof, Vingmed A/S, Oslo, Norway) with a linear array real-time scanner (ADR 2130, Advanced Diagnostic Research Corp., Tempe, Arizona). This initiated systematic studies of intrauterine circulation at Lund University. These studies contributed significantly to development and establishment of obstetric Doppler as an important clinical tool for surveillance of fetal health in complicated pregnancies, especially in those with intrauterine growth restriction and/or pre-eclampsia.

First, normal values were collected for the volume flow in fetal aorta and umbilical vein calculated from the ultrasonically measured diameter of the vessel and mean velocity recorded with Doppler ultrasound (23). Furthermore, reference values were established for waveform parameters of maximum blood velocity recorded from fetal aorta (24) and umbilical artery (25). Based on the material collected from pregnancies with complications, a new semi-quantitative classification of blood velocity patterns in fetal aorta, so called Blood Flow Classes, was developed (26). The Blood Flow Classes were then modified for the Doppler signals recorded from the umbilical artery (27) and proved very useful for antenatal fetal monitoring in clinical context (Fig. 6.7). For maternal uterine artery, an analogical principle was applied and Uterine Artery Score developed (28).

Step by step, evidence was collected to constitute a basis for development of a clinical model for surveillance of growth-restricted fetuses; this model is now widely used both in Sweden and abroad. An important component of the development was the multicentre randomized clinical study comparing the traditional monitoring of fetuses small-for-gestational age using cardiotocography with monitoring based on Doppler examination of umbilical artery, in which four Swedish obstetric departments participated (29). The postnatal development of growth-restricted fetuses from the prospective studies performed in early 1980s in Malmö was followed-up to 23 years of age and related to the intrauterine Doppler findings (30, 31). These follow-up studies that are ongoing, are unique and much appreciated by international experts (32).

More recently, in the research on intrauterine circulation, some new features of modern ultrasound machines are being utilized, e.g. a method was developed for quantification of power Doppler signals representing fetal lung perfusion (33). The active

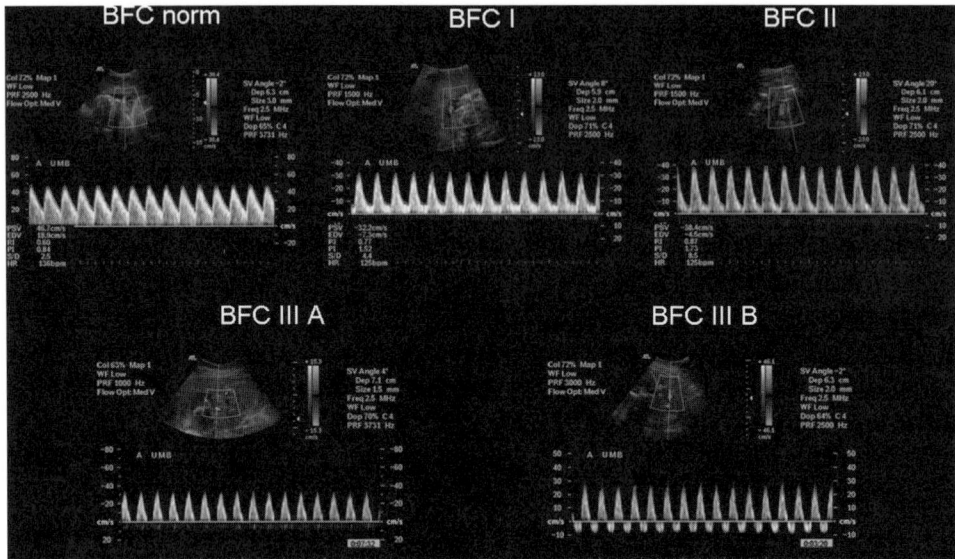

Fig. 6.7 Blood Flow Classes (BFC) of blood velocity waveforms recorded from the umbilical artery. BFC norm, positive diastolic flow velocity, pulsatility index (PI) within mean ± 2 standard deviations (SD) of the reference curve; BFC I, positive diastolic flow, PI > mean + 2SD and ≤ mean + 3 SD; BFC II, positive diastolic flow, PI > mean + 3 SD; BFC IIIA, absent end-diastolic flow velocity; BFC IIIB, reverse end-diastolic flow velocity. (This figure is reproduced in colour in the colour plate section.)

research in obstetric Doppler ultrasound at the perinatal laboratories in Lund and Malmö is now continuing under the leadership of Professor Saemundur Gudmundsson.

Gynaecological ultrasound

Some of the very first transvaginal examinations were performed by Alfred Kratochwil in 1960s (34). Vlasta Václavinková, gynaecologist at the Department of Obstetrics and Gynecology at Sabbatsberg Hospital in Stockholm, visited Professor Kratochwil in Wien in early the 1970s and then used the mechanical rotating transvaginal transducer for evaluation of pelvic capacity (35). To date, the problem of measuring female pelvis with ultrasound has not been solved despite the modern advanced techniques of transvaginal and translabial scanning.

In the 1980s, ultrasound transducers for transvaginal examination became commercially available and were soon widely used in gynaecological outpatient offices. In Sweden, three university centres systematically evaluated the potentials of transvaginal ultrasonography in gynaecology. The research group at Sahlgrenska University Hospital in Gothenburg studied the possibilities of differentiating between malignant and benign processes in endometrium. They lead a Nordic multicentre study that showed in women with postmenstrual bleeding that an endometrium thickness of 4mm or less could exclude malignancy (36). The results of their study elicited a large interest internationally. Wikland et al. (37) in Gothenburg introduced the ultrasonically-guided transvesical collection of oocytes for *in vitro* fertilization.

Andolf and Jörgensen (38) in Lund studied ovarian cysts that often are an accidental finding in women without clinical symptoms. In Malmö, Lil Valentin established a strong research group that evaluated various ultrasound-based models for diagnosing malignancy in female genital organs. Her group systematically investigated the value of gynaecological Doppler ultrasound for diagnosis of endometrial (39) and ovarian (40) cancer.

Safety of diagnostic ultrasound

Diagnostic ultrasound has traditionally had merits of being a non-invasive and safe method. However, ultrasound with high output intensities can potentially interact with biological tissues and might even cause damage. Embryonic/fetal tissues under development would be especially sensitive to such influences. In view of the fact that the modern ultrasound systems might produce very high intensities if not properly managed, it is increasingly important to ensure that the ultrasound operators have the necessary knowledge to use the technique in a correct way. Also, it is of value to follow all reports evaluating possible adverse effects.

In Sweden, the question of ultrasound safety was seriously considered in Sundén's pioneer studies (4) and Sundén was a co-author of the first international follow-up study of infants exposed to ultrasound *in utero* (41). The study did not find any signs of negative effects of ultrasound on the developing fetus. Later, the research group at the Uppsala University performed a follow-up study of infants that were part of the above mentioned randomized study on routine ultrasound examination in mid-pregnancy (15). In agreement with the results of the Norwegian follow-up study, the Uppsala group found a slight increase in the non-right-handedness of boys exposed to ultrasound *in utero* (42). In addition, Kieler et al. (43) performed a register study that gave certain support to the findings of increased left-handedness after fetal ultrasound. No other supporting results were reported and no causal relationship between ultrasound exposure and disturbed development of handedness has been proven. Nevertheless, the findings from the two groups in Sweden and Norway, respectively, should alert the ultrasound researchers to search for any signs of possible adverse effects of diagnostic ultrasound.

The awareness of safety aspects of obstetric ultrasound among Swedish researchers is vindicated by the active participation in the international ultrasound safety committees. Professor Kjell Lindström has participated in a Working Group on Radiation and Ultrasound Safety of the World Health Organization, Professor Karel Maršál has been a member of the European Committee for Medical Ultrasound Safety (ECMUS; the 'watchdogs') for 10 years and he has been succeeded in the committee by Professor Lil Valentin. At present, Maršál is a member of the Safety Committee of the World Federation for Ultrasound in Medicine and Biology (WFUMB).

International standing

The pioneering work in the field of obstetric and gynaecological ultrasound of Swedish researchers has been awarded internationally on several occasions. Bertil Sundén has received the AIUM/WFUMB History of Medical Ultrasound Pioneer Award in 1988 and in 2000, Karel Maršál was been awarded the Ian Donald Gold medal by the International Society of Ultrasound in Obstetrics and Gynecology (ISUOG). Maršál has been a Board member of the European Federation of Societies for Ultrasound in Medicine and Biology (EFSUMB), WFUMB, and ISUOG; he has also served as the President of ISUOG. Lil Valentin has been a member of the EFSUMB Board, responsible for the committee developing education of ultrasound users on European level, and she was a member of the ISUOG Board. For several years, Valentin has been the editor of *Ultrasound in Obstetrics and Gynecology*, the leading international journal of high ranking.

In 2003, Sweden hosted the 14th World Congress on Ultrasound in Obstetrics and Gynecology. The congress took place in Stockholm, the scientific programme was of a very high quality and the meeting attracted 1300 participants from all over the world.

Conclusions

The above account of achievements indicates that research in obstetric and gynaecological ultrasound in Sweden has been very active since the very early days of diagnostic ultrasound and that Swedish researchers have contributed in a significant way to the international development. The activities at many centres in Sweden are ongoing with unchanged intensity, which certainly mirrors the importance of ultrasound in obstetrics and gynaecology. The ultrasound technique has become an indispensable tool for all clinically active obstetricians and gynaecologists and is of great benefit to obstetric and gynaecological patients.

References

1. Leksell L (1956). Echoencephalography I: Detection of intracranial complications following head injury. *Acta Chir Scand* **110**:301–15.
2. Donald I, Mac Vicar J, Brown TG (1958). Investigation of abdominal masses by pulsed ultrasound. *Lancet* **1**(7032):1188–95.
3. Sundén B (1960). Ultraljudsdiagnostik i obstetrik och gynekologi. *Svenska Läkartidningen* **57**(11):769–83.
4. Sundén B (1964). On the diagnostic value of ultrasound in obstetrics and gynaecology. *Acta Obstet Gynecol Scand* **43**(Suppl 6):1–191.
5. Sundén B (1965). Ultrasound in the diagnosis of twins and hydramnios. *J Obstet Gynaecol Brit Cwlth* **72**:952–4.
6. Sundén B (1965). Diagnostic application of ultrasound in obstetrics and gynaecology. *Gynäkol Rundsch* **2**(4):296–309.
7. Sundén B (1970). Placentography by ultrasound. *Acta Obstet Gynecol Scand*, **49**:179–84.
8. Donald I (1974). Sonar–the story of an experiment. *Ultrasound Med Biol* **1**(2):109–17.
9. Maršál K, Gennser G, Lindström K (1976). Real-time ultrasonography for quantified analysis of fetal breathing movements in man. *Lancet* **2**:718–19.
10. Sindberg Eriksen P, Gennser G, Lindström K (1984). Physiological characteristics of diameter pulses in the fetal descending aorta. *Acta Obstet Gynecol Scand* **63**(4):355–63.
11. Grennert L, Persson PH, Gennser G (1978). Benefits of ultrasonic screening of a pregnant population. *Acta Obstet Gynecol Scand Suppl* **78**:5–14.

12. Persson PH, Weldner BM (1986). Intra-uterine weight curves obtained by ultrasound. *Acta Obstet Gynecol Scand* **65**(2):169–73.
13. Maršál K, Persson PH, Larsen T, Lilja H, Selbing A, Sultan B (1996). Intrauterine growth curves based on ultrasonically estimated foetal weights. *Acta Paediatr* **85**:843–8.
14. Selbing A (1983). The pregnant population and a fetal crown-rump length screening program. *Acta Obstet Gynecol Scand* **62**(2):161–4.
15. Waldenström U, Axelsson O, Nilsson S, Eklund G, Fall O, Lindeberg S, et al. (1988). Effects of routine one-stage ultrasound screening in pregnancy: a randomised controlled trial. *Lancet* **332**(8611):585–8.
16. Crang-Svalenius E, Dykes AK, Jörgensen C (1996). Women's informed choice of prenatal diagnosis: early ultrasound examination – routine ultrasound examination – age-independent amniocentesis. *Fetal Diagn Ther* **11**(1):20–5.
17. Saltvedt S, Almström H, Kublickas M, Valentin L, Bottinga R, Bui TH, et al. (2005). Screening for Down syndrome based on maternal age or fetal nuchal translucency: a randomized controlled trial in 39 572 pregnancies. *Ultrasound Obstet Gynecol* **25**(6):537–45.
18. Valentin L, Maršál K, Lindström K (1986). Recording of fetal movements. A comparison of three methods. *J Med Engineering Technol* **10**:239–47.
19. Maršál K (1978). Fetal breathing movements in man – characteristics and clinical significance. *Obstet Gynecol* **52**:394–401.
20. Gennser G, Maršál K, Brantmark B (1975). Maternal smoking and fetal breathing movements. *Am J Obstet Gynecol* **123**:861–7.
21. Stale H, Maršál K, Gennser G, Benthin M, Dahl P, Lindström K (1991). Aortic diameter pulse waves and blood flow velocity in the small-for-gestational age fetus. *Ultrasound Med Biol* **17**(5):471–8.
22. Eik-Nes SH, Brubakk AO, Ulstein MG (1980). Measurement of human fetal blood flow. *Br Med J* **280**:283–4.
23. Eik-Nes SH, Maršál K, Brubakk AO, Kristoffersen K, Ulstein M (1982). Ultrasonic measurements of human fetal blood flow. *J Biomed Engineering* **4**:28–36.
24. Lingman G, Maršál K (1986). Fetal central blood circulation in the third trimester of normal pregnancy. Longitudinal study. II. Aortic blood velocity waveform. *Early Hum Dev* **13**:151–9.
25. Gudmundsson S, Maršál K (1988). Umbilical artery and uteroplacental blood flow velocity waveforms in normal pregnancy – a cross-sectional study. *Acta Obstet Gynecol Scand* **67**:347–54.
26. Laurin J, Lingman G, Maršál K, Persson PH (1987). Fetal blood flow in pregnancies complicated by intrauterine growth retardation. *Obstet Gynecol* **69**:895–902.
27. Gudmundsson S, Maršál K (1991). Blood velocity waveforms in the fetal aorta and umbilical artery as predictors of fetal outcome – a comparison. *Am J Perinatol* **8**:1–6.
28. Hernandez-Andrade E, Brodszki J, Lingman G, Gudmundsson S, Molin J, Maršál K (2002). Uterine artery score and perinatal outcome. *Ultrasound Obstet Gynecol* **19**:438–42.
29. Almström H, Axelsson O, Cnattingius S, Ekman G, Maesel A, Ulmsten U, et al. (1992). Comparison of umbilical artery velocimetry and cardiotocography for surveillance of small-for-gestational-age fetuses. *Lancet* **340**:936–40.
30. Ley D, Laurin J, Bjerre I, Maršál K (1996). Abnormal fetal aortic velocity waveform and minor neurological dysfunction at 7 years of age. *Ultrasound Obstet Gynecol* **8**:152–9.
31. Brodszki J, Länne T, Maršál K, Ley D (2005). Impaired vascular growth in late adolescence after intrauterine growth restriction. *Circulation* **111**:2623–8.
32. Walker DM, Marlow N (2008). Neurocognitive outcome following fetal growth restriction. *Arch Dis Child Fetal Neonatal Ed* **93**(4):F322–F325.

33. Jansson T, Hernandez-Andrade E, Lingman G, Maršál K (2003). Estimation of fractional moving blood volume in fetal lung using power Doppler ultrasound; methodological aspects. *Ultrasound Med Biol* **29**:1551–9.
34. Kratochwil A (1969). A new vaginal method of ultrasonotomography. *Geburtshilfe Frauenheilkd* **29**(4):379–85.
35. Václavinková V (1973). A method of measuring the interspinous diameter by an ultrasonic technique. *A preliminary report. Acta Obstet Gynecol Scand* **52**(2):161–5.
36. Karlsson B, Granberg S, Wikland M, Ylöstalo P, Kiserud T, Maršál K, Valentin L (1995). Transvaginal ultrasonography of the endometrium in women with postmenopausal bleeding – a Nordic multicenter study. *Am J Obstet Gynecol* **172**:1488–94.
37. Wikland M, Nilsson L, Hansson R, Hamberger L, Janson PO (1983). Collection of human oocytes by the use of sonography. *Fertil Steril* **39**(5):603–8.
38. Andolf E, Jörgensen C (1988). Simple adnexal cysts diagnosed by ultrasound in postmenopausal women. *J Clin Ultrasound* **16**(5):301–3.
39. Epstein E, Skoog L, Isberg PE, De Smet F, De Moor B, Olofsson PA, Gudmundsson S, Valentin L (2002). An algorithm including results of gray-scale and power Doppler ultrasound examination to predict endometrial malignancy in women with postmenopausal bleeding. *Ultrasound Obstet Gynecol* **20**(4):370–6.
40. Sladkevicius P, Valentin L, Maršál K (1995). Transvaginal Doppler examination for the differential diagnosis of solid pelvic tumors. *J Ultrasound Med* **14**:377–80.
41. Hellman LM, Duffus GM, Donald I, Sundén B (1970). Safety of diagnostic ultrasound in obstetrics. *Lancet* **1**(7657):1133–4.
42. Kieler H, Axelsson O, Haglund B, Nilsson S, Salvesen KA (1998). Routine ultrasound screening in pregnancy and the children's subsequent handedness. *Early Hum Dev* **50**(2):233–45.
43. Kieler H, Cnattingius S, Haglund B, Palmgren J, Axelsson O (2001). Sinistrality – a side-effect of prenatal sonography: a comparative study of young men. *Epidemiology* **12**(6):618–23.

Chapter 7

A history of ultrasound in obstetrics and gynaecology

Stuart Campbell

Introduction

It is often difficult to know when most developments in medicine actually begin. They tend to evolve and many people will claim the credit of being the first to make the breakthrough. With ultrasound in obstetrics and gynaecology there is no such doubt for it had a very definite beginning with the 1958 classic *Lancet* paper (1) by Ian Donald, John McVicar, and Tom Brown 'The investigation of abdominal masses by pulsed ultrasound'. Actually this is an unfortunate title because it does not identify what was truly unique about the paper which is that it was entirely devoted to ultrasound studies in clinical obstetrics and gynaecology and contained the first ultrasound images of the fetus and also gynaecological masses. The other unique feature was that these were the first images taken with a compound contact scanner which was the first practical scanning machine.

Before Donald

It would be short-sighted to write about the development of medical ultrasound without mentioning some of the great scientists of the 19th and 20th centuries whose conceptual advances paved the way for the modern ultrasound machine. Thomas Young in 1801 described 'phase shifting' in relation to light waves but this concept is used in ultrasound phased array systems to control interference patterns and is used in the production of three-dimensional (3-D) images. Christian Doppler in 1842 described what we now call the 'Doppler effect' in relation to the motion of stars but this principle is now used as the basis for blood flow studies in pelvic vessels and the fetus. Pierre Curie in 1880 described the piezo electric effect whereby mechanical distortion of ceramic crystals would produce an electric charge; the reverse of this effect is used in all transducers to generate ultrasonic waves. Paul Langevin in 1915 built the first hydrophone which used ultrasonic waves to locate the position and distance of submarines and is the principle behind the measurement of the fetus and abdominal masses by ultrasound. The development of Radar by Watson-Watt and his team using electromagnetic waves in 1943 was later adapted for ultrasound to produce two-dimensional (2-D) images.

The first simple A-scan metal flaw detectors and modifications of this equipment were used medically in 1949 by George Ludwig at the Massachusetts Institute of Technology (MIT) to locate gallstones and John Julian Wild at the Technical Research Institute in Minnesota to detect breast masses. In 1953, Inge Edler and Hellmuth Hertz in Lund University adapted a metal flaw detector to obtain M-mode recordings from the adult heart. Wild, together with his engineer John Read, published the first 2-D images in 1952 but his efforts were directed towards tissue characterization especially of breast tumours and the accolade for producing the first tomographic images of human anatomy must go to Douglass Howry in Denver who published his landmark paper (2) in the same year. There was a major problem, however, with the Howry approach which depended on immersing the body part to be examined in degassed water (called water delay scanning) to avoid artefactual echoes from superficial structures. The equipment was inelegant and uncomfortable for the patient and it seems unlikely that ultrasound diagnosis would have made the breakthrough into becoming the most widespread imaging modality in clinical use was it not for the development of the compound contact scanner by Donald and Brown in the late 1950s.

Ian Donald

Donald was a tall, red-haired charismatic Scottish obstetrician gynaecologist with a brilliant mind and a quick temper. He was a most generous and principled man whose anti-abortion stance denied him honours in his own country. He worked feverishly partly because he was a workaholic but principally because he had severe rheumatic heart disease (he needed mitral valve operations on at least three occasions) and every moment was precious to him. It was probably fortunate that Donald knew little of the work being carried out in Denver so armed with some knowledge of radar technology which he learned in the air force, he got together with a very clever engineer called Tom Brown and with help from a local engineering company developed the world's first contact compound 2-D ultrasound scanning machine, called the Diasonograph (Fig. 7.1). He and his team published their seminal pioneering paper in *The Lancet* in 1958. It begins with the physics of ultrasound scanning techniques, safety experiments, ultrasound images of pregnancy, the fetus and gynaecological tumours, and a really detailed description of the strengths, weaknesses, and potential of this new technique. The ultrasound images were crude and bistable (i.e. totally lacking grey-scale) and static with the image being slowly created on a cathode ray tube by rocking the transducer slowly over the abdomen. But the starting gun had been fired and the ultrasound race had begun.

The static scanner years
Equipment development

During the next decade a large number of static scanning machines were made. They were initially built in research centres where it was essential always to have dedicated physicists on hand for these were pre-transistor days and the equipment was prone to develop electronic faults. Compared to today's sleek real-time digital scanning machines, the Diasonograph was the equivalent of Babbage's difference engine to the modern laptop. It was 8ft in height and occupied about one-third of the scanning room. The gantry that

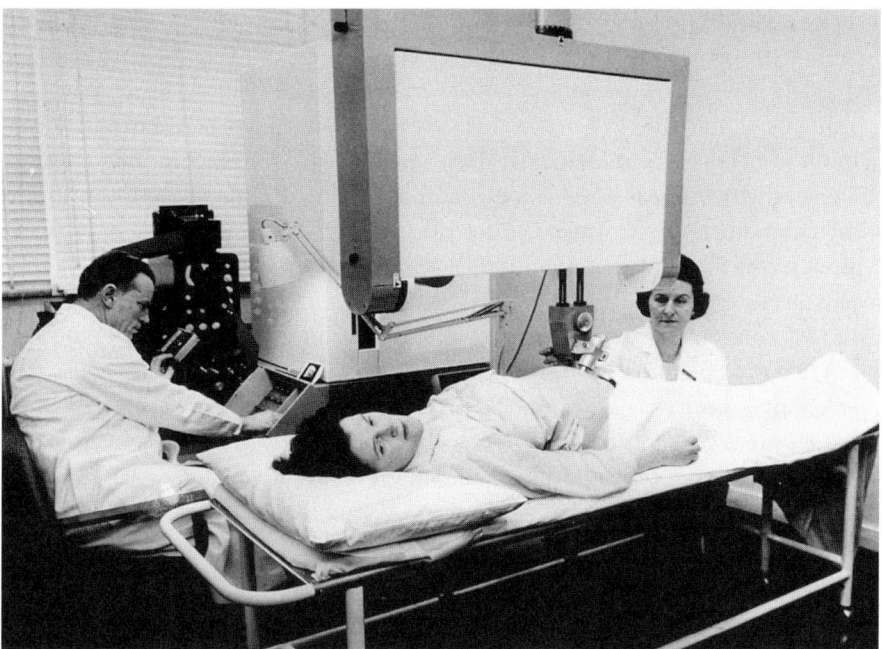

Fig. 7.1 Ian Donald in action with the Mk3 Diasonograph in 1960.

housed the probe was very large and had to be physically shifted with no small effort to alter the scanning plane. Many people, especially the Americans, unkindly called it the Dinosaur. However, it had positive features which allowed users to take an early lead in ultrasound biometry. For example, it had by far the best image resolution compared to its rivals. The rigid gantry frame meant that reproducible scans could be made at any angle and in any plane, although if the fetus moved it meant beginning the lining up process again which could be time-consuming. The probe was on a pulley system and could be skimmed with ease across the woman's abdomen as the static image was built up on the oscilloscope. The first contact machine developed in America was the Physionics (to become the Picker machine) which emanated from Howry's laboratory in Denver and was used for ObGyn scanning by Horace Thomson and Ken Gottesfeld. It had an articulated scanning arm which was easy to manipulate but it made the obtaining of reproducible planes more difficult and the resolution and sensitivity to low-level echoes was initially poor. Similar style machines were built in Vienna by Kretztechnic (used by Alfred Kratochwil), in Copenhagen by Hewlett Packard (used by Jens Bang and Hans Hendrik Holm), and in Japan by Aloka (used by Hsiao Takeuchi). Both Kretztechnic and Aloka developed commercial transvaginal transducers in the mid-1960s but the potential of transvaginal scanning was not realized until the advent of real-time imaging. Two distinctly different machines compared to the static machines described above were also built in the mid-1960s. In Germany, Richard Soldner, an engineer who worked for Siemens, developed the first (almost) real-time scanner which consisted of a very large fluid-filled plastic membrane as the scanning head which housed three rotating transducers in front of a parabolic mirror to produce flickering images at 15 frames per second. Compared to the Diasonograph the image resolution was poor yet this machine was purchased widely in German-speaking countries and by the late 1960s was probably the most commonly used machine in Europe. Initially exponents such as Manfred Hansmann from Bonn and Hans Jurgen Hollander from Munster used the machine like a static scanner but eventually the real-time facility was found to be useful. At the Commonwealth Acoustic Laboratories in Australia George Kossoff one of the most brilliant engineers in the history of medical ultrasound built the Octoson static scanner in 1962. This machine followed the Howry principle of water delay scanning with the patient lying face down on a plastic tank containing a large amount of degassed water. Although there was an absence of artefactual reverberation echoes beneath the skin surface, the images were initially of average quality and it was not until the invention of the scan converter by Kossoff in the late 1960s that gave this equipment especial prominence. The scan converter allowed the display of scattered reflections in shades of grey thus giving an appearance of tissue texture and introducing the concept of grey-scale scanning. The Octoson mark 2 images in the late 1960s were spectacularly good in demonstrating fetal anatomy but the Octoson's time of brilliance was short-lived following the introduction of the scan converter into contact static scanning machines and the convenience of the latter equipment won the day.

Clinical studies

Donald and his team with the benefit of priority made some early breakthroughs and in 1963 had described the early diagnosis of hydatid mole (with its snowstorm appearance), assessment, and growth of the early gestation sac (by the full bladder technique) and the diagnosis of early pregnancy complications (3).

Placentography

Accurate location of the placenta was the holy grail of antenatal diagnosis in the early 1960s for placenta praevia was the cause of significant maternal mortality due to severe haemorrhage in late gestation. Many radioisotope methods were used at this time but they were unable to accurately define the lower placental edge. In 1966 Ken Gottesfeld and the Denver group published the first paper on ultrasound placentography (4) although they were unable to visualize the posterior placenta (posterior praevia was implied by a space posterior to the fetal head) and it was not till 1968 that Donald and Usama Abdulla in a larger study (5) and with their superior equipment were able to demonstrate placenta in all locations including posterior praevia.

Fetal biometry

The initial studies in fetal biometry employed blind A-scan measurements of the biparietal diameter (BPD) and James Willocks from Donald's department published an interesting paper on head growth in the third trimester showing different rates of growth between growth-restricted and normally growing fetuses. The method was intrinsically inaccurate, however, and precision was needed for meaningful biometry. This was provided by one of Donald's registrars, Stuart Campbell who described the B-mode technique in 1968 where the midline echo of the fetal head was visualized in two dimensions and then an A-scan measurement was made between the parietal eminences at the widest point. It was not until on-screen callipers were introduced several years later that A-scan was no longer required. Campbell demonstrated that the midline echo could be seen reliably from 13 weeks' gestation and soon showed that second trimester cephalometry was an effective method of dating pregnancy in women with uncertain dates introducing the concept of an ultrasound expected date of confinement (EDD) (6). Following this he developed the first cephalometry graph from 13–40 weeks and used this to identify the intrauterine growth-restricted (IUGR) fetus by showing a sharp slowing of biparietal diameter growth in the third trimester. Cephalometry graphs were subsequently produced by Manfred Hansmann, Alfred Kratochwil, Rudi Sabbagha, and many others and serial cephalometry became a standard method of measuring fetal growth for many years.

The disadvantage of just measuring the fetal head is that brain is the last structure to be affected in growth restriction and Horace Thompson and Ed Makowsky from Denver in 1971 introduced measurement of the thoracic circumference (TC) and the concept of fetal weight prediction using a combination of this measurement and the BPD (7). Manfred Hansmann in Bonn confirmed these results and demonstrated an asymmetry between the BPD measurement and the thoracic circumference in IUGR fetuses. Stuart Campbell—who had now moved to Queen Charlotte's Hospital in London—believed there were intrinsic problems with reproducibility with TC measurements as the chest is cone-shaped in the fetus and there was no reliable marker to indicate the level of the scan. In 1975 he introduced the abdominal circumference measurement (AC) at the level of the intra-abdominal umbilical vein as a more reliable measurement and this has become a standard measurement ever since (8). As the AC measurement is at the level of the liver which is the most severely affected organ in IUGR, the head circumference to abdomen circumference ratio was introduced as a means of recognizing the brain-spared IUGR fetus.

The value of routine screening of the obstetric population for accurate dating, early detection of twin gestations, and placental location was first demonstrated by Lars Grennert and Per-Håkan Persson from Malmö (9) who described the evolution of a routine screening programme over a 5-year period; 24% of women had an uncertain EDD and 95% of women were delivered within 12 days of the ultrasound prediction. Also 95% of twins were detected in the second trimester as opposed to 70% before the programme was started.

Early pregnancy

Kratochwil using his transvaginal transducer demonstrated fetal cardiac motion by A-scan from 7 weeks' gestation in 1967 but most studies in the 1960s and early 1970s were carried out abdominally by the full bladder technique. For example, Bang and Holm from the Copenhagen school reported identifying the fetal heart beat from 10 weeks' gestation in 1968. The seminal work on early pregnancy assessment came from Hugh Robinson from the Glasgow school. In 1973, using an improved Diasonograph he produced the first detailed biometry charts of the fetal crown–rump length (CRL) from 7–16 weeks' gestation; his measurements were so meticulous that they are still in use today (10). Using the combined A- and B-mode equipment he subsequently produced charts of the fetal heart rate from 7 weeks' gestation and showed that the detection rate was 100%. He was the first to point out the prognostic significance of finding a fetal heartbeat at 8 weeks' gestation in relation to subsequent fetal demise. This work had a profound influence on the management of patients with threatened abortion.

Fetal abnormalities

Anecdotal reports of the prenatal diagnosis of congenital abnormalities in women with polyhydramnios in the late second or third trimester were made by Bertil Sundén in 1964 (a case of anencephaly) and William Garrett in 1970 who described a case of polycystic kidneys. Ultrasound prenatal diagnosis really began with the *Lancet* paper by Campbell and his group who in 1972 reported the diagnosis of anencephaly at 17 weeks which resulted in elective termination of pregnancy (11). Subsequent to this he systematically examined the fetal spine in women with raised serum AFP and reported the diagnosis of spina bifida in 1975. By 1977 he was able to report on 329 high-risk pregnancies examined between 16 and 20 weeks in which ultrasound detected 25 of the 28 neural tube defects; 10 of the 13 cases of spina bifida were detected with the false negatives being low sacral lesions (12). In the United States, John Hobbins and his team at Yale in 1978 described the prenatal diagnosis of several abnormalities including limb reduction defects (13). The widespread use of ultrasound in prenatal diagnosis came with the invention of the real-time scanning machines.

The real-time revolution
Equipment development

Mechanical sector real-time scanners were introduced by several companies such as Aloka and Kretztechnic in the early to mid-1970s but these were quickly superseded by the multi-element linear array and phased array scanners in the mid to late 1970s. Due to the huge advances in integrated circuit technology occurring at this time, the machines were small and moveable and as they were less expensive, a department would have several instead of the single large static scanner. Movements of the fetus could now be followed and the probe angle instantly adjusted to identify the plane of interest. Sonographers and research fellows could be quickly trained and as complete fetal biometry could be achieved in a matter of minutes, screening the whole obstetric population was now feasible. The first commercial linear array real-time scanner was the ADR, a small company founded by Martin Wilcox in Tempe, Arizona. Initially it had only 64 lines so the resolution was poor but the second version, the ADR 2130 in 1975, had over 500 lines and phased focusing and could compete with static scanners in terms of resolution. Most large ultrasound companies produced real-time equipment over the next few years, leapfrogging each other in degrees of sophistication but the development of the Acuson 128 by Sam Maslak in 1983 with its advanced beamforming software (called 'computed sonography') set new standards in both spatial and contrast resolution. In 1985, Kretztechnic produced the first practical endovaginal mechanical sector transducer which was designed to improve the technique of oocyte collection in *in vitro* fertilization (IVF). These transducers provided excellent images but probe vibrations were a disadvantage and by the end of the 1990s most manufacturers had developed small multi-element probes which provided excellent resolution.

By 1985, Aloka had incorporated colour Doppler imaging (originally called colour flow mapping) into their real-time equipment and this was quickly followed by other major manufacturers. By 1990 colour was available on the transvaginal probe for gynaecological investigation. By the end of the 1990s harmonic imaging was introduced which even further improved image resolution. Although early studies on 3-D imaging were begun in Japan by Kazunon Baba in 1984, it was not until the production of the third-generation 530D Voluson in the mid-1990s that the world was convinced that 3-D/4-D ultrasound had a major role to play in both obstetrical and gynaecological imaging. Much of the credit for promoting this new technology must go to Bernard Benoit, a French doctor working in Nice who published stunning 3-D images of the fetus, especially in the first trimester. It could thus be said that (apart from a few refinements) the modern real-time scanning machine with high-resolution abdominal and endovaginal transducers, harmonic imaging, colour and power Doppler facilities with a 3-D/4-D option was on the market by the year 2000 (Fig. 7.2).

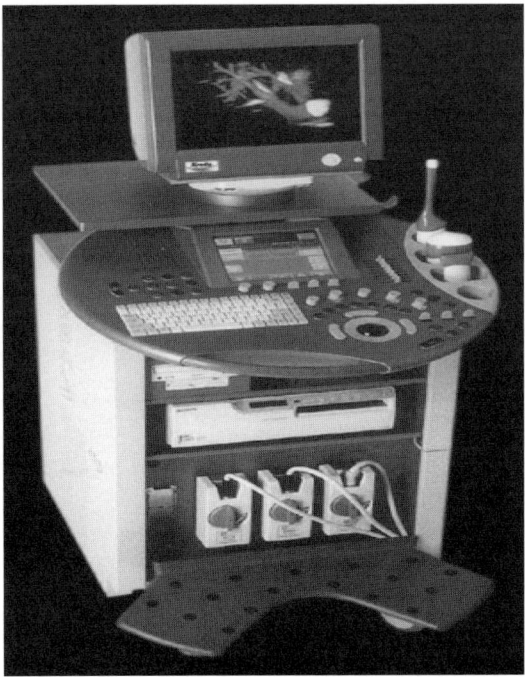

Fig. 7.2 A typical modern scanning machine complete with high-resolution imaging, colour and power Doppler, and a 3-D/4-D option (GE Voluson Expert). (This figure is reproduced in colour in the colour plate section.)

Clinical studies in obstetrics

The development of real-time scanning was a great democratizing influence in obstetric scanning which was no longer confined to an elite group of experts in a few major centres. Real-time scanners being inexpensive were now widely available and many experienced practitioners of static scanning were surprised (and not a little discomfited) at how quickly their junior doctors, midwives, and sonographers became experts in scanning almost overnight (Fig. 7.3).

Fetal biometry

The ease with which the probe could be manipulated meant that many fetal structures were measured and a great number of charts of different planes and organs were developed. For example, charts of interorbital diameter (14), long bones, foot length, ear length, the sizes of virtually every fetal organ, and multiple ratios between parameters like femur to foot were produced within a space of a few years. However, the standard measurements CRL, BPD, head circumference, and abdomen circumference which were developed during the static era remained the standard fetal biometric measurements for assessing growth with only the addition of the femur length (which was now easier to measure) incorporated into equations for fetal weight and growth predictions (15).

Fetal activity

Studies of fetal behaviour were inspired by leaders in development biology such as Geoffrey Dawes in Oxford and Heinz Prechtl in Nijmegan. The ability to follow fetal movements by ultrasound inspired much interest as to whether quantification of these movements and especially fetal breathing movements might be helpful in assessing fetal well-being. In the late 1970s, detailed studies using event markers on a chart recorder were made by groups led by Karel Maršál in Malmö, John Patrick in London, Ontario and Alistair Roberts in London. The time, incidence, and number of movement episodes or fetal breaths were quantitatively assessed and behavioural states identified. Both fetal breathing movements and fetal activity are episodic and are rarely concordant so the concept of

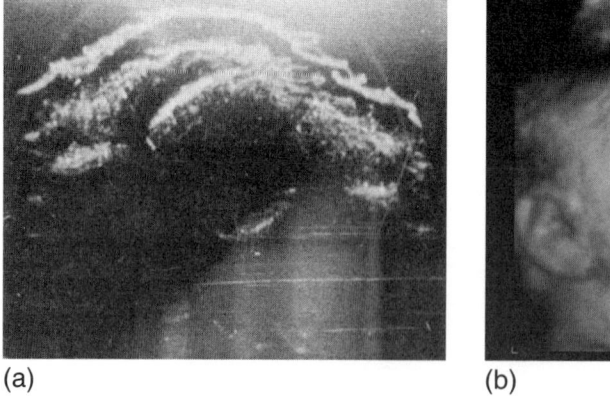

(a)   (b)

Fig. 7.3 Fifty years of progress. (a) Fetal head from Donald's 1958 paper (1). (b) Fetal head by 3-D scan 2008.

measuring total fetal activity over a 30-minute period was employed. Although there was an association between reduced total activity and IUGR, the test had a low predictive value for a positive test due to the large physiological variation in the incidence of both breathing and motor activity (16). For this reason in Europe the measurement of fetal activity fell out of favour as a means of assessing fetal well being. In the United States, however, Frank Manning and Larry Platt in 1980 incorporated both of these measures into a 30-minute fetal biophysical profile test (17) which also included an assessment of amniotic fluid, fetal tone and a non-stress test (cardiotocography, CTG) of the fetal heart. This test with minor modifications became the mainstay of fetal well-being assessment in the United States for over 20 years. In Europe, however, researchers turned increasingly to Doppler ultrasound to solve the problem as to how to effectively assess fetal well-being and optimize the timing of delivery when there is fetal compromise.

Doppler assessment

The demonstration of the umbilical artery waveform using blind continuous wave (CW) Doppler was reported as early as the mid-1960s from Osaka, Japan and in 1977 by D.E. Fitzgerald and John Drumm from Dublin using 2-D static scans to identify where the probe should be placed but neither of these two groups followed-up their observations. Two groups initiated pulsed Doppler studies of the fetus. In Australia, Robert Gill working with the Kossoff group, measured flow velocity in the umbilical vein. However, the long path length of the Octoson prevented the measurement of high velocity arterial flow and this system was impractical for clinical Doppler studies. Sturla Eik-Nes working in Karel Maršál's department in Malmö described the first duplex linear array system (18) where an offset pulsed Doppler probe was attached at a fixed angle of 52°. He measured flow velocities from the fetal aorta and found that they were reduced in IUGR fetuses. Equipment similar to the Malmö duplex Doppler system was used by workers in several academic units in the early to mid-1980s across Europe to define the fetal circulatory response to hypoxia. It was found that absolute velocity measurements were inferior to waveform analysis especially the pulsatility index in the assessment changes in the fetal circulation to hypoxia. Yuri Wladimiroff in Rotterdam was the first to draw attention to the compensatory increase in the cerebral circulation or 'centralization of the fetal circulation' associated with IUGR fetuses (19). Karel Maršál and his Malmö group correlated circulatory changes with behavioural states while Campbell, David Griffin and Kypros Nicolaides at King's College Hospital in London correlated these changes with blood gases obtained by cordocentesis. In Australia, Brian Trudinger and Warwick Giles rediscovered the importance of the umbilical artery waveform and established the significance of absent and reversed end diastolic flow (20). In 1983, Campbell and his group described the uterine artery waveform and the appearance of notching which together with a high resistance index was associated with pre-eclampsia (21). His group subsequently used this finding to screen the pregnant population at 24 weeks' gestation to predict the subsequent development of pre-eclampsia, and IUGR and showed a high sensitivity for the severe forms of these conditions.

The advent of colour Doppler as an integral part of the ultrasound machine made visualization of fetal vessels much easier and studies of virtually every fetal artery (such as the renal, splanchnic, cerebral) was investigated and charts made of the gestational changes of pulsatility index (PI) under different clinical circumstances. In the early 1990s, the principal vessels studied to evaluate fetal well-being were the umbilical artery and middle cerebral artery. Although these were useful they were no better than the antenatal CTG in determining the optimal time of delivery in the compromised fetus. This led to several groups investigating the venous side of the fetal circulation. Initial studies concentrated on the inferior vena cava but in 1991 in a landmark *Lancet* paper, Torvid Kiserud from the Eik-Nes group in Trondheim, Norway described the measurement of the pulsatility of the ductus venosus (22) which has become established as a key measure of cardiac function and indicator fetal asphyxia. With modern equipment, Doppler evaluation of the fetal circulation—especially umbilical and middle cerebral arteries and ductus venosus—is now established as a fundamental requirement in the assessment of fetal well-being and the timing of delivery of the compromised fetus.

The prediction of pre-eclampsia and IUGR by uterine artery Doppler was further explored by Nicolaides in a very large multicentre studies. The Nicolaides group showed that the uterine artery PI performed at 23 weeks predicted 85% of women who would develop severe pre-eclampsia for only a 5% screen positive rate (23). One of the problems is that prevention by agents such as low-dose aspirin does not seem to be effective. Nicolaides and others are now exploring the possibility of screening for pre-eclampsia in the first trimester (when preventive therapy appears to be effective) using uterine artery Doppler and biochemical markers such as placental growth factor (PlGF) and pregnancy-associated plasma protein-A (PAPP-A).

Preterm delivery

Preterm labour is the greatest cause of neonatal death and handicap and the care of the preterm baby is hugely expensive. Although the causes of spontaneous preterm labour are many and not fully understood, a common final pathway is shortening and effacement of the cervix. Several studies in the early 1980s using transabdominal ultrasound drew attention to the association between a short cervix and funnelling with cervical incompetence. Frank Andersen from Ann Arbor, Michigan was the first to draw attention to the superiority of transvaginal scanning (24) and provide a risk for preterm delivery based on a cervical length. Subsequent studies by Jay Iams from Columbus, Ohio and Kypros Nicolaides from King's College, London have confirmed that screening around 23–24 weeks' gestation will predict a large percentage of women who will go into preterm labour. For example, Nicolaides screened over 32 000 women at 23 weeks and was able to identify 50% of women delivering before 33 weeks' gestation by using a cut-off cervical length of 15mm. Unfortunately cervical cerclage does not appear to be effective in extending gestation in these women although there appears to be significant prolongation of gestation in the shortened cervix group with progesterone suppositories.

Fetal abnormality screening

Following the introduction of real-time scanning there was a large number of review papers documenting the experience of tertiary centres in diagnosing a wide range of abnormalities of virtually every organ of the fetal body. By the mid-1980s most hospitals had introduced screening for fetal abnormalities as part of the routine 20-week scan. Many of the studies published at this time were invalid because of low ascertainment of anomalies in the newborn (the prevalence should be between 2% and 3%). A controversial American multicentre study (RADIUS) published in 1993 demonstrated a low detection rate of 17% for the early detection of fetal abnormalities but this was not the experience in European centres. Multicentre studies as a rule had lower detection rates than those from single centres. For example, in Salvator Levi's large Belgian multicentre study conducted between 1990 and 1992, only 40% of fetuses with anomalies were detected before 23 weeks while Carrera, in a single-centre in Barcelona, reported an 85% detection rate in a similar time period.

Fetal cardiac defects

For the first time the diagnosis of cardiac abnormalities was now possible. In 1980, two breakthrough papers on real-time fetal echocardiography were published, by Lindsey Allan from King's College Hospital, London and Charles Kleinman from Yale. In her classic study, Allan (25) was the first to describe the systematic examination of the heart to demonstrate the four-chamber view and outflow tracts and published images of the eight classic ultrasound views together with anatomic correlates and was one of the first to promote routine screening for fetal cardiac abnormalities. In 1997, S.-J. Yoo (26) described an additional classic view, namely the three-vessel view of the outflow tracts. The advent of colour Doppler facilitated studies of intracardiac flow with groups led by Greg DeVore (27), Rabih Chaoui, and Ulrich Gembruch making significant contributions.

Fetal chromosome abnormalities

Before the real-time revolution, amniocentesis was offered to the 'high-risk' group of women over the age of 35 years but this policy failed to diagnose the 70% of babies with Down syndrome who were born to younger women. In 1985, Beryl Benacerraf and her group in Boston first described that an increased nuchal skin-fold measurement in the second trimester was associated with Down syndrome (28) and subsequently described the other classic second trimester markers of shortened femur and pyelectasia. For the first time younger women could be offered amniocentesis on the basis of a combination of markers. The decisive breakthrough came in 1992 when Kypros Nicolaides from King's in London described the first-trimester measurement of nuchal translucency in the diagnosis of Down's syndrome (29). Nicolaides and his group subsequently demonstrated the association of increased nuchal translucency, absence of the nasal bone, tricuspid regurgitation, and increased ductus venosus PI with Down's syndrome. They have combined these markers with the measurement of serum PAPP-A and free beta human chorionic gonadotropin (hCG) to provide a likelihood ratio for the presence of Down's syndrome. With this programme, 90% of Down's syndrome fetuses are detected for a 5% screen positive rate. With chorionic villus sampling (CVS) being offered to women at increased risk, this screening programme has been adopted throughout the world.

Invasive procedures

The importance of identifying the position of the needle during amniocentesis was first highlighted by Jens Bang in Copenhagen in 1973 during the static scan era but few practitioners used his transducer with a central hole and scans at this time were usually used to identify a placenta-free accessible pool of fluid prior to the procedure. The advent of real-time scanning allowed the performance of invasive procedures under continuous vision thus reducing bloody taps and avoiding placental, cord, or fetal injury. In 1974 fetoscopy was introduced by John Hobbins and Maurice Mahoney at Yale for the prenatal diagnosis of haemoglobinopathies (30) from fetal red blood cells obtained from the chorionic plate. Many believed that this technique would supersede ultrasound-guided methods, especially when Rodeck and Campbell at King's in London described the obtaining of pure fetal blood from the umbilical vein by this method and Niels Hahnemann and Jan Mohr with a similar instrument obtained chorionic tissue trancervically for genetic diagnosis. However, in 1983, Fernand Daffos and co-workers from Paris introduced pure fetal blood sampling from the cord insertion by direct ultrasound-guided needling using two operators (31) and subsequently Nicolaides from King's perfected the single operator two-hands method and called it cordocentesis. He and his team used this technique to assess the severity of fetal anaemia in rhesus disease thus supplanting the old method based on bilirubin measurements in the amniotic fluid (32). Nicolaides and others such as Giorgio Pardi in Milan also used this technique to assess aspects of fetal acid–base status and biochemistry in the IUGR fetus. Another nail in the coffin for fetoscopy came with the introduction of transabdominal first-trimester fine needle aspiration of chorionic villi (CVS) by Steen Smidt-Jensen and Hahnemann in 1984 (33), a technique which has been adopted universally for the prenatal diagnosis of fetal genetic and karyotype defects.

Fetal therapy

The treatment of severe rhesus disease in the fetus by intraperitoneal transfusion under X-ray guidance was pioneered by Lilley in 1959. Hansmann, in 1968, used the Vidoson's 'real-time' capability to simplify the technique into an ultrasound-guided procedure (34). Access to the fetal circulation, however, prompted the development of therapeutic procedures by cordocentesis such as fetal blood transfusion in severe rhesus disease (35) and platelet transfusion for alloimmune thrombocytopenia. Ultrasound-controlled needling procedures were also used to insert shunts to decompress obstructions in the urinary tract and cerebral ventricles or to drain fluid from pleural effusions but none of these procedures were found to significantly improve outcome and in the case of ventriculomegaly, the condition was frequently made worse. Two prenatal surgical procedures that have been shown to be useful involve the combined use of ultrasound and fetoscopy. In 1995, Yves Ville and Nicolaides from King's College in London demonstrated the effectiveness of laser ablation to the communicating placental vessels in the treatment of twin-to-twin transfusion syndrome (36) and this technique has been shown to be superior to therapeutic amniocentesis in terms of fetal survival. In 1998, Harrison's group in San Francisco described occlusion of the fetal trachea by ultrasound-guided fetoscopic surgery for the treatment of severe diaphragmatic hernia and subsequently Jan Deprest, Eduard Gratacos, and Nicolaides described temporary endoscopic balloon occlusion for this condition resulting in a significant improvement in outcome.

Clinical studies in gynaecology

Advances in gynaecological scanning were rapid following the introduction of the real-time transvaginal probe in the mid-1980s. Before this, visualization of the pelvic organs required the patient to have a distended bladder which not only frequently caused her distress but often pushed the structure of interest beyond the focal distance of the transducer. Despite this, important studies were made with the static scanners. Following on Donald's original observations of the characteristics of malignant ovarian tumours, Patricia Morley and Ellis Barnett from Glasgow described in 1970 the ultrasound differential diagnosis of ovarian masses. In 1981, Nick Kadar and Roberto Romero from Yale (37) described the discriminatory zone (i.e. the minimal hCG level that should be associated with an intrauterine sac) for the diagnosis of ectopic gestation. In 1979 Joachim Hackeloer, a German doctor working on sabbatical in Glasgow, published his classic paper on the tracking of ovarian follicular growth (38) and showed a correlation between follicular size and serum oestradiol. In 1985, Judith Adams working in Howard Jacobs Unit in London determined the classic ultrasound parameters for the diagnosis of polycystic ovaries (PCO) and subsequently showed that PCO affected 23% of the female population during their reproductive years. However, the advent of transvaginal sonography changed the diagnostic impact of ultrasound in gynaecology.

Early pregnancy disorders

The importance of understanding normal embryogenesis was emphasized by Ilan Timor-Tritsch from Columbia University, New York who pioneered the concept of transvaginal 'sono-embryology' in the late 1980s (39) and subsequently he and other workers described the diagnosis of early embryonic abnormalities. The direct diagnosis of ectopic pregnancy was also revolutionized by transvaginal probe. David Nyberg and Roy Filly from San Francisco (40) and Bruno Cacciatore from Finland in the late 1980s described the many sonographic manifestations of this condition and reported diagnostic success rates of over 90%. In the 1990s virtually every hospital had an emergency diagnostic unit where women with pelvic pain and bleeding were assessed by an expert transvaginal scan and a sensitive beta hCG blood test.

Pelvic masses

Transvaginal sonography (TVS) allowed greater discrimination between benign and malignant masses and there were several attempts to create a scoring system of morphological parameters to better define the differential diagnosis. Sassone and Timor Tritch in New York Hospital first described such a scoring system. The advent of colour Doppler allowed the detection of angiogenesis in tumours and in 1989 Tom Bourne and Campbell at King's demonstrated high vascularity with increased peak velocity flow was associated with malignant masses. Anil Tailor from the same group developed a multiple regression model incorporating morphological and blood flow criteria. More recently a European multicentre trial (IOTA) led by Dirk Timmerman from Leuven and Lil Valentin from Malmö has developed sophisticated models to discriminate benign from malignant masses (41). While these models have provided useful information they have not been shown to be superior to the subjective evaluation by an experienced observer in differentiating benign from malignant tumours

Screening for malignancy

Ovarian cancer has the highest mortality rate of all gynaecological cancers because it is symptom free in its early stages. Campbell and his team at King's in London in 1989 (42) using transabdominal scanning and John Van Nagell in Lexington, Kentucky in 1991 using transvaginal ultrasound both reported a high detection rate for ovarian cancer, most of which were at stage 1 but due to the high number of benign cysts the operation rate per cancer detected was unacceptably high. In 1999, Ian Jacobs at University College London introduced the concept of multimodal ovarian cancer screening in which serial CA125 measurements were used as the screening test backed up by TVS in screen positive cases to reduce the false positive rate. He has since set up a large UK multicentre randomized screening programme (UKCTOCS) which is at present ongoing but initial published data (43) indicates a high detection rate for epithelial cancer with only 2.7 operations per cancer detected.

Reproductive medicine

The advent of TVS transformed reproductive medicine, especially the monitoring and procedures associated with IVF. Traditionally following on the pioneer work of Patrick Steptoe, oocyte collection was made by laparoscopy but in 1990 Susan Lenz from Jens Bang's unit in Copenhagen described the ultrasound guided transvesical aspiration of oocytes (44). At King's John Parsons used the Copenhagen technique to make IVF a totally outpatient procedure. In 1995, Wilfred Feichtinger and Pieter Kemeter from Vienna described transvaginal oocyte aspiration with a needle guide attached to the transvaginal probe (45) and this has now become the standard technique.

Clinical studies in 3-D/4-D ultrasound

The advent of 3-D ultrasound imaging has led to a flurry of publications extolling the virtues of this new modality yet substantial evidence of definitive benefit is hard to obtain. Most fetal anomalies can be detected by high-resolution 2-D ultrasound and most practitioners report that the addition of 3-D is rarely required. Almost all 3-D studies have been carried out with the Voluson originally introduced by Kretztechnic and now made by General Electric. Early workers in the field and strong advocates of 3-D ultrasound are Dolores Pretorius from Los Angeles, Kazunori Baba from Japan, and Eberhard Merz from Germany. Three-dimensional ultrasound is superior in demonstrating superficial fetal defects such as facial clefts and studies from several groups have shown that the technique has a high sensitivity for diagnosing defects of the secondary palate which are rarely detected by 2-D ultrasound (46). In fetal echocardiography the capture of a volume of the beating fetal heart (called STIC) allows the study of tomographic slices of cardiac anatomy and movement in slow motion. Proponents of this technology are Greg DeVore in the United States and Rabih Chaoui in Germany. In gynaecology, Davor Jurkovic from King's in London demonstrated that 3-D imaging of the uterus was superior to 2-D imaging in recognizing and classifying congenital abnormalities of the uterus (47). Volumetric quantification of vascularity and flow (3-D flow indices) offers an alternative to Doppler velocimetry in the assessment of flow within an organ. Nick Raine Fenning from Nottingham has shown interesting data on endometrial flow and implantation of the embryo but as yet the technique has not been shown to be clinically useful. Real-time 3-D ultrasound imaging (i.e. 4-D) is most useful in showing fetal movements and there is evidence that this has real benefit in improving maternal–fetal bonding (Fig. 7.4). Three-dimensional/4-D ultrasound is very much 'work in progress' and further technical developments such as the matrix probe will undoubtedly pave the way for further advances in obstetrical and gynaecological imaging in the future.

Postscript

When a former president of the Royal College of Obstetricians and Gynaecologists was asked what were the three most important advances in his specialty in the 20th century he replied ultrasound, ultrasound, and ultrasound. The brief overview given above cannot do full justice to the huge range of beneficial effects of ultrasound examination in improving

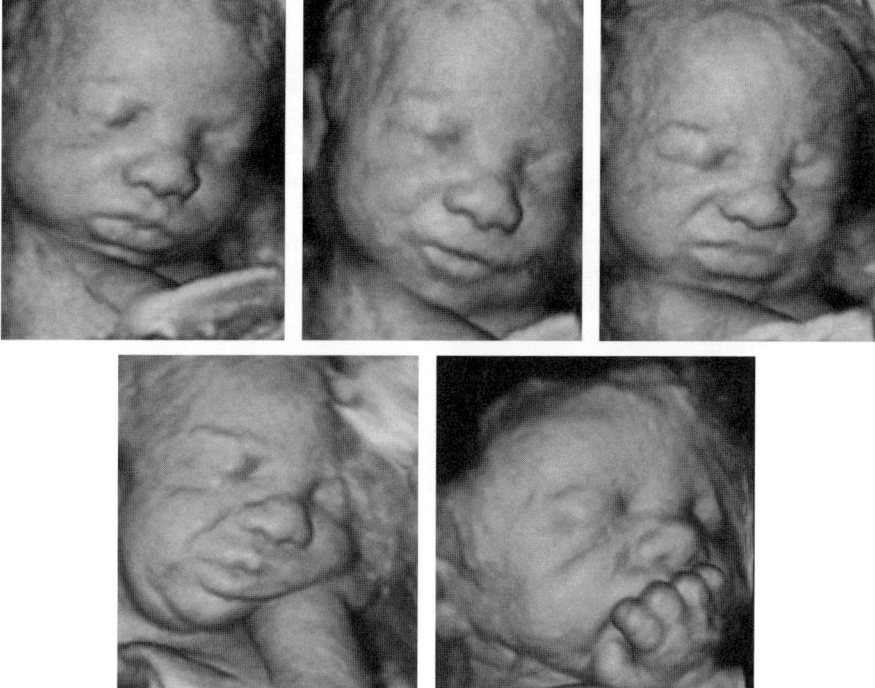

Fig. 7.4 It is believed that a 3-D moving sequence (i.e. 4-D ultrasound) demonstrating the 'humanity' of the fetus can encourage prenatal bonding. (This figure is reproduced in colour in the colour plate section.)

the health of women and babies in the second half of the 20th century. Ultrasound scanning features in almost everything we do in obstetrics and gynaecology. The great advances described in this chapter have come about because of a symbiotic relationship between brilliant engineers and the doctors who exploited each new development for the benefit of their patients and then fed back to the engineers what was next required. Ultrasound is unique in that it is safe even for the smallest embryo and that the examination is convenient and causes no discomfort. Indeed for most patients the ultrasound examination is both enjoyable and instructive. The greatest problem with ultrasound is that the results are still very much dependent on the skill of the operator. Space does not permit me to praise the great teachers of ultrasound or the organizations such as the International Society of Ultrasound in Obstetrics and Gynecology (ISUOG) and Fetal Medicine Foundation (FMF) which are dedicated to improve the knowledge and performance of the clinicians, sonographers, and nurses who use ultrasound equipment in everyday practice. Without these teachers and trainers the advances described in this chapter could never have been introduced into clinical practice.

References

1. Donald I, MacVicar J, Brown TG. Investigation of abdominal masses by pulsed ultrasound. *Lancet* 1958; **1**:1188–95.
2. Howry DH. The ultrasonic visualization of soft tissue structures and disease processes. *J Lab Clin Med* 1952; **40**:812–13.
3. Donald I. Clinical applications of ultrasonic techniques in obstetrical and gynaecological diagnosis. *Br J Obstet Gynaecol* 1962; **69**:1036.
4. Gottesfeld KR, Thompson KE, Holmes JH, Taylor ES. Ultrasonic placentography – a new method for placental localisation. *Am J Obstet Gynec* 1966; **96**:538–47.
5. Donald I, Abdulla U. Placentography by sonar. *J Obstet Gynaecol Br Commonw* 1968; 75(10):993–1006.
6. Campbell S. Prediction of fetal maturity by ultrasonic measurement of the biparietal diameter. *J Obstet Gynaec Brit Comm* 1969; **76**:603–9.
7. Thompson HE, Makowski EL. Estimation of birthweight and gestational age. *Obstet Gynecol.* 1971; 37(1):44–7.
8. Campbell S, Wilkin D. Ultrasonic measurement of the fetal abdomen circumference in the estimation of fetal weight. *Br J Obstet Gynaecol* 1975; **82**:687–9.
9. Grennert L, Persson P, Gennser G. Benefits of ultrasound screening of a pregnant population. *Acta Obstet Gynecol Scand Suppl* 1978; **78**.5–14.
10. Robinson, HP. Sonar measurement of fetal crown-rump length as means of assessing maturity in the first trimester of pregnancy. *BMJ* 1973; **4**:28–31.
11. Campbell S, Johnstone FD, Holt EM, May P. Anencephaly: early ultrasonic diagnosis and active management. *Lancet* 1972; **2**:1226–7.
12. Campbell S. Early prenatal diagnosis of neural tube defects by ultrasound. *Clin Obstet Gynecol* 1977; **20**(2):351–9.
13. Hobbins JC, Grannum PA, Berkowitz RL, Silverman R, Mahoney MJ. Ultrasound in the diagnosis of congenital anomalies. *Am J Obstet Gynecol* 1979; **134**(3):331–45.
14. Mayden K, Tortora M, Berkowitz RL. Orbital diameters: a new parameter for prenatal diagnosis and dating. *Am J Obstet Gynec* 1982; **144**:289–98.
15. Hadlock FP, Harrist RB, Sharman RS, Deter RL, Park SK. Estimation of fetal weight with the use of head, body and femur measurements–a prospective study. *Am J Obstet Gynecol* 1985; **151**(3):333–7.

16. Maršál K. Fetal breathing movements-characteristics and clinical significance. *Obstet Gynecol* 1978; 52:394–401.
17. Manning FA, Platt LD, Sipos L. Antepartum fetal evaluation: development of a biophysical profile. *Am J Obstet Gynecol* 1980; **136**(6):787–95.
18. Eik-Nes SH, Brubakk AO, Ulstein MK. Measurement of human fetal blood flow. *Lancet* 1980; 1:283–5.
19. Wladimiroff JW, Tonge HM, Stewart PA. Doppler ultrasound assessment of cerebral blood flow in the human fetus. *Br J Obstet Gynaecol* 1986; **93**(5):471–5.
20. Trudinger BJ, Cook CM, Jones L, Giles WB. A comparison of fetal heart rate monitoring and umbilical artery waveforms in the recognition of fetal compromise. *Br J Obstet Gynaecol* 1986; **93**(2):171–5.
21. Campbell S, Diaz-Recasens J, Griffin DR, Cohen-Overbeek TE, Pearce JM, Willson K, et al. (1982). New Doppler technique for assessing uteroplacental blood flow. *Lancet* 1983; 1(8326 Pt 1):675–7.
22. Kiserud T, Eik-Nes SH, Blaas HG, Blaas HG, Hellevik LR. Ultrasonographic velocimetry of the fetal ductus venosus. *Lancet* 1991; 338:1412–14.
23. Papageorghiou AT, Yu CK, Bindra R, Pandis G, Nicolaides KH. Multicenter screening for pre-eclampsia and fetal growth restriction by transvaginal uterine artery Doppler at 23 weeks of gestation. *Ultrasound Obstet Gynecol* 2001; **18**(5):441–9.
24. Andersen HF, Nugent CE, Wanty SD, Hyashi RH. Prediction of risk for preterm delivery by ultrasonography measurement of cervical length. *Am J Obstet Gynec* 1990; 163:859–67.
25. Allan LD, Tynan MJ, Campbell S, Wilkinson, JL, Anderson, JH. Echocardiographic and anatomical correlates in the fetus. *Br Heart J* 1980; **44**:444–51.
26. Yoo S-J, Lee YH, Kim ES, Choi HS, Cho KS, Kim A. Three-vessel view of the upper mediastinum: an easy means of detecting abnormalities of the ventricular outflow tracts and great arteries during obstetric screening. *Ultrasound Obstet Gynecol* 1997; **9**(3):173–82.
27. DeVore GR, Horenstein J, Siassi B, Platt LD. Fetal echocardiography. Doppler color flow mapping: a new technique for the diagnosis of congenital heart disease. *Am J Obstet Gynecol* 1987; **156**(5): 1054–64.
28. Benacerraf BR, Barss VA, Laboda LA. A sonographic sign for the detection in the second trimester of the fetus with Down's syndrome. *Am J Obstet Gynecol* 1985; **151**(8):1078–9.
29. Nicolaides KH, Azar GB, Byrne D, Mansur CA, Marks K. Nuchal translucency: ultrasound screening for chromosomal defects in the first trimester of pregnancy. *BMJ* 1992; 304:867–9.
30. Hobbins J, Mahoney MJ. In utero diagnosis of hemoglobinopathies; technique for obtaining fetal blood. *N Engl J Med* **290**:1065–7.
31. Daffos F, Cappella-Pavlovsky M, Forestier F. Fetal blood sampling via the umbilical cord using a needle guided by ultrasound. Report of 66 cases. *Prenat Diagn* 1983; 3:271–7.
32. Nicolaides KH, Soothill PW, Clewell WH, Rodeck CH, Mibashan R, Campbell S. Fetal haemoglobin measurement in the assessment of red cell isoimmunization. *Lancet* 1988; 1:1073–5.
33. Smidt-Jensen S, Hahnemann N. Transabdominal fine needle biopsy from chorionic villi in the first trimester. *Prenat Diagn* 1984; **4**(3):163–9.
34. Hansmann M, Lang N. Intrauterine transfusion controlled by ultrasound. *Klin Wochenschr* 1972; **50**(19):930–2.
35. Nicolaides KH, Soothill PW, Rodeck CH, Clewell W. Rh disease: intravascular fetal blood transfusion by cordocentesis. *Fetal Therapy* 1986; 1:185–92.
36. Ville Y, Hecher K, Ogg D, Warren R, Nicolaides KH. Successful outcome after Nd-YAG laser separation of chorioangiopagus-twins under sonoendoscopic control. *Ultrasound Obstet Gynecol* 1992; 2:429–33.
37. Kadar N, DeVore G, Romero R. Discriminatory hCG zone: its use in the sonographic evaluation of ectopic pregnancy. *Obstet Gynecol* 1981; **58**(2):156–61.

38. Hackelöer BJ. Ultrasonic demonstration of follicular development. *Lancet* 1978; **1**: 941.
39. Timor-Tritsch IE, Monteagudo A, Peisner DB. High frequency transvaginal sonographic examination for the potential malformation assessment of the 9 week to 14 week fetus. *J Clin Ultrasound* 1992; 20:231–8.
40. Nyberg DA, Filly RA, Laing FC, Mack LA, Zarutskie PW. Ectopic pregnancy: Diagnosis by sonography correlated with hCG levels. *J Ultrasound Med* 1987; **6**:145–50.
41. Timmerman D, Testa AC, Bourne T, Ferrazzi E, Ameye L, Konstantinovic ML, *et al*. Logistic regression model to distinguish between the benign and malignant adnexal mass before surgery: a multicenter study by the International Ovarian Tumor Analysis Group. *J Clin Oncol* 2005; **23**: 8794–801.
42. Campbell S, Bhan V, Royston P, Whitehead MI, Collins WP. Transabdominal ultrasound screening for early ovarian cancer. *BMJ* 1989; **299**:1363–7.
43. Menon U, Gentry-Maharaj A, Hallett R, Ryan A, Burnell M, Sharma A, *et al*. Sensitivity and specificity of multimodal and ultrasound screening for ovarian cancer, and stage distribution of detected cancers: results of the prevalence screen of the UK Collaborative Trial of Ovarian Cancer Screening (UKCTOCS). *Lancet Oncol* 2009; **10**(4):327–40.
44. Lenz S. Collection of human oocytes in IVF by ultrasonically guided follicular puncture. *Lancet* 1981; **1**:1163.
45. Feichtinger W, Kemeter P. Transvaginal sector scan sonography for needle guided transvaginal follicle aspiration and other applications in gynecologic routine and research. *Fertil Steril* 1986; 45:722–5.
46. Campbell S. Prenatal ultrasound examination of the secondary palate. *Ultrasound Obstet Gynecol* 2007; **29**(2):124–7.
47. Jurkovic D, Geipel A, Gruboeck K, Jauniaux E, Natucci M, Campbell S. Three-dimensional ultrasound for the assessment of uterine anatomy and detection of congenital anomalies: a comparison with hysterosalpingography and two-dimensional sonography. *Ultrasound Obstet Gynecol* 1995; **5**(4):233–8.

Chapter 8

Eugene Strandness and the development of Doppler ultrasound in vascular disease

David S. Sumner and Kirk W. Beach

This is the story of how a young surgeon, Donald Eugene Strandness Jr (Gene) (Fig. 8.1) was instrumental in the development of the Doppler ultrasonic flow meter, which evolved into the duplex scanner—perhaps the most versatile instrument in the modern vascular lab. He was born in Bowman, North Dakota, in 1928, and attended high school in Olympia, Washington, where he was a football player and a star gymnast. He graduated from Pacific Lutheran University in 1946, studied medicine at the University of Washington (UW), and in 1950 entered the general surgical residency programme.

At the time of the Korean War, Gene was drafted out of his residency; met his 2-year service obligation to the United States Air Force; and in 1959 returned to Seattle, where he hoped to join in the extensive research underway on the gastrointestinal system under the direction of Professor Henry Harkins. Instead, Dr Harkins urged him to change directions and join a small group at the Seattle VA Hospital who were investigating arterial disease. This group included John Bell, Hub Radke, and J.E. Jesseph (1). Strandness, swallowing his initial disappointment at having to give up gastrointestinal research, quickly embraced the vascular challenge.

The 1950s were a particularly exciting time in the history of vascular surgery. Improved sutures, grafts, and anaesthesia made it possible for the first time to perform major arterial surgery, such as resection of abdominal aortic aneurysms, endarterectomy of the carotid bifurcation, and bypass of iliac, femoral, and popliteal arteries. In preparation for major arterial surgery, the need for imaging was keenly felt. Physiological studies to select patients for surgery took a backseat to arteriograms and physical examination—in part because pulse palpation and patient testimony were the only methods readily available for measuring preoperative functional impairment or postoperative success. Invasive methods for studying blood flow were limited to electromagnetic flowmetry, which was performed in the operating room with the patient anaesthetized (2). No effort was made to duplicate normal physiological conditions.

Early vascular laboratories

Prior to the 1960s, a few surgeons and internists maintained rudimentary vascular labs where systolic blood pressure and blood flow were measured plethysmographically.

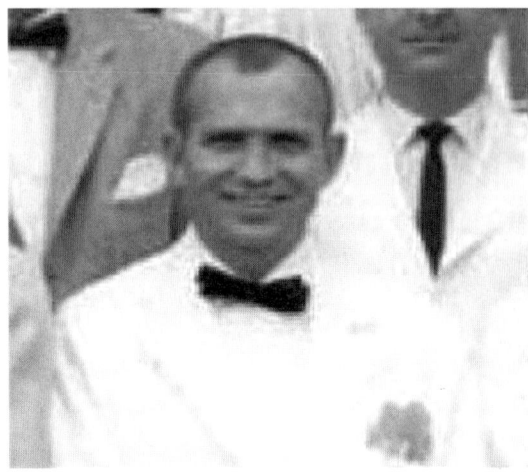

Fig. 8.1 Surgery Instructor D. Eugene Strandness with the UW Department of Surgery Faculty, 1962.
Reproduced from Beach KW. D. Eugene Strandness Jr, MD and the revolution in noninvasive vascular diagnosis. Part 1: Foundations. *J Ultrasound Med* 2005; **24**:259–72, with permission.

Included in this small group were Jack Cranley, Robert Linton, F.A. Simeone, and Travis Winsor (3, 4). Plethysmographs measure volume changes only. Flow rates can only be inferred from the rate at which the body part expands when venous outflow is occluded (venous occlusion plethysmography). Although they may provide valuable information, these methods are difficult to use, require skilled personnel, are applicable only to the limbs, and are not suitable for evaluating flow in individual arteries or veins. Carotid arteries cannot be studied.

In 1961, I (DSS) was an assistant resident at Harborview Hospital on First Hill overlooking Puget Sound. Strandness was the Chief resident. We became close friends. One dreary Saturday morning, he asked me to come across the street to the residents' quarters: he had something he wished to show me. What he had was a small black plastic box with a large knob. Called the 'Rudy Box' (Fig. 8.2a) after its maker and designer, Rudolph Helmer, this unimposing device proved to be an impedance matching circuit used to couple mercury strain gauges to Hewlett Packard recorders (5). Devised by Whitney in 1953, the mercury strain gauge had many advantages over air and water plethysmographs (6). The gauges were simple, but relatively rugged, consisting of a small rubber (later silastic) tube filled with mercury (later a non-toxic liquid alloy). They were quite sensitive and accurate and could be used to measure volume flow or pulse contours with equal accuracy in fingers, toes, arms, or legs (7). With this instrument, Gene studied finger and toe pulses and measured segmental arterial pressure in pre- and postoperative patients (8). In a number of papers, he demonstrated the frequent failure of reconstructive surgery to fully correct the physiological defect even when grafts were patent and peripheral pulses were present (9, 10). He emphasized the increased sensitivity of studies made when the circulation was stressed by exercise on a treadmill (11). Even as a resident, Gene's work gained attention

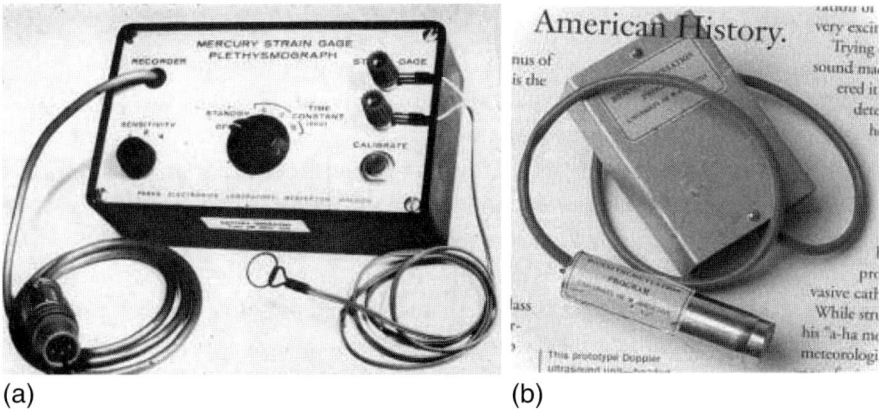

Fig. 8.2 'Rudy Box' strain gauge plethysmograph and CW Doppler. (a) The loop of elastic tube containing mercury (lower centre) was placed around a finger (or, in a larger version, placed around a leg), increasing in electrical resistance by 0.1% when the leg volume expanded by 0.1%. (b) CW Doppler developed by Don Baker in UW Bioengineering with transistorized electronics in the box and the transducer pair (transmitter and receiver) at the end of the tubular 'probe'.
Reproduced from Beach KW. D. Eugene Strandness Jr, MD and the revolution in noninvasive vascular diagnosis. Part 1: Foundations. *J Ultrasound Med* 2005; **24**:259–72, with permission.

in the vascular world. Of more importance, this hands-on experience provided a wealth of information that guided the development of the Doppler.

Across town

Robert Rushmer (1915–2001) was trained as a paediatric cardiologist and circulatory physiologist. He was also Chief of Biomedical Engineering at the University of Washington. He believed that cardiovascular physiology should be studied with the subject intact, and with all organs *in situ* as part of a functioning system, rather than as individual organs isolated from the rest of the body. And he wanted the studies conducted in unanaesthetized, free-living conditions that could be used in human epidemiology. He also was adamant that quantitative measurements should be used to characterize the cardiovascular system. Rushmer led animated discussions to identify which parameters were essential to describe cardiovascular dynamics: blood pressure, blood flow, and blood volume seemed to be likely candidates. Measuring key parameters required assembling an alliance of collaborating engineers. Among the first was Richard Ellis, who provided technology to study the dynamics of the heart and blood flow in real-time (12–15). Such studies, however, required invasive methods which could only be used in animals. For human studies, non-invasive techniques were required. For measuring blood flow, a likely candidate was ultrasound, which appeared to be innocuous and which had been studied extensively as a method for defining the limits of subcutaneous structures by time-gating echoes. Another possibility was to measure the time required for an ultrasonic pulse to move from one site to another along the flow stream; but this is best accomplished with the vessel surgically exposed.

Doppler ultrasound

The change in pitch of a train whistle as the train passes by has been known as long as trains have been in existence. As the train approaches an observer standing beside the track, the pitch of the whistle increases and then decreases as the train passes the observer and recedes into the distance. In his youth, young Gene Strandness thrilled at the effect as the transcontinental *Milwaukee Road* trains rushed through Bowman, North Dakota on the express run from Minneapolis to Tacoma. This wonderful phenomenon is known as the *Doppler effect,* in honour of the Austrian mathematician and physicist, Christian Johann Doppler (1803–53), who in 1842 (before an audience of only five people), presented his work on the colour of starlight relative to the speed of stars in space (16). The presentation had the rather formidable title: 'Uber das farbige Licht der Doppelsterne und einiger anderer Gestirne des Himmels' ('On the coloured light of the binary stars of the heavens'). Doppler thought the principle could be applied to waves in air, water, and 'ether'. That the Doppler effect is valid in air was confirmed in 1845 by the Dutch scientist Buys Ballot, who employed skilled observers to evaluate the tone played by trumpets on a train passing by at 40 miles per hour (16).

Physics of continuous wave Doppler

When a beam of ultrasonic energy generated by vibration of a piezoelectric crystal encounters an acoustic interface (such as a red blood cell), part of the energy is backscattered toward the probe where it can activate another crystal adjacent to the first. If the red cells are moving toward the probe, the frequency (f) of the backscattered signal exceeds that of the transmitted signal (f_o). If, on the other hand, the red cells are moving away from the probe, the reflected signal will have a lower frequency than that of the transmitted wave. The transmitted and reflected frequencies are added electronically to obtain a beat frequency equivalent to the difference between the two frequencies (Δf)

$$\Delta f = \frac{2 f_o\, u\, \cos \theta}{c} \quad \text{(Equation 1)}$$

As shown in equation 1, the observed frequency shift (Δf) is directly proportional to the velocity of red blood cells (u). The cosine of the angle of intersection ($\cos \theta$) between the ultrasonic beam and the direction of blood flow is introduced to correct for over-prediction of the frequency shift by geometric projection. Rearranging the terms of equation 1 gives equation 2, the velocity of red blood cells as a function of frequency shift:

$$u = \frac{c\, \Delta f}{2\, f_o\, \cos \theta} \quad \text{(Equation 2)}$$

To complete these equations, the speed of sound in blood ($c = 1.56 \times 10^5$ cm/s) must be included.

An interesting observation is that the human ear is sensitive to sound frequencies of about 20Hz to 20kHz, which correspond to velocities of 0.312–312cm/s for a 10MHz ultrasound transmitter at a Doppler angle (θ) of 60° (0.5 = cos60) and to 1.25–1250cm/s for a 2.5MHz transducer. This means that velocities in the audible range can be returned as sound. This, in turn, is a decided advantage to the sonographer in tracing the vessel being studied and in identifying sites of vascular disease.

Japan

Credit for constructing the first clinically applicable Doppler ultrasonic flow detector goes to Shigeo Satomura of Japan (17). He was born in Osaka (1919), received his PhD degree from Osaka University School of Physics in 1944, and worked at Osaka Institute of Scientific and Industrial Research. In 1960, he died suddenly from a subarachnoid haemorrhage and was promoted to Professor after his death.

His initial research concerned the measurement of vibrations in wooden boards using microwaves and ultrasound. At the suggestion of his supervisor, he applied his methods to measurements of heart motion and peripheral artery pulsations. His first paper, entitled 'A new method of the mechanical vibration measurement and its application' was published in 1955. It demonstrated that 3MHz Doppler signals can be retrieved from heart motion. Beginning in 1958, Satomura and Professor Ziro Kaneko demonstrated that transcutaneous flow recordings were feasible. In 1959, Satomura presented a paper entitled 'Study of the flow patterns in Peripheral arteries by ultrasonic'. Although this, like all his previous work, was published in Japanese, the paper included a summary in English (18). Prior to this the Western world had taken little or no notice of Satomura's work. After Satomura's death, his work was carried on by Kaneko and Kato, Professor in the Division of Acoustics. Early on, the group believed that turbulent flow was responsible for the recorded flow patterns (like noise heard through a stethoscope); but, by 1962, they concluded that reflections from red blood cells moving at different velocities simultaneously were responsible for different Δf's as mentioned above. This led to spectral analysis.

Seattle

Meanwhile at the University of Washington, parallel studies by Dean Franklin led to the development of a 'pulsed ultrasound flowmeter' which was an invasive instrument that had to be attached directly to the blood vessel wall. The Japanese flowmeter, on the other hand, was not only non-invasive but also transcutaneous. Because Japanese reports were almost exclusively written in Japanese with little in English, the benefits of shared data were not realized. American researchers developed a parallel programme and the Japanese were content to go their own way. Robert Rushmer expanded his interest to include cardiovascular physiology under normal conditions in unanaesthetized animals. To do this required the development of a method for measuring blood flow non-invasively.

As founder of the division of biomedical engineering at the UW, Rushmer set out to accomplish this goal by recruiting well-trained and enthusiastic young electronic engineers. These included Don Baker, who after serving 4 years in the United States Air Force, spent an additional 2 years working on detection of low-flying aircraft using radar. After discharge from the air force in 1955, Baker obtained a BScE degree from the UW. In 1958, while still a student, he started working under Rushmer. Together with Dean Franklin and Dick Ellis, Baker designed a multichannel transit-time flowmeter that had to be attached to the animal's blood vessel. There followed work on pulsed Doppler in 1959. The opportunity to design and construct new flow-measuring instruments and the availability of improved barium titanate transducers attracted many postdoctoral fellows to the University of Washington ultrasound programmes.

Dr Rushmer organized and conducted an intense 3-month course on electronic engineering for advanced postgraduate students. Strandness took the course in July of 1964. His meeting with Rushmer was one of those seemingly minor events that had a major impact on the direction of non-invasive studies. Strandness also arranged to be tutored in calculus, so that he could more readily comprehend mathematical analysis of blood flow. Strandness maintained close contact with Rushmer and his biomedical engineers. Most of the effort at this period was focused on devising transit time flowmeters as well as Doppler flowmeters (Fig. 8.2b). Dean Franklin was the pioneer in this work.

A Doppler—at last

In 1962, Strandness joined the faculty at the UW as an assistant professor in the Department of Surgery. His research prospered, attracting senior residents (such as Dick Schultz) to spend their research time in his laboratory.

In 1965, Eugene Hokanson, a young physicist who had grown tired of working on the tail section of Boeing aircraft, applied to Strandness for a job. Within minutes, he found himself a member of Strandness' team. At first, his duties were ill-defined. Strandness often said that Hokanson could do anything and did not hesitate to take advantage of this. Although Hokanson's knowledge of biology was limited, he was a rapid learner. At any rate, his association with Strandness launched a very successful career in medical electronics before his untimely death from an airplane accident in 2005.

In a chance meeting in the hall of the VA Hospital, Strandness invited me (DSS) to join him in a research capacity beginning in July 1966. With Vietnam looming over the horizon, and no firm job offers, I said yes without a moment's hesitation. My joining the team coincided with Gene's promotion to associate professor and to our commitment to write *Hemodynamics for Surgeons*, a major review of vascular physiology (19).*

People often remember where they were and what they were doing at the time of an important event. For me, the first time I (DSS) saw a Doppler was such an event. I was sitting in the little office that Gene Strandness and I shared with his secretary, a treadmill, some plethysmographic equipment, and a clock. It was a day in the summer of 1966. For a change, bright sunlight was streaming through the window and Mount Rainier was in view. I was proofreading Gene's 'Little Brown Book'† while fighting off a nap. It was

---

* Editor's Note (Bo Eklöf): David's and Gene's classical book *Hemodynamics for Surgeons* was the bible (Koran?) in my office in Kuwait. Unfortunately the book was lost when Iraq invaded Kuwait in August 1990.
† Strandness, DE Jr. *Peripheral Arterial Disease, A Physiologic Approach*. Boston: Little, Brown, and Company, 1969, p. 285. The book had a reddish brown cover and was relatively small, hence its

approaching high noon when Gene burst into the room carrying an unimpressive metallic box with only one knob, a speaker, and a cylindrical probe on the end of which two piezoelectric crystals were mounted. This, he said, was the long awaited device that detects blood flow transcutaneously.‡ Moments later we 'listened' to the triphasic signals from our radial and brachial arteries. This was the first time I had heard the characteristic arterial Doppler flow signal—a combination of sounds soon destined to become indelibly etched in our minds; almost as recognizable as the thump-thump heart sounds heard through a stethoscope. Perhaps it is only through the lens of the retro-spectroscope that this simple event becomes important; but my life and career were modified from that day on.

That afternoon, in what was to become a routine, we took the Doppler with us on rounds, listening to normal and abnormal arterial and venous signals. We learned to trace vessels longitudinally and to observe the effect of externally applied pressure on flow patterns. Although preliminary trials had confirmed that prototype instruments would work, there was insufficient experience on which to base recommendations (20, 21). Every observation, therefore, was potentially important. Within a short period, Strandness and his entourage accumulated enough data for a descriptive report, which Gene submitted to the prestigious *New England Journal of Medicine*. The paper was rejected by the editors and promptly returned. Without missing a beat, Gene transferred the manuscript to another envelope with a cover letter to the *American Journal of Surgery*. The manuscript was immediately accepted for publication and became one of Gene's most quoted papers (22).

From these humble beginnings, came the directional Doppler, the pulsed Doppler, the ultrasonic arteriograph, and ultimately the duplex scanner, one of the most versatile diagnostic instruments in use today (23–25). Most of the early work on the simple continuous wave (CW) Doppler was carried out in the Biophysics Laboratories of the UW; but who deserves credit for hands-on construction of the first CW Doppler? The field is crowded; but certainly Don Baker should be close to the beginning of the line with Dean Franklin and Ellis figuring prominently in the pack. The symbiotic relationship between clinical and engineering arms of this study fostered a practical approach to instrument design and development. Collaboration among clinical research services of university-affiliated hospitals was equally important in determining methods used to evaluate Doppler diagnostic procedures.

Reception

Early on there was a significant amount of interest in clinical application of Doppler ultrasound, especially in young research-minded surgeons and their European counterparts (16, 26). But this assessment was not matched by the rank-and-file. For example,

---

nick-name 'Little Brown Book.' It is a summary of Dr Strandness' clinical observations and studies using mercury strain gauge plethysmographs.

‡ Doptone® manufactured for the University of Washington by Smith-Kline instruments. It was built for detecting fetal blood flow; cost about $300; and was never a commercial success.

the most common question is 'How is this better than feeling the pulses?'. The difference between an arterial pressure pulse and a flow signal may be hard to explain. Also, the advantage of objective data versus subjective opinion in evaluating the severity of vascular disease may not be apparent to some. As late as 1980, Jack Wylie in his presidential address to the SVS said: 'I am concerned about the spreading fallacy that noninvasive vascular testing is an essential component of the clinical evaluation of the patient with known or suspected vascular disease ... It is important to remind young surgeons, who are insidiously made to feel insecure, that their fingers, eyes, and ears are still the best noninvasive devices available' (27). His statement has not withstood the test of history.

Problems encountered on the way to the Duplex scanner

Strandness was pleased with CW Doppler, but felt that further improvements with respect to equipment were necessary (28). The problems concerned presentation of data, flow sampling, and colour assignment. Strandness not only identified the problems but often proposed solutions.

Continuous wave Doppler initial experience

The audible signal from simple CW machines was found to be surprisingly informative. It could be used much like the physician uses a stethoscope. Normal peripheral arteries have a characteristic triphasic signal, with the first phase representing forward flow in systole; the second, reversed flow in early diastole; and third, a low-grade forward diastolic flow. The reader is reminded that early CW Dopplers were not direction sensitive, so that the deflections of the three waves are in the same direction. When an artery feeds a low-resistance vascular bed (like the internal carotid or renal arteries), or a vascular bed dilated by exercise or reactive hyperaemia, reversed flow disappears and only one or two phasic sounds are heard.

As expected, no flow is detected over a totally occluded artery. Above or below an occluded artery, the signal volume is variably attenuated, depending on the collateral resistance. Over a stenotic artery, flow velocity is increased and the signal quality may become noisy. In the hands of a skilled technologist, a CW Doppler can be a powerful diagnostic tool.

Findings on venous examination were especially new and exciting (29). With the patient supine, blood flow velocity in leg veins decreased on inspiration and increased on expiration. The presence of phasic flow proved to be good evidence of a normal venous circulation. Gentle squeezing of an arm or leg vein may prove the presence or absence of thrombus or valvular incompetence. Reversal of blood flow in response to cuff inflation or to a Valsalva manoeuvre are among the more reliable signs of valvular incompetence.

Recording and displaying output

Analogue recordings of the Doppler output using zero crossing circuitry are satisfactory for some uses, but the two-directional channels are not accurately separated in the presence of bidirectional flow (30). In normal arteries, as mentioned above, flow is often negative during part of the cardiac cycle, and flow may be present in both directions at the same time. Although flow in both directions is registered, the apparent flow is less in each direction than it really is. Fran McCleod addressed this problem with some success but the forward and reversed channels were not independent (30). Five years later in 1975, Jurgen Nippa, working in Strandness' lab used phase rotation to accurately separate forward and reverse blood flow (31).

Spectrum analysis

The audio-output provides information not readily available from analogue recordings. The problem was how to extract and display these data preferably in real time. From the first days with the Doptone, Strandness thought that sound spectrum analysis was the way to go. At that time, he had to record a 2s segment of audio output to send to the east coast for analysis. After the analysis, the analyzed segment was sent back to Seattle (express mail) for study. The analysis was extremely complex and roundtrip transportation required several weeks. Clearly, this method of study was going the wrong way and should be abandoned. Gene was referred to the Honeywell Corporation where he met with an expert in the evaluation of acoustic patterns of torpedoes. Development of a spectrum analyzer incorporating Fast Fourier Transform (FFT) technology was recommended (28). This worked quite well, showing time on the longitudinal axis, frequency shift (velocity) on the vertical scale, and the number of red blood cells travelling at any velocity–time combination—all of this in real-time.

Pulsed Doppler, selective sampling

CW Dopplers insonate all of the tissue in the sound beam. In the ideal situation, when the velocity profile is parabolic, the mean velocity obtained by simultaneous insonation of the entire cross-section of the vessel turns out to be exactly half of the maximum velocity, which is located at the centre. Spectral analysis would show equal distribution of red cells for each frequency shift. If instead of sampling flow over the entire cross-section of the vessel, the flow velocity was interrogated only at the centre of the flow stream, spectral analysis would show activity paralleling the maximum velocity envelope throughout the entire cardiac cycle. This would leave a prominent 'window' under an envelope representing the peak velocity during systole. If, however, the flow pattern were not laminar but disturbed, the window would decrease in width, a phenomenon known as 'spectral broadening'. These changes in the Doppler spectrum are sensitive to low-grade stenosis. Thus, Gene and others recognized the value of selective sampling of velocities in a limited 'sample volume'.

This problem was solved by Don Baker, who used radar principles to construct a 'pulsed Doppler' (28). Unlike the CW Doppler, which has a separate crystal for transmitting and receiving a continuous beam of ultrasonic energy, the pulsed Doppler uses only one crystal to transmit and receive the ultrasonic information. By time-gating the interval between transmission and receipt of a small packet of ultrasonic energy, one can control the distance of the sample volume from the probe. Since the speed of sound in tissue (c) is constant, distance is proportional to the time required to travel to the sample site and back.

Ultrasonic arteriography

One afternoon in 1971, Gene Hokanson and Doctors Mozersky, Barnes, and Sumner were enjoying a routine coffee break at the Seattle VA hospital. The conversation drifted into the area of non-invasive methods for imaging the arterial lumen. Mozersky proposed making a flow map using a pulsed Doppler attached to a position-sensing arm to scan the tissues over a superficial artery. When blood flow was encountered, a dot was to appear in the proper place on an oscilloscope screen; no dot would appear in the absence of flow. Hokanson rushed back to his lab, put odds and ends together, and within a short time emerged with the first Doppler ultrasonic arteriograph. This device, once refined, became commercially available (32). Richard Miles, a bioengineer working in Sumner's laboratory in Springfield, Illinois, took advantage of the full range of data captured by a multigate version of the pulsed Doppler arteriograph system to produce a separate flow map in a plane orthogonal to the skin. The result was an image in two planes (33). This 'computerized' arteriograph proved to be reasonably accurate for surveying carotid arteries. Elsewhere in Seattle, Merrill Spencer and Jack Reid devised a CW arteriograph that traced a line on an oscilloscope whenever flow was detected by the operator.

Colour Doppler

Colour was introduced in 1980 (34) to identify direction of flow and velocity on a two-dimensional image. Most manufacturers use red for flow in arteries and blue for flow in veins, with the intensity of colour being proportional to the velocity of flow. Depending on the anatomical site, flow away from the probe may be blue and that toward the probe red, or vice versa. Because of turbulence, tortuosity, or stenotic plaques, areas of blue may appear in an otherwise red artery. Colour must be interpreted conservatively in conjunction with the flow image. Colour has proved useful in diagnosis of deep venous valvular incompetence.

Timeline

The vision of Gene Strandness has guided over half a century of vascular diagnosis evolution at the UW. Many people have contributed to the development and testing of non-invasive methods (Fig. 8.3). The cadre of Strandness students has continuing worldwide impact developing and providing superior cost-effective vascular diagnosis.

Epilogue

By the mid-1970s, Gene entered a new phase in his life: Sumner moved to Illinois, Beach came on board at the University Laboratory, *Hemodynamics for Surgeons* was published (19), the Doppler had been adopted around the world, and the duplex scanner was well

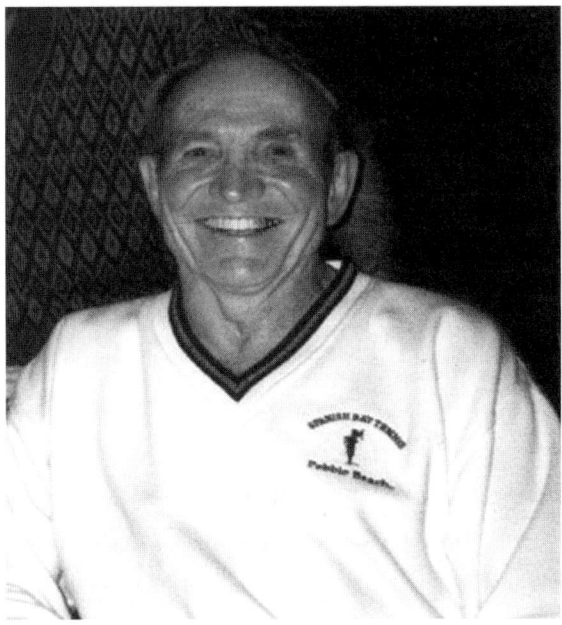

Fig. 8.3 Strandness smiles after another tennis victory at Pebble Beach.

on its way to becoming a functioning reality (23–25). Working with Gene had been an inspiration: exciting and intellectually stimulating. Every week, he spent one morning in the vascular lab at the Seattle VAH, discussing research and whatever else came to mind. Almost every evening he would call me (DSS) at home (invariably during the evening meal) to discuss—well, practically anything. A bibliography of 15 books, 176 book chapters, and 451 scientific papers testify to his academic accomplishments. Conquering a 'fear of flying' phobia, Gene became known as a world traveller, captivating lecturer, and outspoken panellist—warmly received throughout Europe and Asia. He had no magic formula for success, attributing it to hard work while others are playing. Yet, Gene did allow himself some relaxation. On the tennis court, he was a formidable opponent (Fig. 8.4).[§]

Gene was also an avid reader, especially of history and biography. Among the many honours bestowed on him were the Cid Dos Santos Prize in Coimbra, the Pioneer Award of the Society of Vascular Technology, The Albion O. Bernstein Award from the Medical Society of New York, and an Honorary Doctorate of Medicine from Lund University. He died, prematurely, on 7 January 2002, at home with his family after a long debilitating illness.

About the authors (Fig. 8.5)

David Sumner moved from the Seattle VA Hospital in Seattle to Southern Illinois University School of Medicine in 1975 where he rose to the Chair of Vascular Surgery.

[§] Editor's Note (Bo Eklöf): Gene was indeed a ferocious competitor on the tennis court. I had many opportunities to play with him. It often turned into national fights between Norway (Gene) and Sweden (Bo), where Norway most of the time took the victory.

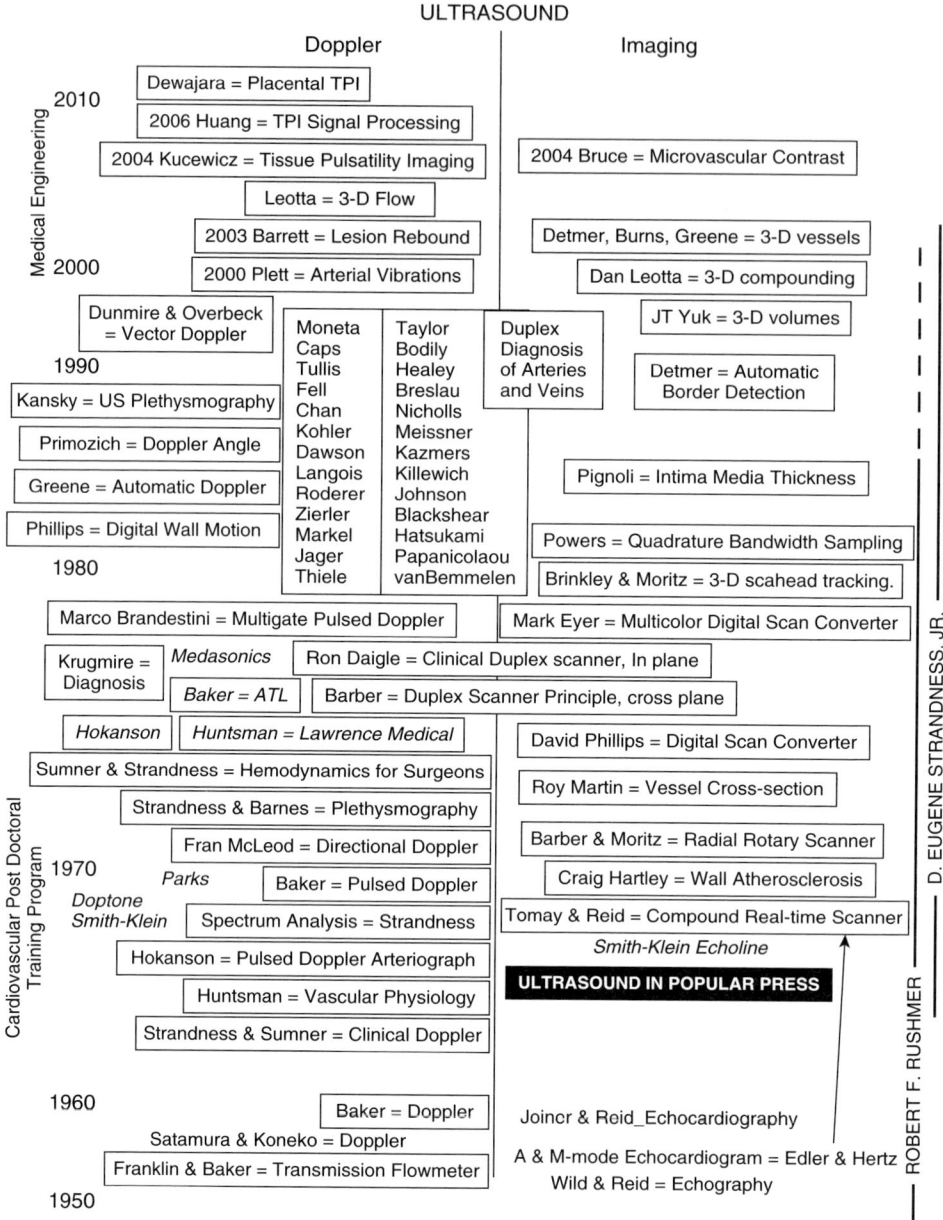

Fig. 8.4 Some of the researchers and programmes contributing to non-invasive diagnosis.

He was awarded the Society for Vascular Surgery's (SVS) Lifetime Achievement Award, the society's highest honour, in 2010.

Kirk Beach joined the Strandness Vascular Lab in 1976 where he continues to play via telecommuting since 'retirement'.

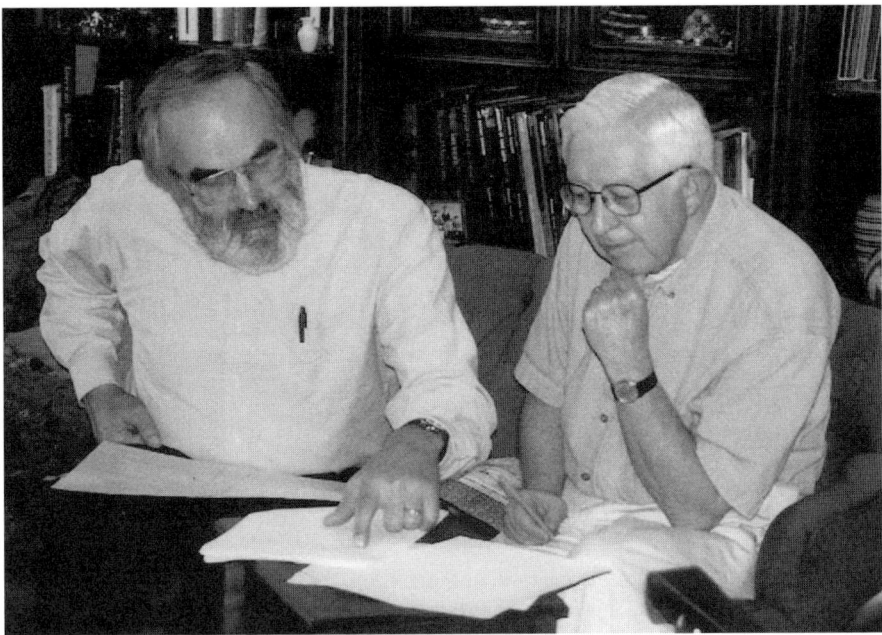

Fig. 8.5 Beach and Sumner ponder a circuit model of the cerebral circulation.

References

1. Radke HM, Bell JW, Strandness DE Jr, Jesseph JE. Monitor of digit volume changes in angioplastic surgery: use of strain gauge plethysmography. *Ann Surg* 1961; **154**:818–25.
2. Cannon JA, Lobpries El, Herrold G, Frankenberg HL. Experience with new electro-magnetic flow-meter for use in blood flow determinations in surgery. *Ann Surg* 1960; **152**:635–47.
3. Cranley JJ, Buchanan JL, Simeone FA, Linton RR. A critique of laboratory methods in peripheral vascular disease. *Surgery* 1952; **31**:74–87.
4. Winsor T. Influence of arterial disease on the systolic pressure gradients of the extremity. *Am J Med Sci* 1950; **220**:117–26.
5. Parrish D. Appendix. In: Strandness DE Jr, Bell JW (eds) Peripheral vascular disease: diagnosis and objective evaluation using a mercury strain gauge. *Ann Surg* 1965; **161**(Suppl.4):32–5.
6. Whitney RJ. The measurement of volume changes in human limbs. *J Physiol Lond* 1953; **121**:1–27.
7. Gibbons GE, Strandness DE Jr, Bell JW. Improvements in design of the mercury strain gauge plethysmograph. *Surg Gynecol Obstet* 1963; **116**:679–82.
8. Strandness DE Jr, Bell JW. Peripheral vascular disease: diagnosis and objective evaluation using a mercury strain gauge. *Ann Surg* 1965; **161**(Suppl.):1–35.
9. Strandness DE Jr. Abnormal exercise responses after successful reconstructive arterial surgery. *Surgery* 1966; **59**(2):325–33.
10. Strandness DE Jr, Bell JW. Ankle pressure responses after reconstructive arterial surgery. *Surgery* 1966; **59**(4):514–16.
11. Strandness DE Jr, Bell JW. An evaluation of the hemodynamic response of the claudicating extremity to exercise. *Surg Gynecol Obstet* 1964; **119**:1237–42.

12. Rushmer RF. Continuous measurements of left ventricular dimensions in intact, unanesthetized dogs. *Circ Res* 1954; **2**(1):14–21.
13. Rushmer RF, Crystal DK, Wagner C, Ellis RM. Intracardiac impedance plethysmography. *Am J Physiol* 1953; **174**(1):171–4.
14. Ellis RM, Franklin DL, Rushmer RF. Left ventricular dimensions recorded by sonocardiometry. *Circ Res* 1956; **4**(6):684–8.
15. Franklin DL, Ellis RM, Rushmer RF. Aortic blood flow in dogs during treadmill exercise. *J Appl Physiol* 1959; **14**:809–12.
16. Bollinger A, Partsch H. Christian Doppler is 200 years young. *VASA* 2003; **32**:225–333.
17. Satomura, S. Ultrasonic Doppler method for the inspection of cardiac function. *J Acoust Soc Am* 1957; **29**(11):1181–5.
18. Satomura S. Study of flow patterns in peripheral arteries by ultrasonics. *J Acoust Soc Jpn* 1959; **15**:151–7.
19. Strandness DE Jr, Sumner DS. *Hemodynamics for Surgeons.* New York: Grune and Stratton; 1975.
20. Rushmer RF, Baker DW, Stegall HF. Transcutaneous Doppler flow detection as a nondestructive technique. *J Appl Physiology* 1966; **21**:554–66.
21. Strandness DE Jr, McCutcheon EP, Rushmer RF. Application of a transcutaneous Doppler flowmeter in evaluation of occlusive arterial disease. *Surg Gynecol Obstet* 1966; **122**:1039–45.
22. Strandness DE Jr, Schultz RA, Sumner DS, Rushmer RF. Ultrasonic flow detection: a useful technique in the evaluation of peripheral vascular disease. *Am J Surg* 1967; **113**:311–20.
23. Beach KW. D. Eugene Strandness Jr, MD and the revolution in noninvasive vascular diagnosis. Part 1: Foundations. *J Ultrasound Med* 2005; **24**:259–72.
24. Beach KW. D. Eugene Strandness Jr, MD and the revolution in noninvasive vascular diagnosis. Part 2: Progression of vascular disease. *J Ultrasound Med* 2005; **24**:403–14.
25. Beach KW. D. Eugene Strandness Jr, MD and the revolution in noninvasive vascular diagnosis. Part 3: Seeking precision. *J Ultrasound Med* 2005; **24**:567–81.
26. Yao ST, Hobbs JT, Irvine WT. Ankle systolic pressure measurements in arterial disease affecting the lower extremities. *Br J Surg* 1969; **56**:676–9.
27. Wylie EJ. Presidential address vascular surgery – reflections of the past three decades. *Surgery* 1980; **88**:743–7.
28. Strandness DE Jr. History of ultrasonic duplex scanning. *Cardiovasc Surg* 1996; **4**:273–80.
29. Sumner DS, Baker DW, Strandness DE Jr. The ultrasonic velocity detector in a clinical study of venous disease. *Arch Surg* 1968; **97**:75–80.
30. McLeod FD Jr. Progress reports, directional Doppler blood flow meter. NRG 33–010–074. New York: Cornell University; 1969.
31. Nippa JH, Hokanson DE, Lee DR, Sumner DS, Strandness DE Jr. Phase rotation for separating forward and reverse blood velocity signals. *IEEE Trans Sonics Ultrasonics* 1975; **22**(5):340–6.
32. Mozersky DJ, Hokanson DE, Sumner DS, Strandness DE Jr. Ultrasonic visualization of the arterial lumen. *Surgery* 1972; **72**:253–9.
33. Miles RD, Russell JB, Sumner DS. Computerized ultrasonic arteriography: a new technique for imaging the carotid bifurcation. *IEEE Trans Biomed Eng* 1982; **29**:378–81.
34. Phllips DJ, Powers JE, Eyer MK, Blackshear WM Jr, Bodily KC, Strandness DE Jr, *et al*. Detection of peripheral vascular disease using the duplex scanner IIIa. *Ultrasound Med Biol* 1980; **6**:205–18.

Chapter 9

The development of ultrasound in vascular disease in Sweden

Tomas Jogestrand and Olav Thulesius

The famous British scientist Sir Cyril A. Clarke in 1975 wrote the introduction for a new book, *Arteries and Veins*, with the following words:

> In spite of all advances, mortality remains a steady 100 per cent and it is disorders of the arteries and veins which claim the majority of us. We sclerose, we clot, arrhythmias hit us, or our tubing wears out. By way of consolation, however, more of us now go the way of all flesh properly diagnosed and there are many ways of cheating the ancient enemy (1).

Clark at the time did not realize what advances were ahead of him, and the book he introduced with these dark lines included a chapter by R.G. Gosling and D.H. King which described a new promising technique of ultrasound angiography. Cyril Clark himself died at the age of 93!

New techniques

Blood flow measurements during resting conditions fail to detect any reduction of volume flow in patients with occlusive vascular disease, therefore for quantitative evaluation of the functional capacity of the peripheral circulation various functional tests implying increased circulatory demands needed to be introduced. The most useful clinical information could be obtained from peak-flow values after a period of obstruction and exercise followed by volume plethysmographic measurements of blood flow. Olav Thulesius introduced a foot ergometer in 1963 which allowed detection of maximal blood flow after graded muscular exercise (2). Its use was complicated and time-consuming when applied in conjunction with blood flow measurements with a water-filled volume plethysmograph. Therefore a faster and easier method for determination of peripheral blood flow was desirable.

In 1967, the ultrasound scanning method for the detection of arterial blood flow signals in the diagnosis of fetal life during pregnancy was introduced in Sweden. This same principle became the method for detecting blood flow in peripheral blood vessels. The method used was a hand-held instrument which included two piezoelectric elements, one to transmit ultrasound signals and the other to receive the returning echoes back-scattered from the blood vessels. The instrument used for the detection of peripheral blood flow was the same as that for the detection of the fetal blood flow in pregnancy. It was called 'Doptone' and introduced to be used to find sound signals for the detection of fetal heart beats. The change in frequency observed from what is sent out and received is known as the Doppler shift (3).

This equipment was used for the detection of pulsatile flow signals in arteries to determine peripheral blood flow. The technique employed was for measuring peripheral arterial blood pressure after releasing compression of flow with a blood pressure cuff in the arm and after a period of time in the lower extremity. The instrument transmitted high-frequency, 5MHz, ultrasound waves that were reflected from flowing erythrocytes and the movements of the arterial wall. The first study was done on patient data from 126 legs and performed by Olav Thulesius and Jan Erik Gjöres (4).

Model experiments

In order to apply the method for measurements of arterial blood flow, Olav Thulesius started performing a series of *in vitro* tests. The first measurements were model experiments to detect flow from a short segment of a small latex tube (with an inner diameter of 3mm) perfused by pulsatile and/or constant flow of blood ejected by a Sigma-motor pump (used as a blood pump in open heart surgery). The recorded wave signals were printed out on an electrocardiogram (ECG)-recorder and gave rise to pulsating flow signals to down to 7cm/s and constant flows to 20cm/s as shown in Fig. 9.1.

The perfusion experiments not only were performed with blood but also dextran, long-chain polymers of glucose in isotonic sodium chloride solution used clinically as plasma volume expander. These model experiments with perfusion of blood created signals very

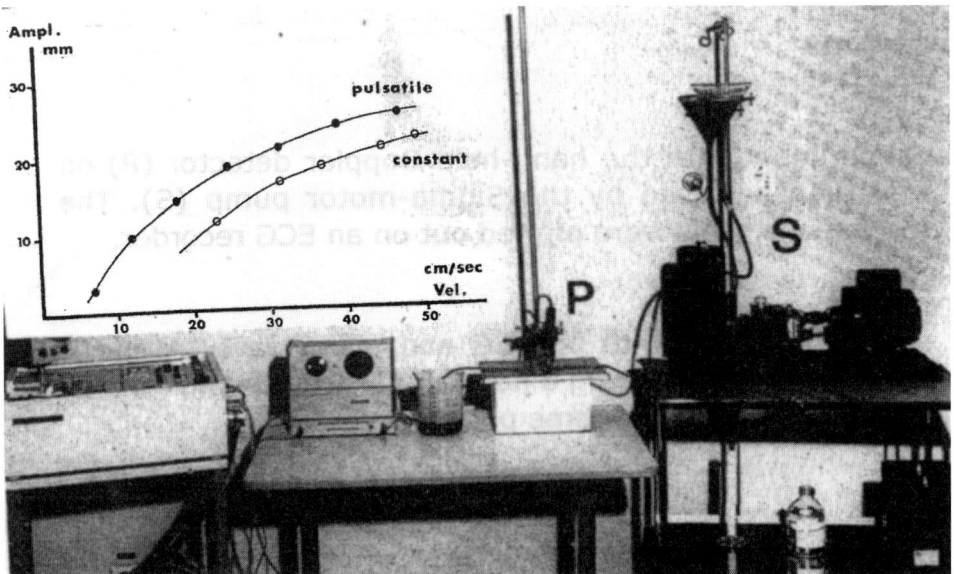

Fig. 9.1 Model experiment with the hand-held Doppler detector (P) on the latex tube perfused by the Sigma-motor pump (S). The recorded wave signals were printed out on an ECG recorder. Modified from Läkartidningen 1969; **66**:1106, with permission.

similar to those obtained *in vivo* but dextran perfusion only gave rise to small signals, depending solely on movement of the vessel wall.

The Doppler technique in arterial disease

The new method introduced in Sweden was able to determine the degree of blood flow in peripheral blood vessels. The normal sound waves are high-pitched usually biphasic signals but a single sound is usually seen in post-stenotic vessels of the lower extremity, and also on normal toe vessels. By semi-quantitative grading of sound waves we can see that normally they are characterized by a large double amplitude in proximal vessels and single short waves in distal vessels compared to small amplitudes after proximal occlusion.

Olav Thulesius correlated sound signals from the lower extremities with the post-exercise maximal blood flow values obtained from plethysmographic maximal flow values in (ml/100g/min). Reduced perfusion pressure of peripheral blood vessels could be detected in diseased lower limb extremity arteries by application of blood pressure cuffs at various locations and measuring perfusion pressure, comparing it with the central systemic blood pressure in both of the upper arms. Now the degree of blood flow reduction could be given in fractions of the systemic blood pressure as presented in Fig. 9.2.

The reduction in blood flow was proportional to distal perfusion pressure. In these tests maximal blood flow capacity was estimated after 5 minutes of arterial occlusion plus

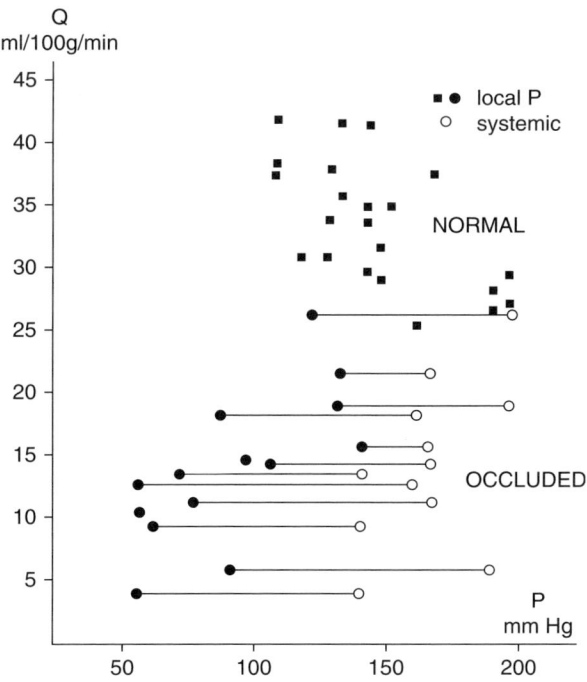

Fig. 9.2 Correlation of local blood pressure (P) and maximal blood flow (Q) in 12 patients with occlusive arterial disease and 21 normals.
Modified from *Läkartidningen* 1969; **66**:1106, with permission.

1 minute of exercise. This enabled a critical assessment of the quantitative diagnostic value of the new ultrasound method for detection of occlusive arterial disease. Previously the functional determination of advanced arterial disease had been based solely on the use of the complicated venous occlusion plethysmography or xenon-133 tissue clearance technique for determination of the degree of arterial perfusion in the diseased extremities. It was now possible to demonstrate the correlation between blood flow levels in diseased limbs with the peripheral perfusion blood pressure to prove the relevance of the new method.

With this method therefore the blood pressure difference between the upper and lower extremities was estimated and called ABPI (ankle–brachial pressure index). Normally it is 1 and in cases with mild disease 0.85 and in severe cases less than 0.4. In vascular medicine this information obtained by Doppler analysis is now the common practice of grading arterial obstructive disease (5).

The Doppler method can also be applied in newborn infants to exclude or determine coarctatio aortae. The method has the advantage over oscillometry that ultrasound investigation is much more accurate and can exclude the fallacy of wrong results in cases where normal pulsations had been detected with a normal A. tibialis anterior but occlusion in the nearby A. tibialis posterior.

Moreover care must be taken when interpreting ABPI measurements from diabetic patients because here the arterial walls of the calf arteries are often calcified and rigid which can lead to falsely elevated recordings.

Ultrasound in carotid arterial disease

Continuous wave Doppler (CW Doppler) as a non-invasive screening method for the diagnosis of extracranial carotid artery stenosis/occlusion was introduced in Sweden in the middle of the 1970s (6) and in 1981, the reliability of this diagnostic approach was demonstrated by two studies, one from Linköping and the other from Lund (7, 8). However, by that time, the combined use of B-mode ultrasonography and pulsed Doppler, known as the duplex technique, had been introduced as an alternative. The first Swedish report on the accuracy of this method in discriminating between carotid artery stenosis and occlusion was published in 1982 (9). Three years later Vera Zbornikova defended her PhD thesis 'Carotid artery disease assessed by ultrasonic duplex scanning—A methodological and clinical study' in Linköping (10). This thesis may be regarded as the starting point for the introduction of the ultrasound duplex technique in Sweden and the method has since then become an important diagnostic tool in patients with TIA (transient ischaemic attack) and minor stroke.

One of the reasons for the introduction of the method to the clinical praxis was the increased interest in a more active approach to diagnosis and treatment of patients with cerebrovascular disease at that time. This interest was manifested by the collaboration of eight Swedish hospitals in the European Carotid Surgery Trial that started in 1981 (11). The aim of the above-mentioned multicentre study was to evaluate the role of carotid surgery in the prevention of stroke in patients with TIA and carotid stenosis. To reduce the number of angiographies in patients with normal carotid arteries, the ultrasound technology was gradually introduced in the participating centres and the final results of the study was presented in 1991 (11), almost simultaneously with the presentation of a similar North American study (12). Both studies showed that carotid endarterectomy was indeed highly beneficial in patients with recent TIA/minor stroke and severe ipsilateral carotid artery stenosis. These results prompted a rapid introduction of the ultrasound duplex technique for detection of carotid stenosis in patients with transient cerebral ischaemic attacks in Sweden. The results of an inquiry investigation during February 1992 published in an expert report from the Swedish National Board of Health and Welfare showed that as many as 25 out of 29 departments of clinical physiology performed carotid duplex examinations. The expert group made a recommendation that each carotid centre have access to the ultrasound duplex technique for rapid screening of the carotid arteries (13).

Replacing carotid angiography?

The development of the ultrasound technique soon led to the discussion whether this non-invasive method also could replace angiography for preoperative investigations (14). Among several studies on the reliability of duplex sonography during the 1990s, one was performed in Malmö and showed that the duplex technique was a valid method for evaluation of stenoses in the carotid arteries (15). During the last year of the century another study was initiated by the Swedish Quality Board for Carotid Surgery with the aim to compare prospectively the results of ultrasound and angiography. The main intention was to establish on a national basis whether the diagnostic accuracy of the duplex technique was sufficient enough to justify carotid surgery without preoperative angiography. Ten Swedish hospitals accepted to participate and 134 patients were included. The study showed that the ultrasonographic duplex technique identified high-grade internal carotid artery stenosis with a high degree of accuracy (16). Furthermore, for the first time it was demonstrated that the method could be further improved by the application of small Doppler angles and the use of angle range-specific peak systolic velocity cut-points (Fig. 9.3). In a recent survey the results of these two Swedish studies were found to be the most (16) and the second most (15) often applied as diagnostic criteria in Swedish vascular laboratories (personal communication).

Duplex ultrasound in arterial disease in the lower extremity

The successful introduction of the ultrasound duplex technique into the diagnosis of carotid artery stenosis/occlusion during the 1980s inspired the attempts to use the method in diagnosis of arterial disease in the lower extremity as well. A source of inspiration was the activity of Eugene Strandness' vascular laboratory in Seattle, United States. Strandness' pioneering work with the ultrasound duplex technique was well known and recognized in Sweden as in many other countries, and several Swedes visited Strandness' laboratory during the 1980s and 1990s. One expression of the Swedish appreciation of Eugene Strandness' achievement was an Honorary Doctorate Degree bestowed on him by Lund University in 1999.

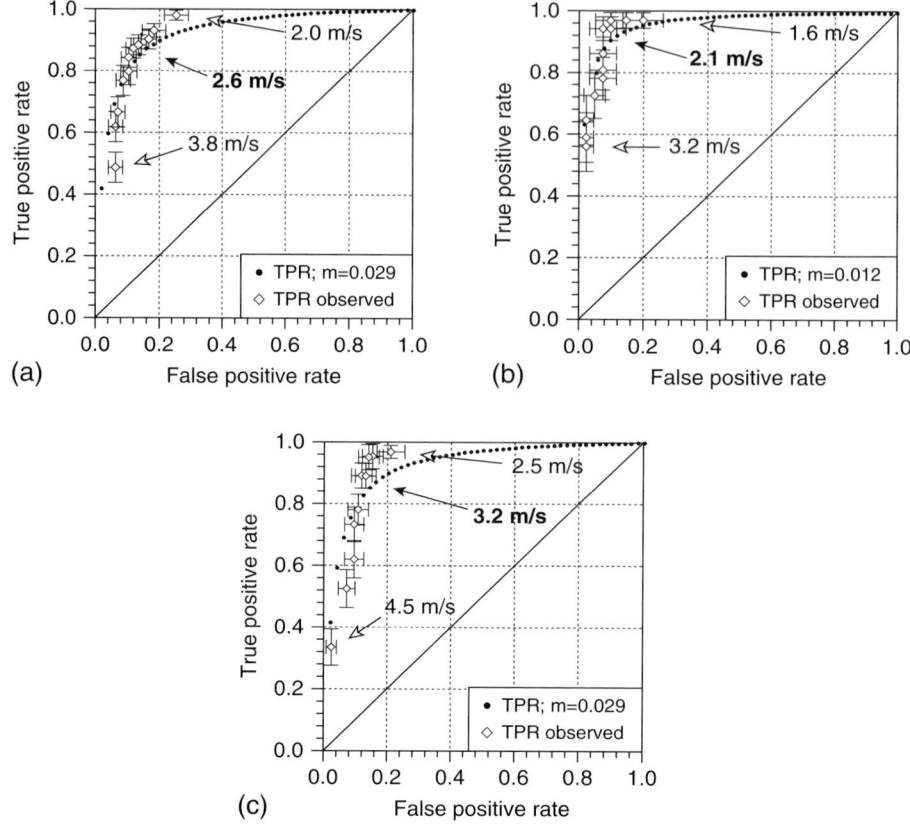

Fig. 9.3 ROC (receiver operating characteristic) curves based on the data from measurements of peak systolic velocity in the internal carotid artery (PSV_{ICA}) in both right- and left-sided ICA for identification of ≥80% ICA stenosis. (a) ROC curve for PSV_{ICA} measured with the Doppler angle 0–62°; (b) ROC curve for PSV_{ICA} measured with the Doppler angle 0–49°; and (c) ROC curve for PSV_{ICA} measured with the Doppler angle 50–62°. The fitted curves defining true-positive rate (TPR) at increasing false-positive rate are described by a slope, m. The individual data points represent the actual true-positive (TPR observed) and corresponding false-positive rates ±SD at the tested PSV_{ICA} cut-off values for the diagnosis of ≥80% ICA stenosis (ECST method). The cut-off values marking the boundaries of the tested cut point range and the optimal cut point values (bold style) for the respective ROC curves are indicated.
Reproduced from Jogestrand T, Lindqvist M, Nowak J, on behalf of the Swedish Quality Board for Carotid Surgery. Diagnostic performance of duplex ultrasonography in the detection of high grade internal carotid artery stenosis. *Eur J Vasc Endovasc Surg* 2002; **23**:510–18, with permission from Elsevier.

Duplex ultrasound for the control of infrainguinal bypass grafts was introduced in Sweden during the end of the 1980s (17). During the following 15 years, the infrainguinal graft surveillance with the duplex technique was advocated in several Swedish hospitals. This development was inspired i.a. by a randomized study from Malmö showing that a programme with duplex scanning led to a significantly higher secondary patency compared with routine follow-up examination (18). Later on, Fischer-Colbrie and colleagues in Stockholm reported that volume flow estimations significantly improved the prognostic capacity of the duplex technique regarding infrainguinal graft patency (19). However, during the last 5 years the importance of the ultrasound-based surveillance programmes has been questioned and the number of ultrasound examinations of infrainguinal bypass grafts has decreased.

The duplex technique was also introduced for evaluation of pelvic and leg arteries. In a study from St Görans Hospital in Stockholm, Rosfors and colleagues found that the ultrasound technique was feasible and accurate in detecting and grading lesions in the aortoiliac region (20). This experience was later confirmed and expanded by Karacagil and colleagues in Uppsala. They found in two of their studies that the duplex technique was feasible and reliable not only in detecting lesions in the aortoiliac arteries but also in detecting femoropopliteal, crural, and pedal arteries in patients with severe ischaemia (21, 22).

A few years ago, a Swedish systematic review concerning methods for diagnosis and treatment of arterial disease in the lower extremity was presented (23). One of the conclusions was that duplex ultrasonography has the same high reliability as conventional angiography when it comes to confirming or ruling out vascular disease in the lower abdominal aorta, as well as the arteries of the pelvis, thigh, and knee. The reliability of the method for diagnosing changes in the lower leg and foot is, however, weaker (23). A survey of clinical practice showed that 23 out of 25 departments of clinical physiology performed duplex scanning of arteries of the pelvis and leg. A little more than 6600 examinations were performed in these departments during 2003 (23).

Duplex ultrasound in venous disease

The ultrasound duplex technique for diagnosis of venous incompetence and deep venous thrombosis in the leg was introduced in Sweden at the end of the 1980s. The first Swedish report on the accuracy of duplex scanning in patients with venous incompetence was published in 1990 (24). The authors concluded that duplex scanning was an accurate method of evaluating deep venous valvular function. In a later study from Gothenburg, colour Doppler was found to be a suitable technique for non-invasive screening of patients with suspected venous insufficiency. The accuracy of the procedure for the superficial and deep femoral veins as well as for the popliteal vein and the great and small saphenous vein was found to be 70–90% (25). It is then, not surprising that this diagnostic modality has become an important instrument in the decision-making and preoperative preparation of the patient with venous insufficiency in Sweden.

Even more so, the ultrasound duplex technique has been established as the method of choice in patients with suspected deep venous thrombosis. Here are some of the diagnostic parameters for B-mode ultrasound:

- Non-compressible vein with a clot.
- No flow in a visualized vein.
- Visible clot.
- No changes in blood flow with respiration (26).

In the guidelines from the Swedish National Board of Health and Welfare from 2004 it is stated that the ultrasound technique should be the first method of choice when venous thrombosis is suspected (27). The statements in this document were based on a report from the Swedish Council on Technology Assessment in Health Care (28). The results of the literature review performed by the working group showed that ultrasound examination (including examination of the veins of the lower leg) has equally high diagnostic certainty as phlebography.

A questionnaire completed 1 year before the publication of the report revealed that nearly 40 000 examinations on clinically suspected deep venous thrombosis were performed in Swedish departments of radiology with a slight preponderance of phlebographies (29). However, if the yearly 8000 ultrasound examinations performed at the departments of clinical physiology were added, the net result already showed a slight predominance of ultrasonography at that time (29).

Duplex ultrasound in clinical studies

The duplex ultrasound technique has been used to a great extent in clinical vascular studies worldwide. One particular area has been in focus, i.e. the possibility to detect and quantify early atherosclerotic changes in the arterial wall. A research team that explored the ultrasound technique early in atherosclerosis research was a Swedish group led by John Wikstrand at The Wallenberg Laboratory for Cardiovascular Research in Gothenburg. They described a computerized analysing system for the measurement of wall thickness in the carotid arteries (30). Furthermore, their *in vitro* experiments indicated that the intima–media thickness in the carotid artery could be measured in a valid way in the far, but not in the near wall of the vessel (30). This was demonstrated in an intact carotid artery mounted in an organbath with buffer solution. The artery was ligated at one end, while the other end was connected to a syringe filled with buffer solution with admixture of air, the latter one being introduced into the vessel so that an air bubble was slowly created along the intima–buffer solution interface of the near wall. It was found that the leading edge of the echo created by the vessel wall–air bubble interface corresponded to the leading edge of the inner near wall echo (echo zone 3) (Fig. 9.4). This result is strong evidence that the inner echo of the near wall is created by the interface between the vessel wall and the blood, and not by the intima itself (30).

Another Swedish research group led by Tomas Jogestrand in Stockholm introduced a method of calculating the circumferential intima–media area by taking into account changes in vessel diameter when evaluating changes in the thickness of the inner layers of the artery (31). The rationale for this approach was the assumption that changes in artery width might cause changes in arterial wall thickness. Thus, secondary to a widening of the artery due to increased blood pressure, a thinning of the arterial wall might occur with a consequent thinning of the intima and media layers (compare with an expanded rubber band). The methodological problem described above has been shown to be a reality and can be overcome by calculating the cross-sectional intima–media area (32). Intima–media complex measurements have been used in several Swedish studies of early atherosclerosis during the last 15 years.

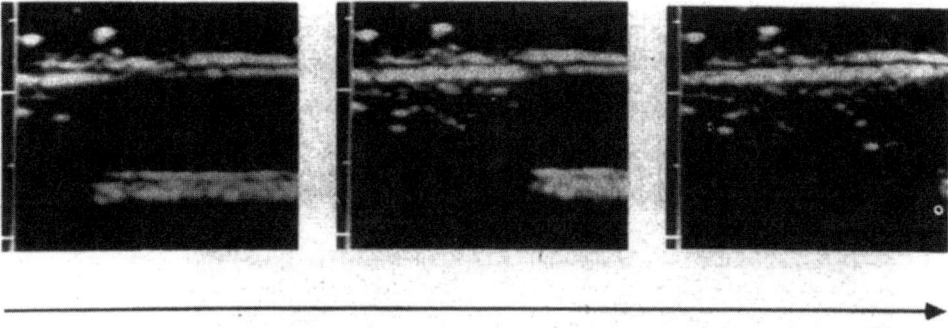

Fig. 9.4 Illustration of an ultrasound image in which an air bubble is created between the vessel wall and the liquid solution in the lumen. The image shows how the leading edge of echo zone 3 coincides with the leading edge of the echo from the air bubble, when the air bubble extends to the right. Also observe the echo shadow below the air bubble.
Reproduced from Wendelhag I, Gustavsson T, Suurkula M, Berglund G, Wikstrand J. Ultrasound measurement of wall thickness in the carotid artery: fundamental principles and description of a computerized analysing system. *Clin Physiol* 1991; **11**:565–77, with permission from John Wiley and Sons, Inc.

Quality control of duplex ultrasound

Clinical physiology, an independent academic and clinical discipline in Sweden since 1954, has been responsible for the non-invasive vascular diagnostic methods in most regions of the country. Over the years the Swedish Society for Clinical Physiology has organized courses in vascular diagnostics, including ultrasound techniques, for physicians and technicians and also published textbooks in the subject, the latest one in 2002 (33). In a cooperation between the Swedish Society of Clinical Physiology and the Swedish Board of Accreditation and Conformity Assessment (SWEDAC) accreditation of the departments of clinical physiology was introduced in 1995. In order to further improve the quality control in vascular diagnostics, a web-based quality control programme with digitized ultrasound examinations to be interpreted by a user was introduced together with the national organization EQUALIS (External Quality Assurance in Laboratory Medicine in Sweden) in 2004. This programme also includes education and training at annual user meetings.

Acknowledgements

The authors would like to thank the following for permission to reproduce copyright material: Läkartidningen (Figs. 9.1 and 9.2), Elsevier (Fig. 9.3), and John Wiley and Sons, Inc. (Fig. 9.4).

References

1. Harcus AW, Adamson L. *Arteries and Veins*. Edinburgh: Churchill Livingstone; 1975.
2. Thulesius O. A foot ergometer for graded muscular exercise. *Scand J Clin Lab Invest* 1963; **15**: 550–2.

3. Larsson J, Malmqvist R, Thulesius O. Ultraljuddiagnostik av fosteraktivitet i tidig graviditet. *Läkartidningen* 1968; **65**:3401–6.
4. Thulesius O, Gjöres JE. Ultraljudregistrering av perifert blodflöde. Report at the 1968 Swedish Meeting of Physicians in Stockholm. *Nordisk Medicin* 1969; **82**:1219.
5. Thulesius O, Gjöres JE. Use of Doppler shift detection for determining peripheral arterial blood flow. *Angiology* 1971; **22**:594–603.
6. Thulesius O, Svendler CÅ, Söderlundh S, Gjöres JE. *Doppler-sonografi av kranialkärlen vid transitoriska ischemiska attacker.* Medicinsk Riksstämma, 1976.
7. Eriksson S-E, Zbornikova V, Johansson I, Link H. Comparison between directional Doppler and angiography in the diagnosis of internal carotid artery disease. *Acta Neurol Scand* 1981; **63**:1–5.
8. Norrving B, Cronqvist S. Doppler examination of the carotid arteries. A comparative study with angiography. *Acta Neurol Scand* 1981; **64**:241–52.
9. Zbornikova V, Åkesson J-Å, Lassvik C. Diagnosis of carotid artery disease–comparison between directional Doppler, Duplex scanner and angiography. *Acta Neurol Scand* 1982; **65**:335–46.
10. Zbornikova V. *Carotid artery disease assessed by ultrasonic duplex scanning. A methodological and clinical study.* Linköping University Medical Dissertations, No. 197. Linköping, Sweden 1985.
11. European Carotid Surgery Trialist's collaborative group. MRC European carotid surgery trial: Interim results for symptomatic patients with severe (70–99%) or with mild (0–29%) carotid stenosis. *Lancet* 1991; **337**:1235–43.
12. North American Symptomatic Carotid Endarterectomy Trial Collaborators. Beneficial effect of carotid endarterectomy in symptomatic patients with high-grade stenosis. *N Engl J Med* 1991; **325**:445–53.
13. Wahlgren NG, Bergqvist D, Holm J, Jogestrand T, Lindqvist M. Karotiskirurgi i Sverige. Bakgrund och förslag till verksamhet. *SoS-rapport* 1994; **14**. Stockholm: Socialstyrelsen; 2004.
14. Jogestrand T, Bygdeman S. Ultraljudsdiagnostik av carotisstenoser. Kirurgi möjlig utan angiografisk kontroll? *Läkartidningen* 1994; **91**:505–7.
15. Hansen F, Bergqvist D, Lindblad B, Lindh M, Mätzsch T, Länne T. Accuracy of duplex sonography before carotid endarterectomy–a comparison with angiography. *Eur J Vasc Endovasc Surg* 1996; **12**:331–6.
16. Jogestrand T, Lindqvist M, Nowak J, on behalf of the Swedish Quality Board for Carotid Surgery. Diagnostic performance of duplex ultrasonography in the detection of high grade internal carotid artery stenosis. *Eur J Vasc Endovasc Surg* 2002; **23**:510–18.
17. Eriksson M, Rosfors S, Bygdeman S. Duplexultraljud bra metod för kontroll av infrainguinala bypass-graft. *Läkartidningen* 1991; **88**:2865–6.
18. Lundell A, Lindblad B, Bergqvist D, Hansen F. Femoropopliteal–crural graft patency is improved by an intensive surveillance program: a prospective randomized study. *J Vasc Surg* 1995; **21**:26–33.
19. Fischer-Colbrie W, Jogestrand T, Takolander R. Ultrasonographic surveillance of infrainguinal bypass grafts–the value of volume flow measurement. *J Vasc Invest* 1996; **2**:41–8.
20. Rosfors R, Eriksson M, Höglund N, Johansson G. Duplex ultrasound in patients with suspected aorto-iliac occlusive disease. *Eur J Vasc Surg* 1993; **7**:513–17.
21. Karacagil S, Löfberg AM, Almgren B, Granbo A, Jonsson ML, Lorelius L, et al. Duplex ultrasound scanning for diagnosis of aortoiliac and femoropopliteal arterial disease. *Vasa* 1994; **23**:325–9.
22. Karacagil S, Löfberg AM, Granbo A, Lörelius LE, Bergqvist D. Value of duplex scanning in evaluation of crural and foot arteries in limbs with severe lower limb ischaemia–a prospective comparison with angiography. *Eur J Vasc Endovasc Surg* 1996; **12**:300–3.
23. The Swedish Council on Technology Assessment in Health Care. *Peripheral arterial disease–diagnosis and treatment. A systematic review.* Report no 187E. Sweden: Stockholm; 2007.
24. Rosfors S, Bygdeman S, Nordström E. Assessment of deep venous incompetence: a prospective study comparing duplex scanning with descending phlebography. *Angiology* 1990; **41**:463–8.

25. Magnusson M, Kälebo P, Lukes P, Sivertsson R, Risberg B. Colour Doppler ultrasound in diagnosing venous insufficiency. A comparison to descending phlebography. *Eur J Vasc Endovasc Surg* 1995; **9**:437–43.
26. Thulesius O. *Diagnos av ventromboser*. In Norgren L (ed) *Vensjukdomar*. Lund: Studentlitteratur; 2004, pp.225–33.
27. Socialstyrelsen. *Socialstyrelsens riktlinjer för vård av blodpropp/venös tromboembolism 2004 – Faktadokument och beslutsstöd för prioriteringar*. Stockholm: Socialstyrelsen; 2004.
28. The Swedish Council on Technology Assessment in Health Care. *Prevention, diagnosis and treatment of venous thromboembolism. A systematic review. Report nr 158/I-III*. Sweden: Stockholm; 2002.
29. Björgell O, Kieler H, Hedenmalm K, Rosfors S, Blomqvist P, Persson I. Striking differences in the diagnostic procedures relating to deep venous thrombosis in Swedish departments of radiology. *Läkartidningen* 2002; **99**:4469–71.
30. Wendelhag I, Gustavsson T, Suurkula M, Berglund G, Wikstrand J. Ultrasound measurement of wall thickness in the carotid artery: fundamental principles and description of a computerized analysing system. *Clin Physiol* 1991; **11**:565–77.
31. Lemne C, Jogestrand T, de Faire U. Carotid intima-media thickness and plaque in borderline hypertension. *Stroke* 1995; **26**:34–9.
32. Jogestrand T, Nowak J, Sylvén Ch. Improvement of common carotid intima+media complex measurements by calculating the cross-sectional area. *J Vasc Invest* 1995; **1**:193–5.
33. Jogestrand T, Rosfors S (eds). *Klinisk fysiologisk kärldiagnostik*. Lund: Studentlitteratur; 2002.

Chapter 10

Ultrasound in vascular disease—state of the art

Kimon Bekelis and Nicos Labropoulos

The current use of ultrasound in vascular disease extends from diagnosis of several disorders to guidance of operative intervention (1). Duplex ultrasound (DU) is the main diagnostic modality used in patients with carotid disease, deep venous thrombosis (DVT), peripheral arterial disease, monitoring patients with subarachnoid haemorrhage for vasospasm transcranially, and many other routine examinations. The introduction of new technology is permitting the expansion of these applications. New interventions such as carotid stenting and endovascular aneurysm repair have necessitated the use of DU for detecting in-stent restenosis or endoleaks. In preparation for lower extremity bypass, arterial mapping of the lower extremity by DU is used as the sole imaging modality for lower extremity bypass procedures (1). DU is also used intraoperatively in evaluating carotid endarterectomy, endovenous procedures such as laser and radiofrequency ablation, and the patency of *in situ* vein bypasses.

Most recently, the breakthroughs in bioengineering have resulted in a plethora of applications for vascular ultrasound. Three-dimensional ultrasound has been used in the assessment of carotid plaque volume together with the monitoring of its evolution with time and its response to various treatments. The use of microbubbles as contrast agents during ultrasound imaging allows the assessment of microcirculation and can be used for ultrasound-guided delivery of drugs and genetic therapies (2). In addition the assessment of brachial flow mediated dilatation and carotid intima–media thickness by DU has provided a non-invasive way of assessing the arterial wall behavior and to evaluate these patients' risks of adverse cardiovascular events (3). Finally, the development of intravascular ultrasound has given birth to the field of virtual histology and has opened new frontiers in the measuring intimal thickness and assessing vulnerable plaques (4).

Expanding use of duplex ultrasound in arterial mapping of lower extremities

In recent years, the 'gold standard' of angiography for arterial mapping of the lower extremities has been challenged by DU. It has been supported as the sole method for evaluating patients undergoing lower extremity interventions by a number of authors (5) (Fig. 10.1). However, scanning the whole arterial tree is time-consuming, and might be obscured in obese patients or patients with tortuous or heavily calcified vessels (1).

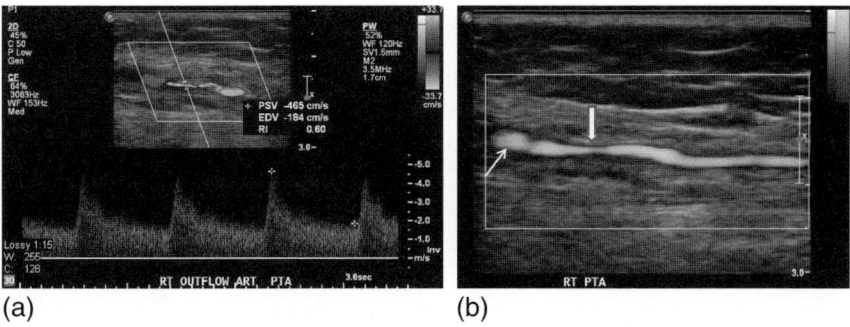

Fig. 10.1 Stenosis of the outflow artery in a patient with femoral to posterior tibial artery saphenous vein bypass. The bypass was patent without a significant stenosis. The posterior tibial artery had a tight stenosis 1cm distal to anastomosis as seen in (a) by the colour aliasing and the high velocities (PSV 465cm/s and EDV 184cm/s). The V2/V1 was >4 indicating a >75% diameter reduction. In (b) the narrowing of the artery (solid arrow) distal to the anastomosis (arrow) is seen with power Doppler which is less angle dependent. (This figure is reproduced in colour in the colour plate section.)

Mazzariol et al. (6), have shown that an abnormal common femoral artery waveform was highly predictive for detecting stenosis greater than 50% proximal to it and many reports support these findings. They concluded that DU was able to provide adequate information for operative planning in 83% of the patients. Proai et al. (7) have confirmed these results.

Although the sensitivity of DU is lower than conventional angiography or magnetic resonance angiography (MRA), its simplicity and safety for the patients makes this technique very attractive as a first line of defining inflow and outflow vessels when planning bypass surgery of the lower extremities (1). At the same time vein mapping is performed and then the best available conduit is chosen making the planning for the treatment easier.

Intraoperative and postoperative ultrasound

To avoid the risks associated with completion angiographies after bypass procedures, intraoperative DU has been proposed as a completion technique (8). After its completion the anastomosis is scanned to detect anatomic and flow abnormalities.

Radiofrequency or laser energy is being used for percutaneous ablation of the greater saphenous vein (1). The use of DU to place a catheter under direct guidance close to the saphenofemoral junction has revolutionized this technique. This has permitted these procedures to be performed under local anaesthesia.

DU has also been used as the sole modality to assist inferior vena cava filter placement or balloon angioplasty and stent placement in peripheral arteries and particularly in dialysis access patients (1).

With the widespread use of endovascular stenting in the treatment of aneurysms and vascular stenosis, DU has acquired a major role in these patients' follow-up. DU assessment of aneurysms for endoleak is now standard in all patients undergoing endovascular aneurysm repair (Fig. 10.2). Restenosis in patients undergoing carotid stenting is also monitored by serial ultrasound examinations (1).

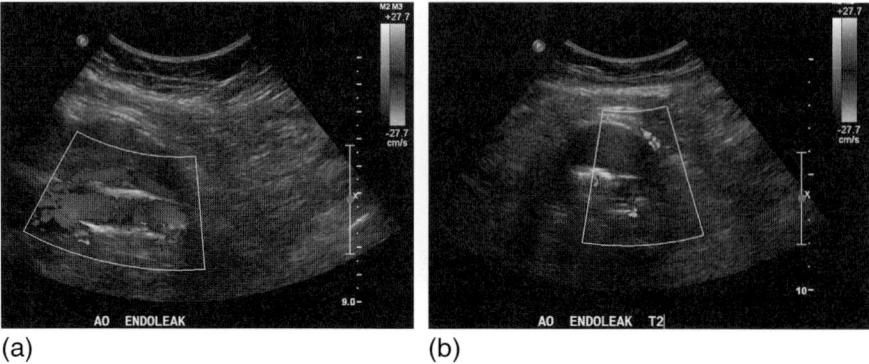

Fig. 10.2 Colour flow imaging or abdominal aortic aneurysm endoleaks after endovascular repair. A type 3 endoleak is seen in (a) as blood coming through the graft components. A smaller type 2 endoleak is seen on the same patient (b). Blood enters the aneurysm sac from a lumbar artery on the posterior wall. (This figure is reproduced in colour in the colour plate section.)

Expanding use of ultrasound in diagnostic applications

DU has recently been used as the primary modality in the diagnosis of various pathologies, substituting modalities like angiography that have been the gold standard for years. DU has been used to select patients for carotid interventions and currently is the main modality in the diagnosis of subclavian steal syndrome and can guide therapeutic decisions without other modalities (9). Flow phenomena and degree of stenosis can be assessed with planimetric methods alone or in combination with velocity measurements (Fig. 10.3).

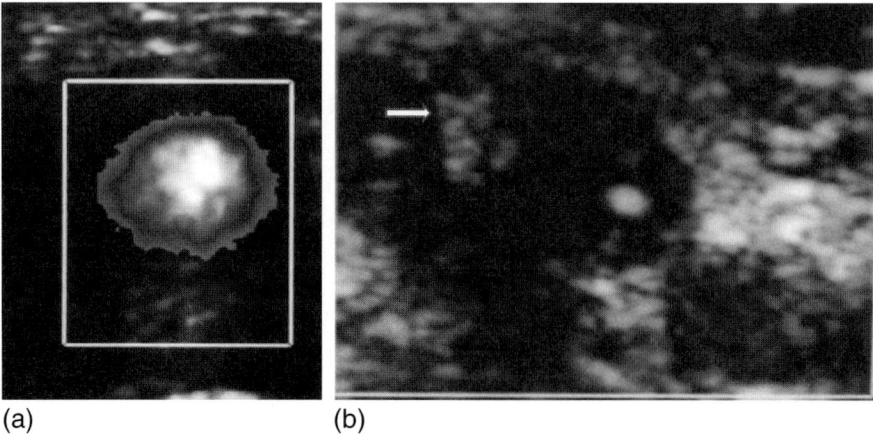

Fig. 10.3 Power Doppler imaging of the carotid arteries in a cross-sectional view. Laminar parabolic flow is seen in a normal subject in (a) with higher velocities in the centre of the lumen that decrease going towards the wall; (b) shows a very tight internal carotid artery stenosis in a patient who presented with transient ischaemic attack appropriate to the plaque side. This is a type 2 plaque as most of the content is echolucent. Calcification at 10 o'clock position produces an acoustic shadow posterior to the calcium (arrow). The image was taken with real-time high definition zoom. (This figure is reproduced in colour in the colour plate section.)

In addition, in the field of venous disease ultrasound has contributed extensively to our understanding of its pathophysiology and its natural history. DU studies have established that progression in venous reflux occurs slowly (10). In a similar way, the extensive study of the natural history of varicosities and their distribution in the lower extremities has established that they usually occur in tributaries of the saphenous trunk, justifying the use of saphenous vein for bypass procedures even in patients with varicosities (11). Particularly in the field of DVT, DU is the sole diagnostic modality in most centres and also provides very good differential diagnosis (Figs. 10.4 and 10.5). Its natural history has been studied with the use of ultrasound establishing that the higher risk of recurrent DVT is associated with unprovoked DVT and age greater than 65, whereas prior surgery and trauma are associated with decreased risk (12). Recently, conditions such as thrombus neovascularization have been investigated in several DU studies (13).

Contrast-enhanced ultrasound and molecular imaging

Gramiac (14) gave the first description of contrast-enhanced ultrasound in 1969, using air bubbles in the aorta (15). With the introduction of microbubble contrast agents, diagnostic DU has entered a new era that allows the dynamic detection of tissue flow of both the macro- and microvasculature. Contrast agents for ultrasound are microbubbles of different gases, 1–7μm in diameter (16). The gas can be air, which has the disadvantage that it dissolves quickly in water, or blood resulting in the loss of its contrast effect. Newer contrast agents therefore use sulphurhexafloride, perfluorocarbons, or other heavy gases, which minimally dissolve in water and behave chemically inactive with biological systems (15). In order to reach the systemic circulation with an intravenous contrast injection and

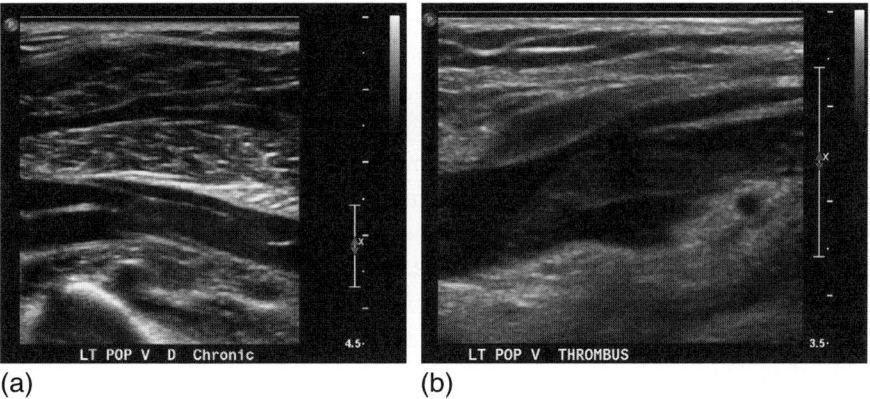

(a)   (b)

Fig. 10.4 Examples of vein thrombosis in the lower extremity veins. In (a) echogenic intraluminal material is seen in the popliteal vein in a patient who presented with chronic leg pain and swelling which was worst at the end of the day. The patient was not aware of having a previous deep vein thrombosis but did undergo joint arthroplasty 4 years ago. The findings of chronic thrombosis with partial recanalization and reflux can explain his symptoms. In (b) a free-floating thrombus is seen in the left popliteal vein. The patient was diagnosed with a peroneal vein thrombosis a week earlier and was on a surveillance protocol as he did not receive anticoagulation.

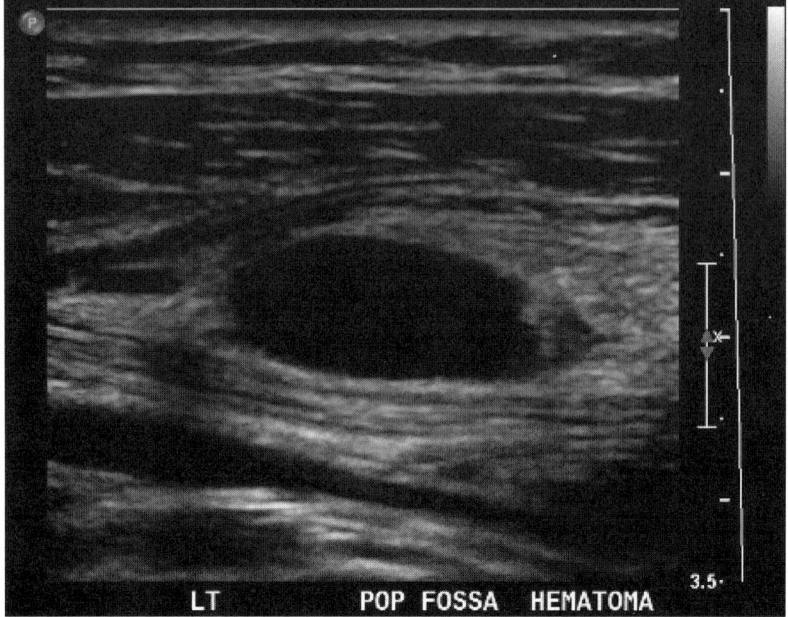

Fig. 10.5 B-mode imaging of the left popliteal fossa in a patient that presented with acute swelling, pain, and tingling sensation. A haematoma is seen superior to the neurovascular bundle compressing the tibial nerve and the popliteal vein. The diameter of the vein is significantly reduced at the site of the compression. Duplex ultrasound not only is helpful in diagnosing thrombosis in the veins but it is an excellent method to provide differential diagnosis and therefore optimize the patient's management.

for longer contrast persistence in the circulation, the microbubbles need to be stabilized with a biodegradable shell. Albumin, simple phospholipids micelles, bilayered membranes, as well as biocompatible polymers have been used *in vivo* and *in vitro* (15).

The limitations of conventional ultrasound that are being addressed with the addition of contrast are: the organ movement creating artefact; the presence of air-containing organs absorbing too much of the ultrasound beam; multiple stenoses or occlusions, which cause the blood velocity to fall below the threshold for blood flow detection by the Doppler system; the presence of anatomical structures like bone or arterial calcifications preventing the passage of the ultrasound beam.

The development of contrast ultrasound was possible because gases are compressible, and thus the microbubbles expand and contract in the alternating pressure waves of the ultrasound beam, while tissues are almost incompressible. Special software using multiple pulse sequences separates these signals from those of tissue and displays them as an overlay. This can be done on low acoustic frequencies so that the microbubbles are not destroyed and scanning can continue in real-time. Therefore, microbubbles act as blood pool markers and significantly enhance the blood–tissue border detection, even in conditions where artefact or low attenuation would make the results of unenhanced ultrasound unreliable (17).

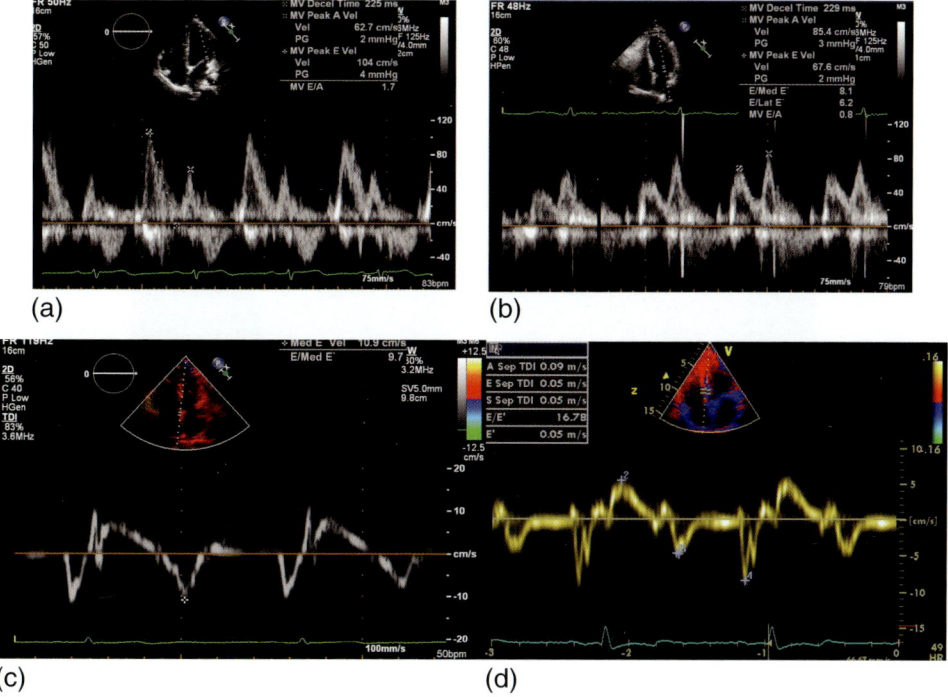

Fig. 3.2 Doppler flow tracings of a normal individual (a) and a patient with impaired relaxation (e<a) (b). Doppler myocardial imaging obtained at the septal part of the mitral ring in a normal individual (c) and a patient with impaired e' velocities (d).

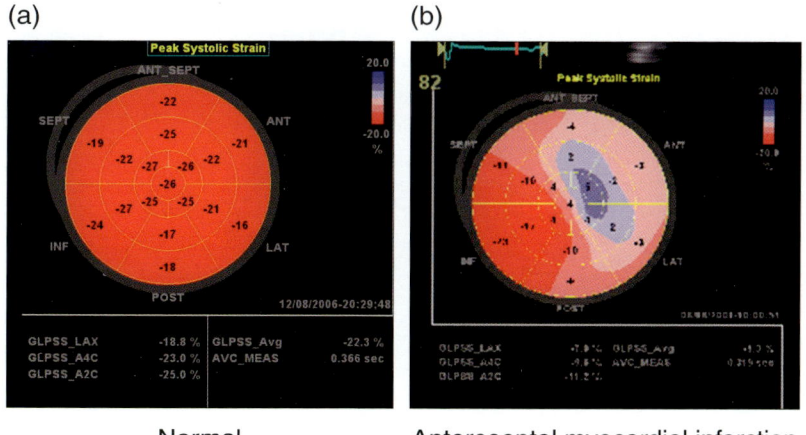

Normal   Anteroseptal myocardial infarction

Fig. 3.3 Automatic functional imaging (AFI) with a bull's eye display of a normal individual (a) and a patient who suffered an anteroseptal infarction, with the corresponding segmental abnormalities (b).

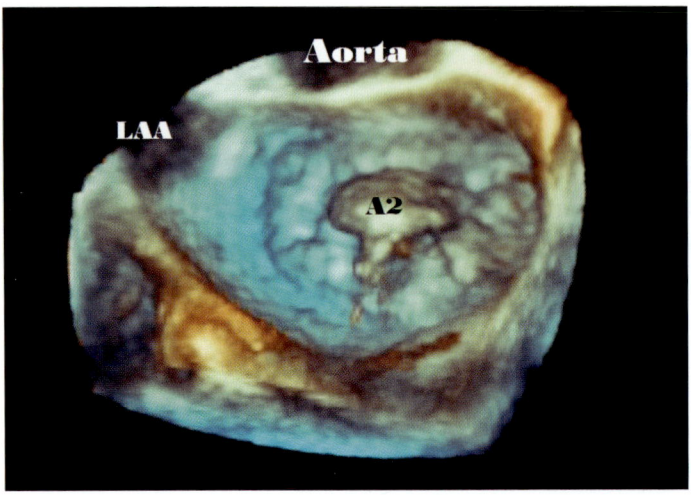

Fig. 3.4 Transoesophageal three-dimensional echocardiogram of a patient with a mitral valve prolapse involving the middle scallop of the anterior leaflet (A2).

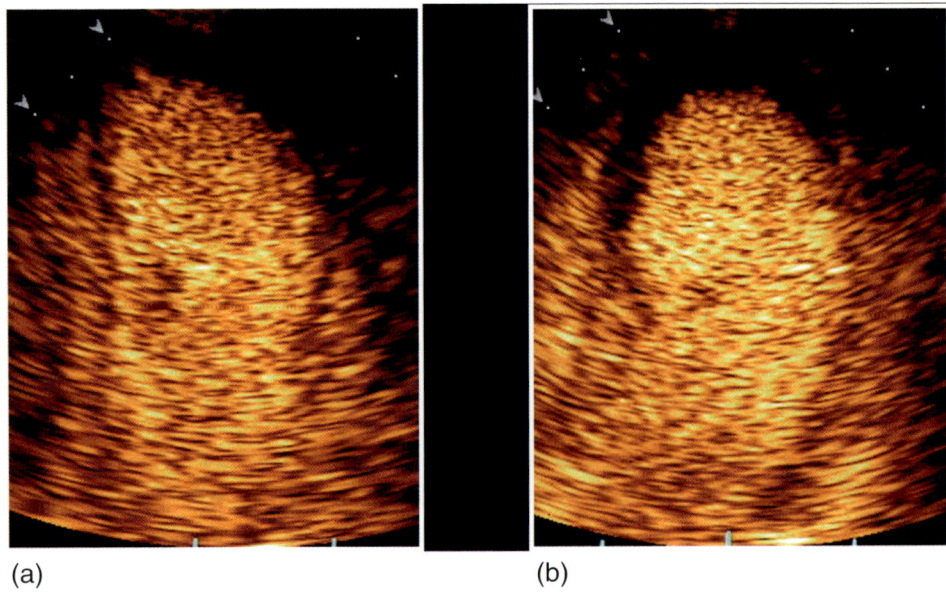

Fig. 3.5 Myocardial perfusion imaging using contrast echocardiography showing a perfusion defect in the distal septum and apex in a patient with a tight left anterior descending lesion. (a) Two- and (b) four-chamber views denote different projections of the image.

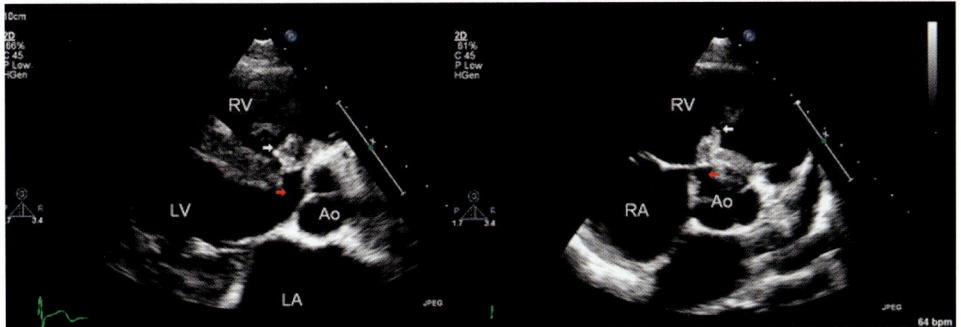

Fig. 4.1 Transthoracic imaging. Left: transthoracic parasternal long-axis view. Patient with small perimembranous ventricular septal defect (VSD; lower arrow) and a large vegetation (upper arrow) due to infective endocarditis. Right: parasternal short axis view. The ventricular septal defect (lower arrow) can be imaged in the perimembranous region of the interventricular septum, partially shrouded by tricuspid valve tissue. There is a large vegetation that extends from the VSD to the right ventricular outflow tract.

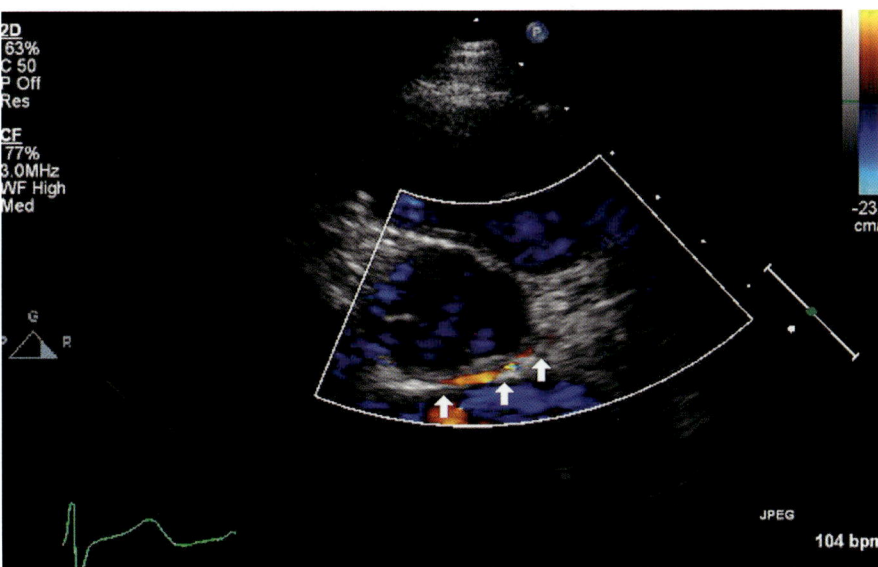

Fig. 4.2 Transthoracic imaging of abnormal coronary artery origin. Use of colour Doppler. Image obtained in 11-year old girl presenting with chest pain and ST-segment changes on ECG. An abnormal course of the left coronary artery (LCA) could be demonstrated by colour Doppler (arrows). The LCA originates from the right coronary sinus and runs posterior to the aorta to the left. The size of the LCA is small and on coronary angiography this segment was shown to be stenosed and hypoplastic. This demonstrates the high resolution of transthoracic echocardiography.

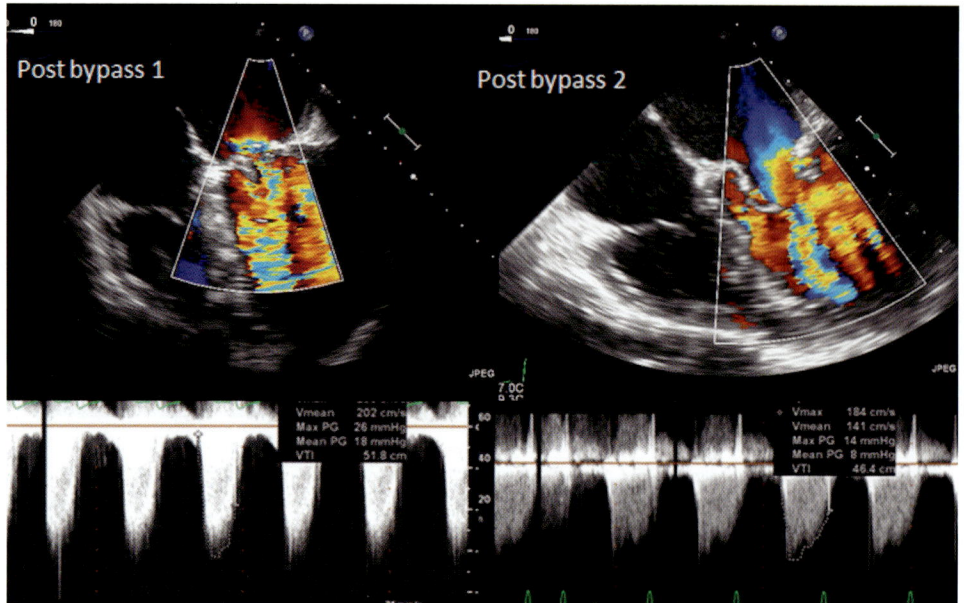

Fig. 4.3 Transoesophageal echocardiography (TOE). Use of perioperative TOE in a 13-year-old boy who underwent mitral valve repair for severe mitral regurgitation secondary to rheumatic fever. Left: after the first bypass TOE showed an immobile posterior leaflet with a narrow inflow jet and a mean gradient of 18mmHg. Right: after the second bypass the posterior leaflet mobility improved, the jet became wider, and the mean gradient was reduced to 8mmHg.

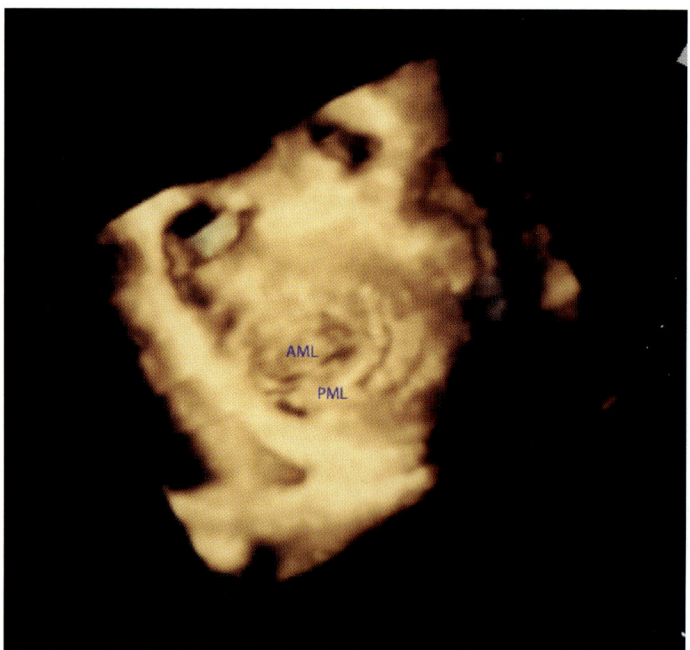

Fig. 4.4 3-D Transoesophageal echocardiography (TOE). In this 3-D picture the mitral valve imaged by 2-D in Fig. 4.3 the mitral valve is imaged from the atrial aspect. The leaflets could be imaged well by 3-D TOE. AML: anterior mitral leaflet; PML: posterior mitral leaflet.

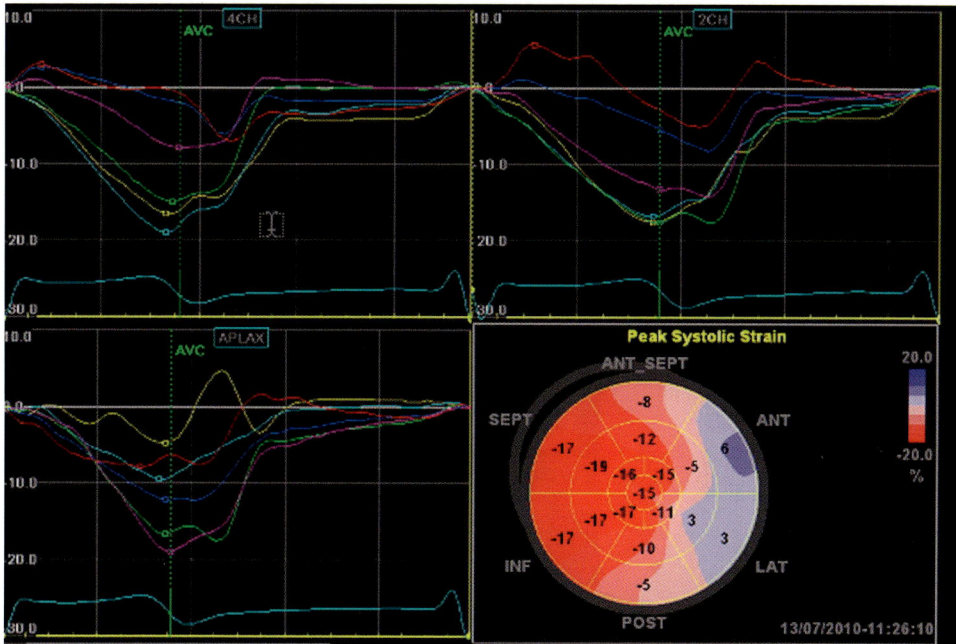

Fig. 4.5 Longitudinal strain measurement using automatic functional imaging. Images obtained in the girl presented in Fig. 4.2 with the abnormal origin of the left coronary artery from the right coronary artery with posterior looping. Longitudinal strain curves were obtained from apical four-chamber, three-chamber, and two-chamber views and were analysed using automatic functional imaging. Severely reduced peak systolic strain measurements were obtained in the anterolateral segments consistent with ischaemic changes in the left anterior descending coronary artery territory. The girl underwent coronary bypass surgery. This illustrates how current technology allows quantification of regional myocardial function.

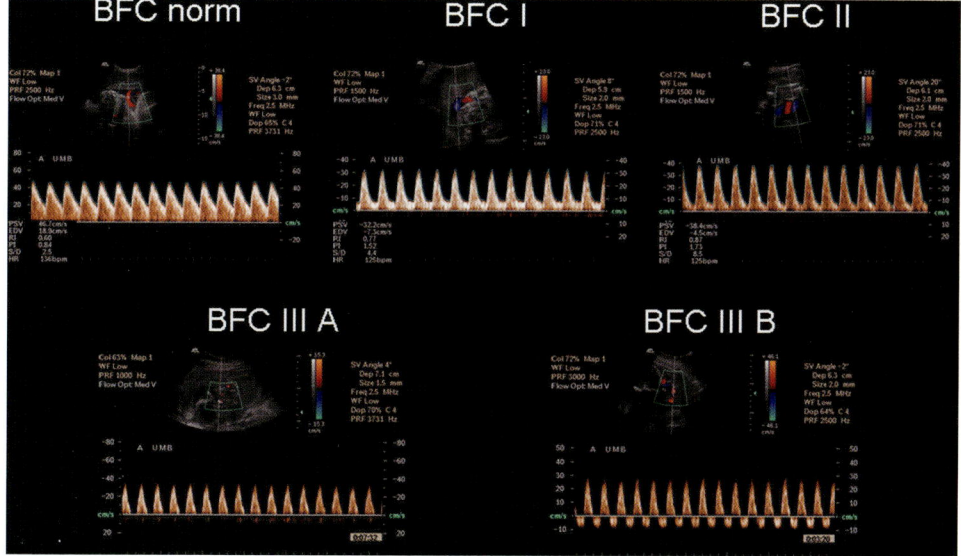

Fig. 6.7 Blood Flow Classes (BFC) of blood velocity waveforms recorded from the umbilical artery. BFC norm, positive diastolic flow velocity, pulsatility index (PI) within mean ± 2 standard deviations (SD) of the reference curve; BFC I, positive diastolic flow, PI > mean + 2SD and ≤ mean + 3 SD; BFC II, positive diastolic flow, PI > mean + 3 SD; BFC IIIA, absent end-diastolic flow velocity; BFC IIIB, reverse end-diastolic flow velocity.

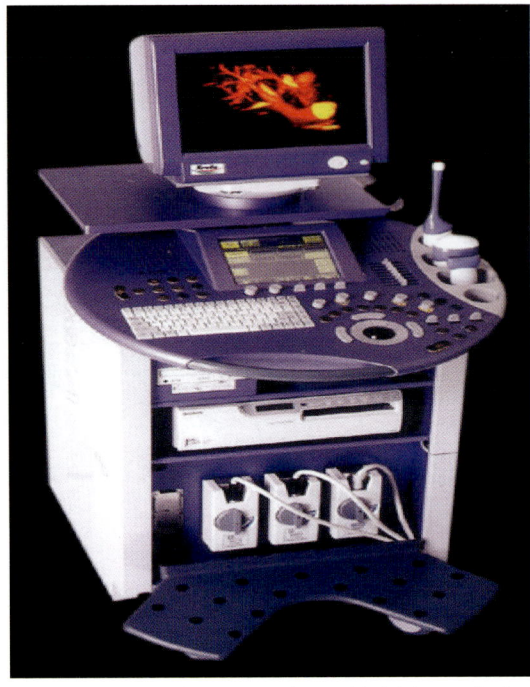

Fig. 7.2 A typical modern scanning machine complete with high-resolution imaging, colour and power Doppler, and a 3-D/4-D option (GE Voluson Expert).

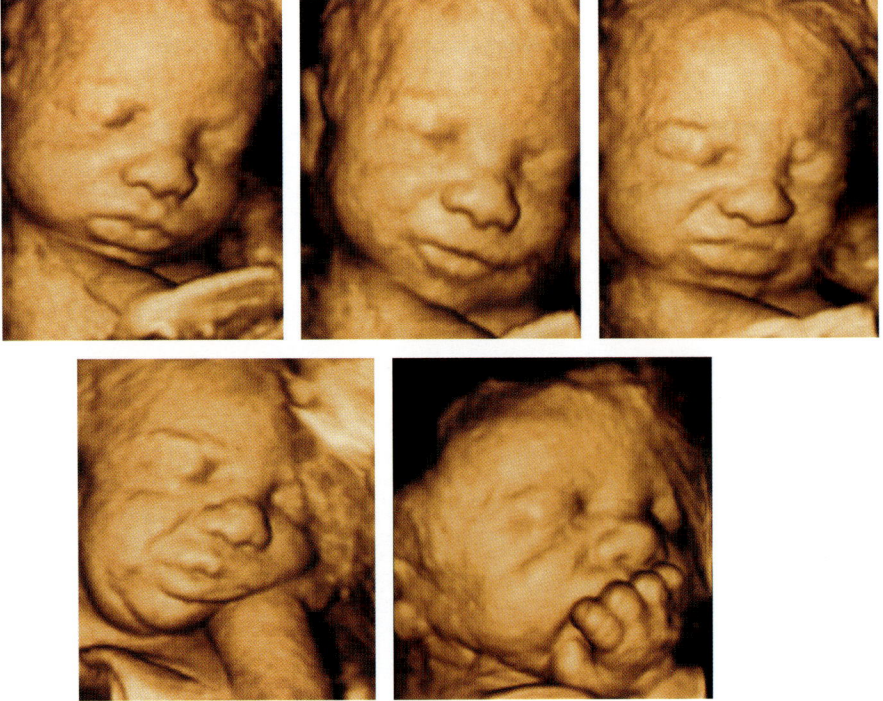

Fig. 7.4 It is believed that a 3-D moving sequence (i.e. 4-D ultrasound) demonstrating the 'humanity' of the fetus can encourage prenatal bonding.

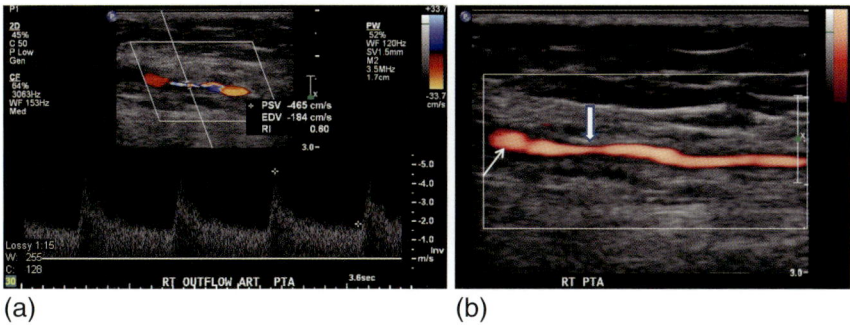

Fig. 10.1 Stenosis of the outflow artery in a patient with femoral to posterior tibial artery saphenous vein bypass. The bypass was patent without a significant stenosis. The posterior tibial artery had a tight stenosis 1cm distal to anastomosis as seen in (a) by the colour aliasing and the high velocities (PSV 465cm/s and EDV 184cm/s). The V2/V1 was >4 indicating a >75% diameter reduction. In (b) the narrowing of the artery (solid arrow) distal to the anastomosis (arrow) is seen with power Doppler which is less angle dependent.

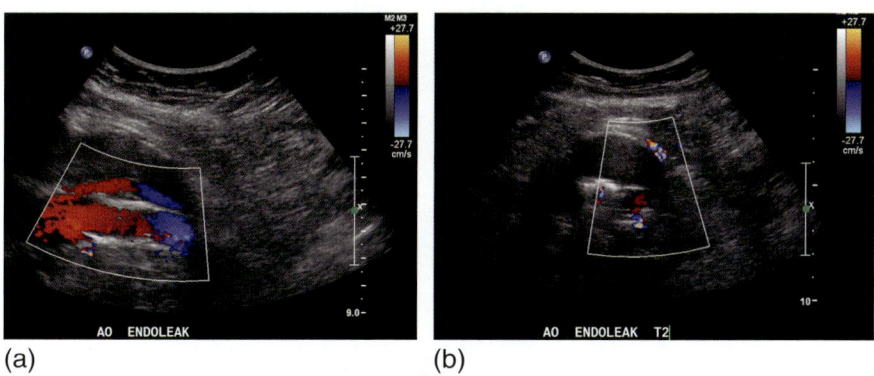

Fig. 10.2 Colour flow imaging or abdominal aortic aneurysm endoleaks after endovascular repair. A type 3 endoleak is seen in (a) as blood coming through the graft components. A smaller type 2 endoleak is seen on the same patient (b). Blood enters the aneurysm sac from a lumbar artery on the posterior wall.

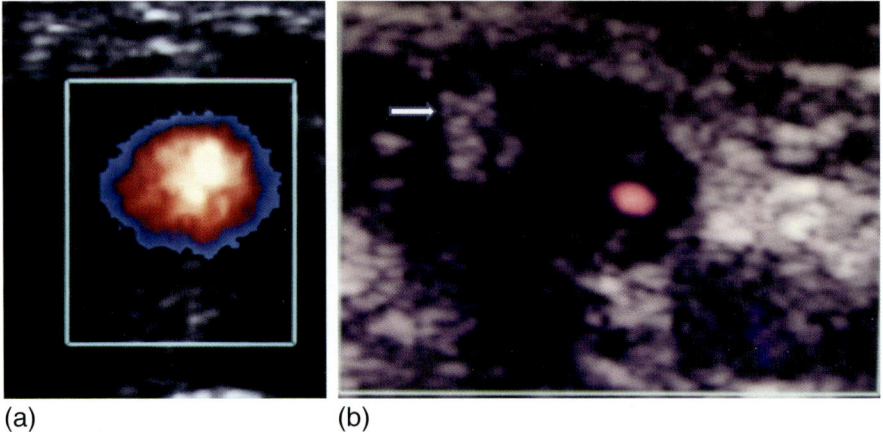

Fig. 10.3 Power Doppler imaging of the carotid arteries in a cross-sectional view. Laminar parabolic flow is seen in a normal subject in (a) with higher velocities in the centre of the lumen that decrease going towards the wall; (b) shows a very tight internal carotid artery stenosis in a patient who presented with transient ischaemic attack appropriate to the plaque side. This is a type 2 plaque as most of the content is echolucent. Calcification at 10 o'clock position produces an acoustic shadow posterior to the calcium (arrow). The image was taken with real-time high definition zoom.

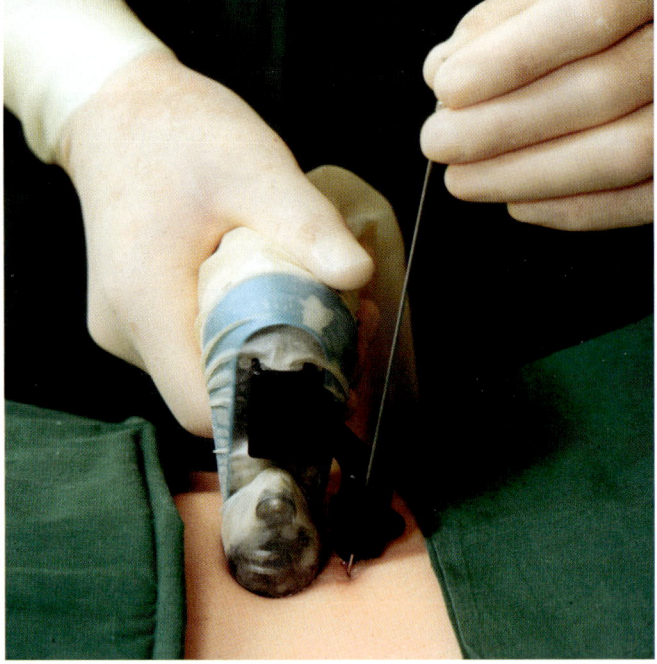

Fig. 11.1 The first needle guide unit designed by P.G. Lindgren for the ATL mechanical sector scanner.

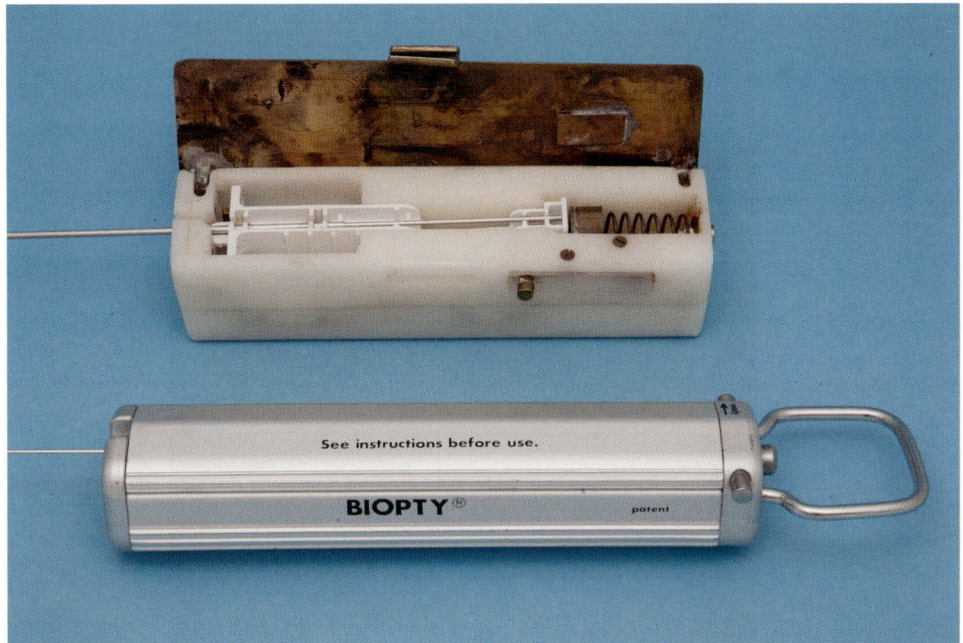

Fig. 11.3 The first semiautomatic biopsy device prototype used by Lindgren and designed for the manual Travenol TruCut® needle (top). Below is the commercial biopsy gun, Biopty® also designed by P.G. Lindgren.

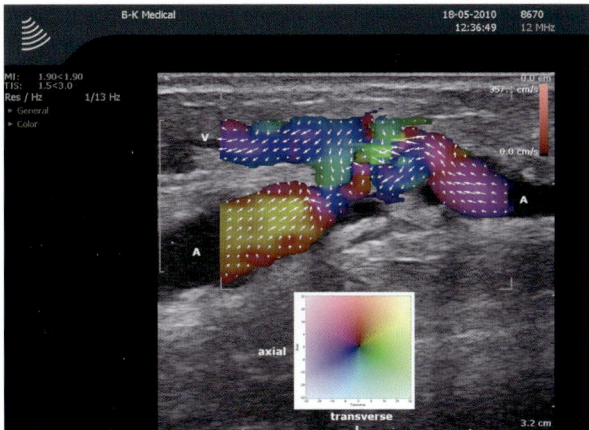

Fig. 13.2 Vector Flow Imaging. This scan of an arterio-venous shunt in a patient receiving haemodialysis shows the very complex anatomy that is readily displayed by non-directional Doppler. The arrows indicate the flow direction which goes from the afferent artery (A) to the vein (V) along a twisty fistula path. In normal colour Doppler the directional dependence would produce uninterpretable colour changes and dropouts at the 90° angles. The colour wheel indicates the coding for direction, lighter shades indicating faster flow. Image courtesy of Dr Stefen Ellebæk Pedersen.

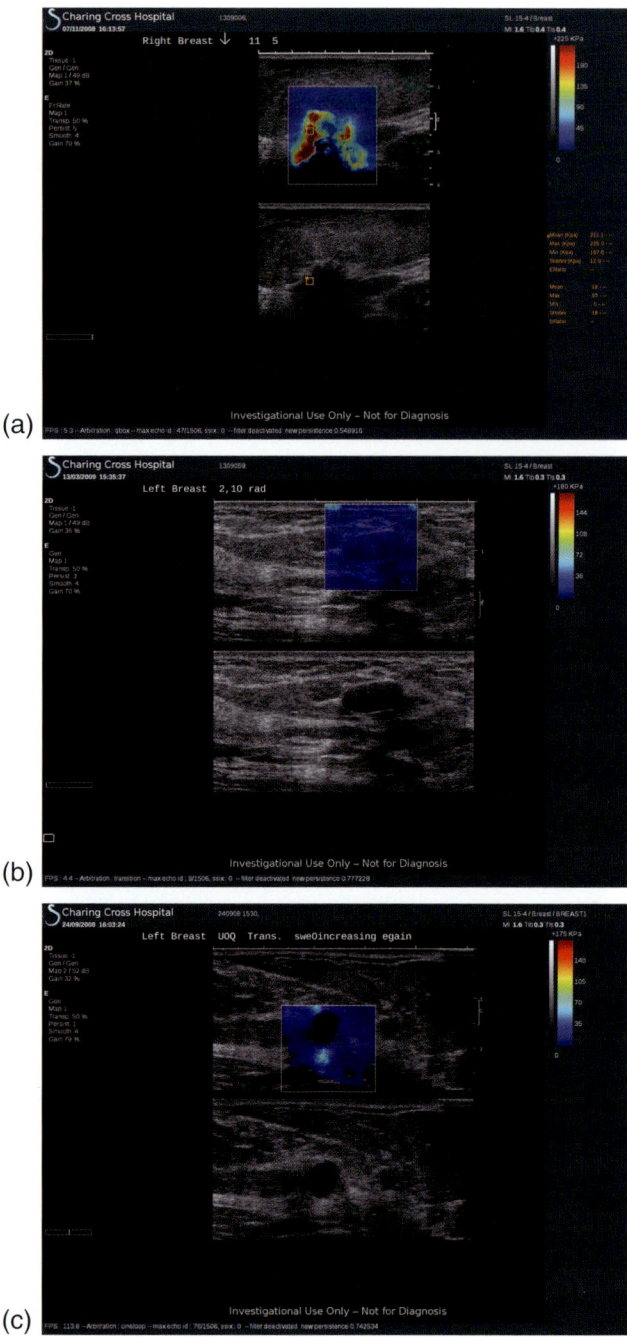

Fig. 13.4 Shear wave elastograms (SWEs) of breast lesions. In these images the SWE is shown as an overlay on the B-mode image in the upper pane; the lower pane shows the B-mode image in its original form. A carcinoma (a) shows a very stiff periphery with a maximum kPa reading of 221, corresponding to a reddish-brown colour code. The stiffness is very typically distributed around the periphery of the mass. A fibroadenoma (b) by comparison, shows low stiffness values and is depicted as a blue tint. Cysts vary in their appearance—this example (c) shows no reading at all and is depicted as a black space. If the cyst fluid is very thick, some signal may be seen.

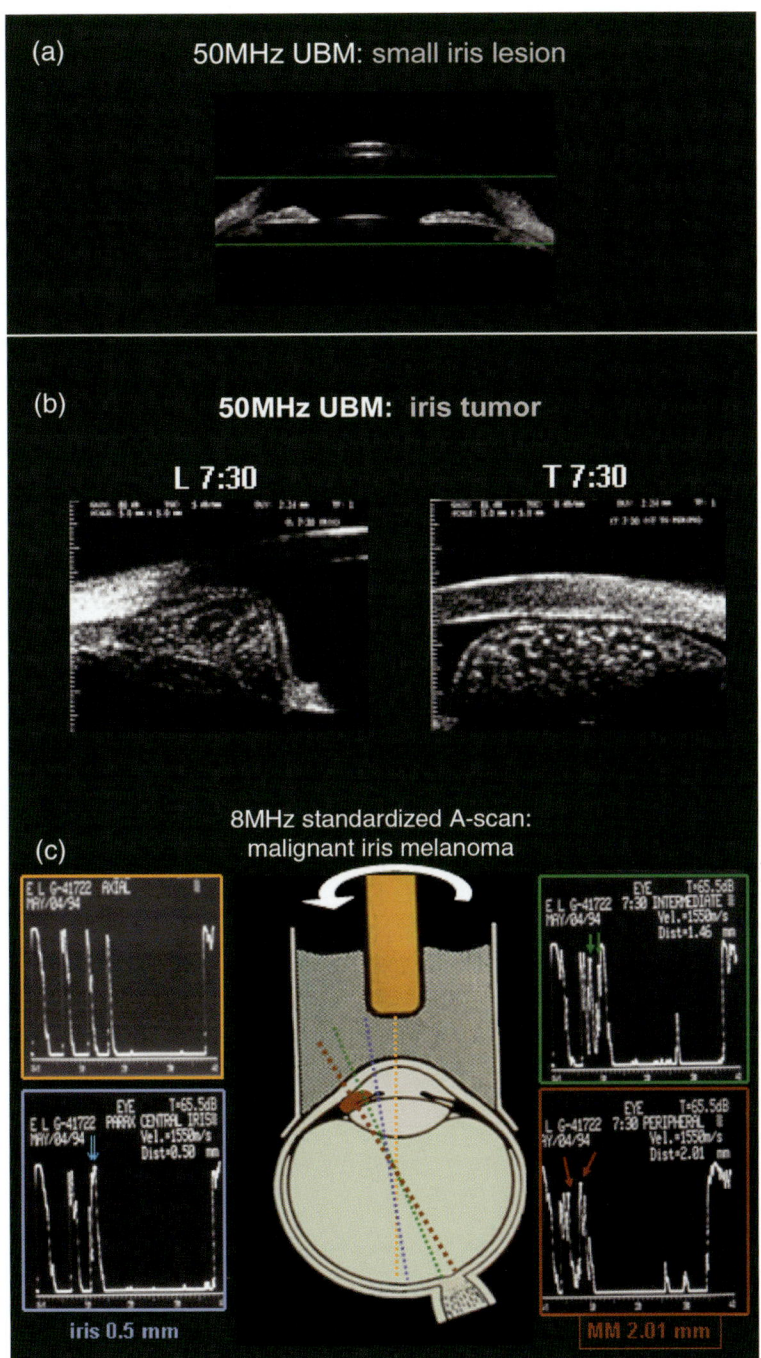

Fig. 15.1 (a) Iris tumour (benign nevus by A-scan). (b) Longitudinal (L), transverse (T) high-frequency ultrasonic biomicroscopy sections of a larger solid iris tumour. (c) Standardized A-scan (immersion technique) proves this iris tumour to be a malignant melanoma.

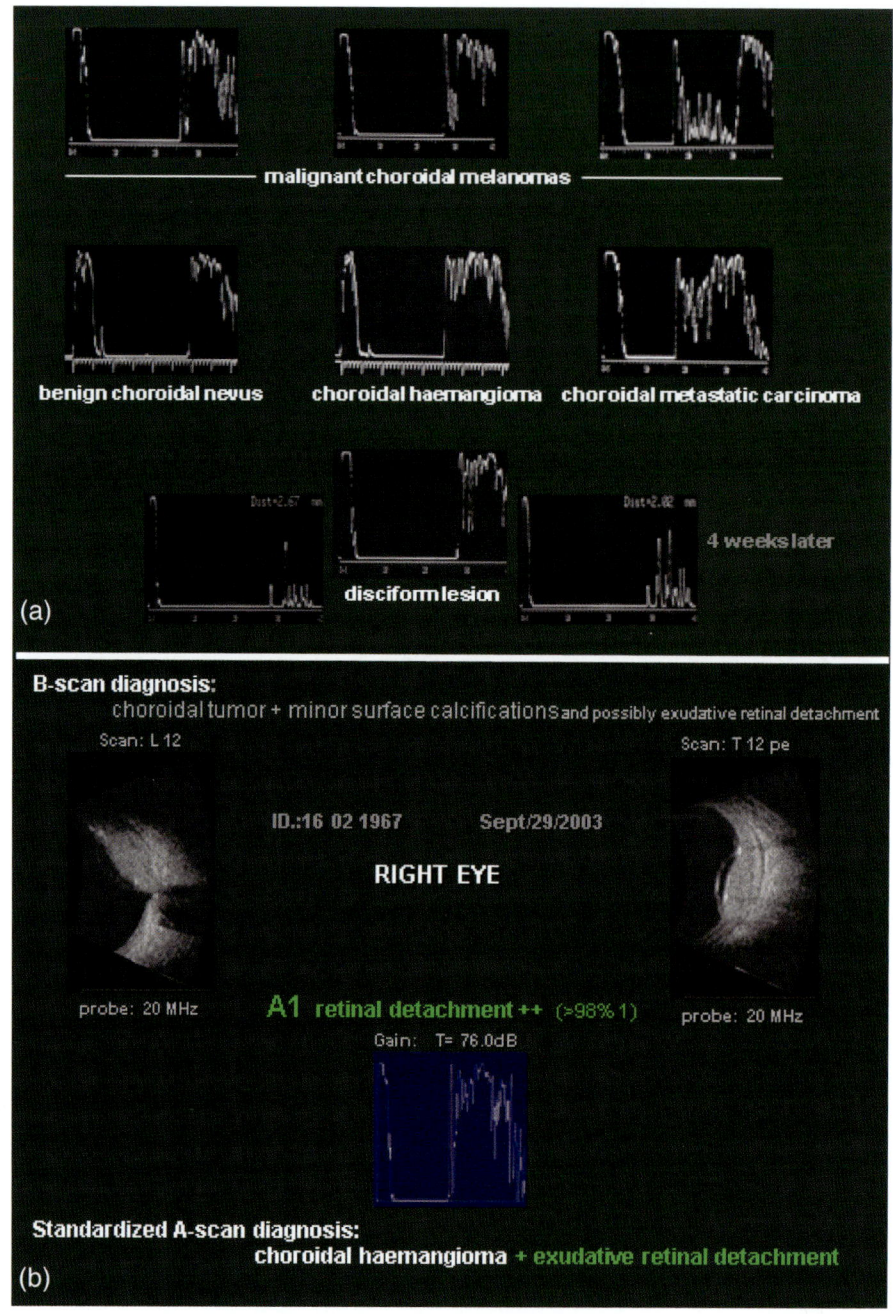

Fig. 15.2 (a) Acoustic patterns typical for different intraocular tumours. (b) Longitudinal (L) and transverse (T) 20MHz B-scans from intraocular tumour with small superficial calcifications producing shadows and overlying the tumour what probably is an exudative retinal detachment. Standardized A-scan confirmed choroidal haemangioma and proved (through an A_1 procedure) the overlying large surface to be retina; this diagnosis was automatically displayed and in parenthesis the reason for retina ++ is given: (reflectivity >98% + great smoothness of surface).

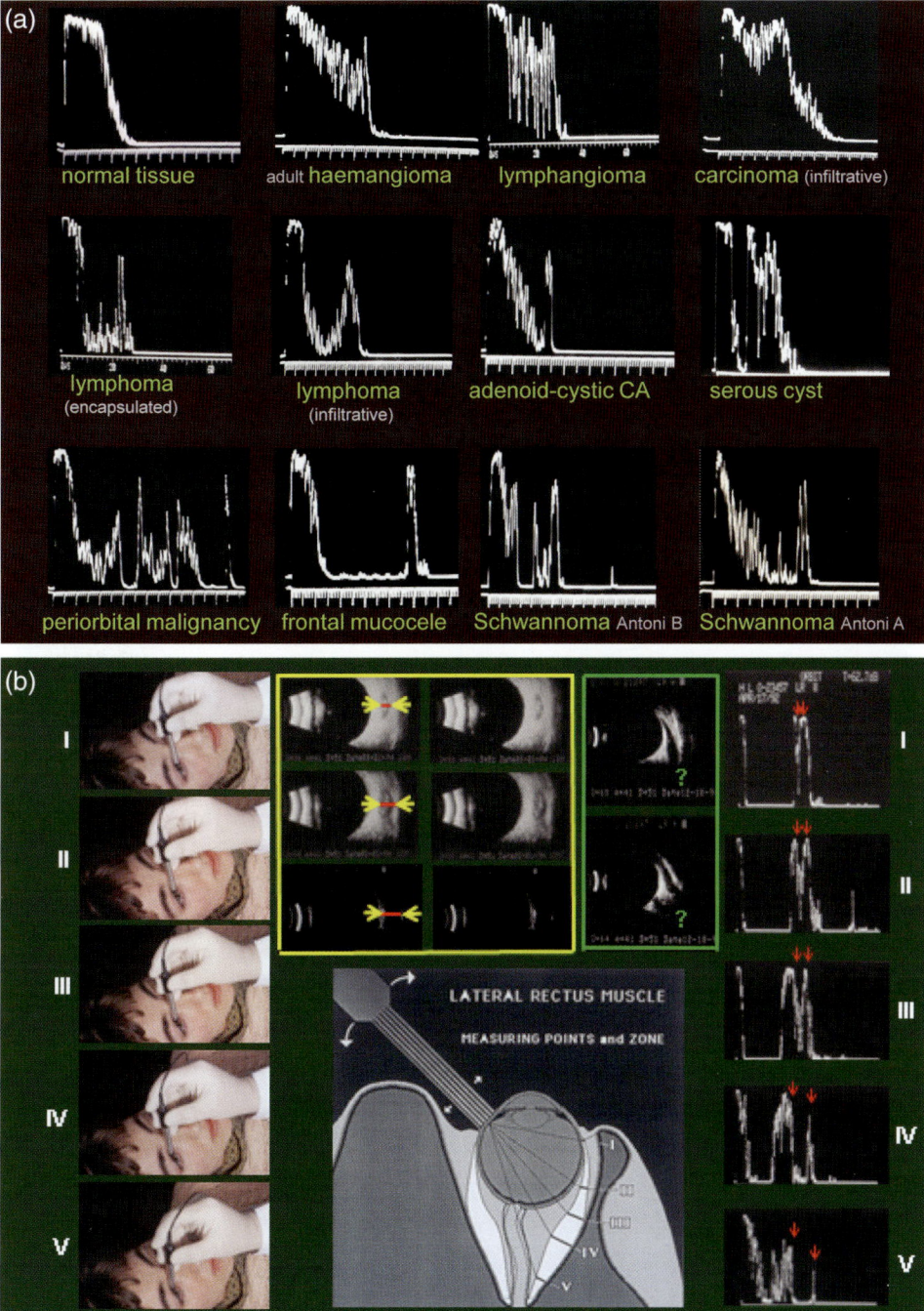

Fig. 15.3 (a) Acoustic patterns typical for different orbit tissues. (b) Illustration of the measurement of the thickness of an extraocular muscle in five different well-defined measuring points.

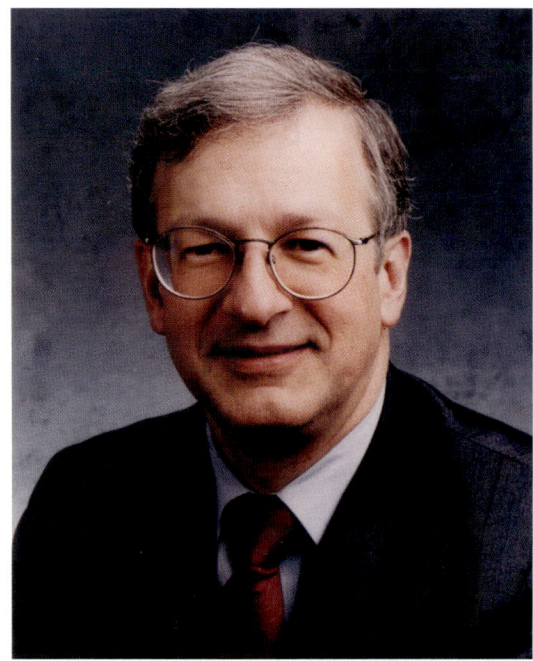

Fig. 17.1 Sam Maslak, founder, President, and Chief Executive Officer, Acuson Corporation 1979–2000.

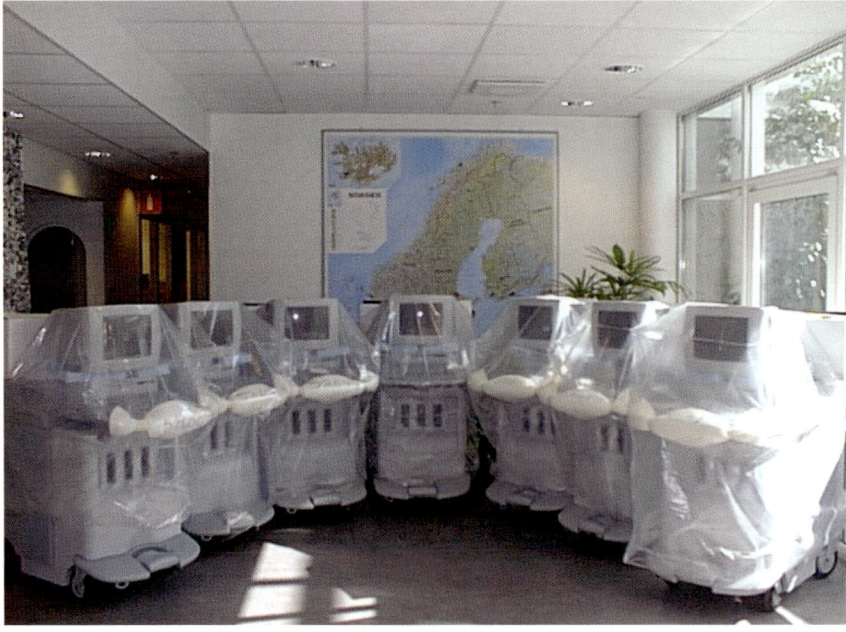

Fig. 17.2 Acuson Sequoia systems waiting for delivery to different Swedish hospitals at Eurostop Arlandastad office in June 1999.

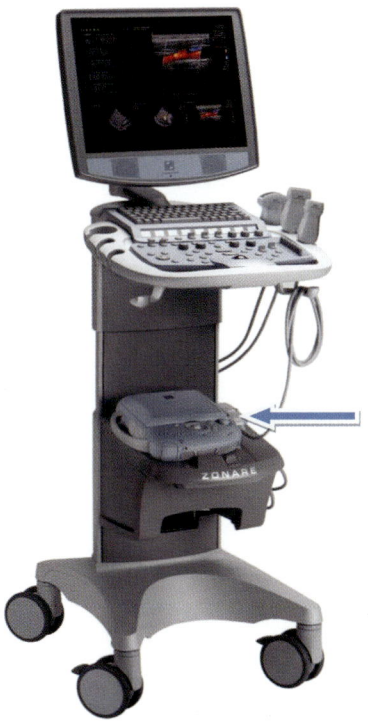

Fig. 17.3 Zonare 2.5kg Hand Carried System (HCU). Reproduced with permission from ZONARE.

The adverse reactions most frequently reported with contrast agents in clinical trials were headache, injection site pain, bruising, burning, and paraesthesias.

Diagnostic applications

The change in density at the surface of a bubble in plasma represents a major impedance mismatch and the echogenicity this produces is exploited in the uses of microbubbles to improve Doppler studies, in a technique called 'Doppler rescue' (16). This is particularly useful when flow information makes conventional studies difficult. Common applications of contrast agents include studies of the basilar and vertebral arteries, transcranial ultrasound examinations in patients with severe hyperostosis of the skull, and measurement of internal carotid stenosis in calcified arteries (16). Most notably, in acute stroke it can differentiate subtotal stenosis from occlusion when blood flow velocity is very slow in nearly occluded vessels (18). In the same setting contrast-enhanced ultrasound can also detect small collaterals. The microbubbles are smaller than regular red blood cells but have similar behaviour. This allows contrast-enhanced technology to image microcirculation and to differentiate occlusion from severely compromised flow (18). This technology appears promising in the accurate delineation of intra- and extracranial blood vessel anatomy avoiding the risks inherent to conventional angiography. Seidel et al. (18) have shown that it can detect middle cerebral artery occlusion with a sensitivity of 100% and a specificity of 83% as compared with conventional cerebral angiography. The positive and negative predictive values were 86% and 100% respectively.

Other applications include studying renal artery stenosis and difficult portal and hepatic artery examinations (e.g. in cirrhosis, in tips shunts, or after liver transplantation) (2). The study of microcirculation has significant applications in oncology, especially for the liver where a three-phase approach studying the arterial, portal, and sinusoidal sequence is used (19).

In addition, the emerging application of intraoperative contrast-enhanced ultrasound using phase inversion harmonic imaging in neurosurgery allows for visualization and morphological assessment of vascular pathologies (20). With these tools, middle cerebral artery aneurysms and arteriovenous malformations can be assessed in real-time, while the use of contrast agent, can reveal the flow dynamics of these lesions allowing appropriate surgical planning (20).

While the current contrast-enhanced ultrasound applications are expanding there is an area of future clinical potential that includes targeting microbubbles for expanding vascular imaging (17). The microbubbles, after attachment of antibodies or other ligands to their shell can bind to specific cell receptors in areas of disease (15). In fact, the acoustic radiation force of ultrasound itself has been shown to enhance targeting of ultrasound contrast agents (21). Because of their ability to reflect ultrasound, the area and the extent of concentration, the timing and spatial extent of the bubbles can provide information about the stage of the disease (15). Research in this field has given birth to the field of molecular imaging with ultrasound. Because microbubbles are pure intravascular tracers, the disease processes must be characterized by antigens that are expressed within the blood vessels. Several *in vitro* and *in vivo* studies have targeted pathological processes with contrast-enhanced ultrasound (15, 22). The pathological states that have been targeted include angiogenesis (by targeting the endothelial integrin $\alpha v\beta 3$) (23), inflammation (by targeting ICAM-1, VCAM-1, P- and L- selectin), thrombus (by targeting IIbIIIa receptors (24) or fibrinogen), plaque (by targeting ICAM-1, VCAM-1, and several angiogenesis markers) (15). Especially the last of these has the potential for future applications in the assessment of atherosclerotic plaque stability and may be of potential clinical use for the identification of patients who are at high risk for atherosclerotic cardiovascular events before stenosis can be detected by angiography (15, 22). In fact, by targeting plaque inflammation and neovascularization, as well as adventitial vasa vasorum and intimal angiogenesis 'vulnerable plaques' can be recognized and the need for their early treatment can become apparent (25).

Therapeutic applications

The therapeutic applications of microbubbles consist in the localized delivery of genes, siRNAs, drugs, and molecules in general designed to treat disease or modify biologic functions (17). Therapeutic agents can be attached to or dissolved within the surface shell, or deposited within the bubbles themselves (26). These applications are based on the local adherence of bubbles to targets of interest. This is the result of the chemical properties of the shell or its attachments that bind to specific cell surface antigens expressed in the region of disease. The localized effect of ultrasound causes the microbubbles to oscillate, collapse, and disintegrate (26). This releases the therapeutic agent and creates pores in the adjacent tissue (sonoporation) enhancing the delivery of the agents into the cells. One interesting application of this property that has been studied in animal models is the transient disruption of the blood–brain barrier and the delivery of drugs and genes to specific areas of the brain treated with ultrasound (27).

Local cavitation due to microbubble destruction can produce other mechanical effects, such as clot fragmentation, which, when combined with local thrombolytic delivery, can enhance thrombolysis (28). Trubestein et al. (29) reported the potential for high-frequency ultrasound to dissolve intra-arterial thrombus. This technique, called sono-thrombolysis, has proven effective in combination with thrombolytic agents at lower frequencies causing less heating and a broader acoustic field. In fact, continuous transcranial Doppler has been shown to augment the tissue plasminogen activator (tPA) induced arterial recanalization in stroke patients (30). Recently, studies demonstrating that intravenously administered microbubbles were able to enhance the thrombolytic effect of ultrasound often resulting in complete vessel recanalization, progressed from *in vitro* and *in vivo* experimentation to clinical trials (28). Clinical trials now in progress may bring this technology into broad clinical application in clot dissolution from dialysis grafts to stroke or myocardial infarction (28, 31).

The use of microbubbles as a tool for drug delivery enhancement and penetration into tissues such as the brain and as a means of rapid and minimally invasive clot lysis has an enormous clinical potential but is met with several challenges. These include the ideal shell composition, the choice of the molecular targets, ideal method of substance incorporation and concentration, and their safety profile. Despite these difficulties, this technique will help improve the therapeutic index, and lower the incidence of adverse events, associated with the current systemic treatments.

Intravascular ultrasound and virtual histology

Angiography is considered to be the 'gold standard' in the assessment of vascular morphology (32). However, it depicts only the contrast agent-filled lumen, giving little information on the vessel wall. In addition, atherosclerotic lesions are usually irregular affecting the final vessel contour with the presence of plaque remodelling. Intravascular ultrasound is a rapidly evolving technique that provides high-quality images of the lumen and vessel wall in high resolution (33).

Using high-frequency catheter-based transducers, physicians have been able to demonstrate the cross-sectional luminal size, shape, and wall thickness, and to identify the various layers of the wall, including the intima, media, adventitia, and perivascular structures (32). Depending on how easily the three arterial layers can be discerned, intravascular ultrasound (IVUS) helps classify the arteries as elastic (central components of the arterial tree) or muscular (peripheral arteries). Hyperechoic areas demonstrate calcifications, whereas hypoechoic regions within an atheroma may correspond to haemorrhage or fat deposition. By providing this information it allows for *in vivo* visualization of the atheroma and quantitative analysis of the plaque, evaluating the extent and composition of the plaque based on the differential acoustic properties of its characteristics (lipid, and calcified tissue, and fibrous) (32).

Besides these properties provided by conventional grey-scale intravascular sonography, several other modes have enhanced the effect of IVUS (4). Colour-flow intravascular sonography provides greater understanding of intraluminal blood flow, lumen size, and the success of endovascular treatment. Virtual histology intravascular sonography takes advantage of the fact that the components of the vessel wall reflect the sonography signal intensity at different frequencies creating an opportunity for histological details to be detected through the generation of a virtual histology intravascular sonography map. With analysis of radiofrequency signals, real-time dynamic assessment of plaque morphology can be performed. A histological classification of the plaque can be produced as a result of the comparison of virtual histology maps with the true histological sections of diseased coronary arteries. Similar to the virtual histology sonography, integrated backscatter intravascular sonography reflects the tissue characteristics but by using a different algorithm.

Therefore, IVUS provides the potential for 'virtual histology' that allows the physician to characterize the properties of the plaques and to tailor his treatments without the need for histology (34, 35). In fact, several studies have shown strong correlation between IVUS plaque characteristics and histopathological specimens. Potkin et al. (36) compared IVUS with histological sections using coronary arterial specimens, to show that fibrous and calcified plaques were identified with good precision. The CAPITAL study validated the use of IVUS in the carotid arteries by showing strong correlation of virtual histology IVUS findings with endarterectomy specimens.

Consequently, patients with vulnerable plaques, heavy in fat deposition, would be considered at higher risk for cardiovascular events and more aggressive treatment might be sought. In addition, the patients' response to anti-atherogenic treatments, e.g. statins, can be monitored by the use of serial IVUS. Several recent studies, including ASTEROID (37), METEOR (38), REVERSAL (39), and STRADIVARIOUS (40) have shown excellent plaque regression in response to statins and lipid-lowering therapies in various arterial beds. IVUS has also helped in the identification of atherosclerosis as a dynamic process. The literature has demonstrated the phenomena of positive and negative remodelling (enlargement or decrease in the vessel diameter) in the setting of an atheroma (32). Identification of these disease processes provides a prognostication tool, since patients demonstrating positive remodelling are believed to have a survival benefit. In addition, it can allow early characterization of restenosis (due to a combination of intimal hyperplasia and negative remodelling) after angioplasty and stenting and prompt more immediate re-treatment (32).

Methods such as IVUS elastography (34) have been introduced to assess the mechanical properties of the vessel wall, which may relate indirectly to the histopathological composition of the atherosclerotic plaque. Intravascular elastography is obtained from cardiac IVUS images associated with intraluminal pressures during the cardiac cycle. The images provide vessel wall strain information and demonstrate the mechanical properties of the tissue.

Intravascular ultrasound has protean clinical applications that have been well studied in several vascular beds. A plethora of clinical trials have shown the superiority of IVUS to angiography (32), that in general underestimates the plaque burden, especially for the detection of concentrical lumen narrowing. IVUS has played a major role in the understanding of the effects of percutaneous transluminal angioplasty on the vascular structure. IVUS has provided direct visualization of the stretching, compression, and redistribution of the plaque as well as tearing processes that are associated with lumen expansion by balloon dilation. Overall about 80% of the increase in the lumen area is due to an increase in vessel size, and 20% is due to a reduction in plaque area (presumably due to axial plaque redistribution) (32). The literature also supports the use of IVUS as a means of planning and evaluating the effects of vascular brachytherapy in the treatment of post-stent restenosis (41). In a similar fashion the use of IVUS for peripheral vascular disease allows the appropriate intervention procedure to be chosen and the correct balloon size to be selected. Furthermore, during endovascular aneurysm repair (EVAR), IVUS can provide imaging information that can reduce the contrast load during angiography in patients with compromised renal function (42). IVUS can provide risk stratification and can be used to optimize selection of the atherosclerotic plaque, which would be most appropriate and least risky for carotid stenting (32).

IVUS has been a relatively safe procedure in the extracranial and intracranial circulation. The most important risk is that in heavily stenotic or tortuous lesions, the catheter is difficult to manoeuvre and can disrupt a plaque, releasing material that may lead in embolic stroke. Most of the series of IVUS have reported no apparent complications.

Three-dimensional ultrasound

Three-dimensional (3-D) ultrasound imaging is a recent development that holds promise for improving the visualization and quantification of complex anatomy and pathology as well as monitoring progression of atherosclerosis (43). The first attempts to create 3-D reconstructions occurred in 1970. The problems inherent to two-dimensional (2-D) ultrasound include (43): conventional images are 2-D leading to variable and at times incorrect quantification of plaque morphology, difficult localization, and significant operator dependence. Although studies based on the reconstruction of 2-D images demonstrated the importance of 3-D imaging in several disease processes, the complexity of the reconstruction was limiting it in research applications. The recent development of matrix array transducers capable of real-time 3-D imaging managed to overcome many of the above problems (17). Consequently, 3-D ultrasound permits shorter scanning time. However, the widespread use of real-time 3-D ultrasound has been prevented by the slow frame rate, the lengthy analysis time, and the limited spatial resolution (17).

Three-dimensional imaging of atherosclerotic plaques will allow reproducible quantitative monitoring of plaque progression and regression, and provide important information about the plaque's natural history response to therapy (17).

The use of contrast in conjunction with 2-D imaging is well established and has improved border recognition in difficult subjects. The combination of contrast with 3-D imaging will likely partially compensate for the limited spatial resolution of the technique and should enhance its value in areas such as stress echocardiography (32).

The development of 3-D IVUS imaging offers a unique method for assessment of normal and diseased vascular structures (32). With this technique, the vascular branches and accessory vessels, as well as their relationships to each other, can easily be demonstrated. Three-dimensional IVUS is useful in the diagnosis of arterial dissections and aneurysms. The complex flaps associated with aortic dissections can easily be depicted with 3-D IVUS, much better than with conventional angiography.

With improved strategies to treat atherosclerosis non-surgically, reproducible non-invasive 3-D imaging techniques allowing direct plaque visualization and quantification are becoming more important in serial monitoring of disease progression and regression. Monitoring plaque morphology and geometry can provide important information about the effects of anti-atherosclerotic therapies.

Assessment of flow-mediated dilatation by ultrasound

Appreciation of the central role played by endothelium in the pathogenesis of the atherosclerotic process has led to the development of a wide range of methods to assess endothelial dysfunction, based on the role of endothelium on vascular tone modulation (44). The degree of vasodilation is considered a measure of endothelial function. The greater the vasodilation, the higher the endothelial function.

The most widely used technique for assessing endothelial function is 'flow-mediated dilatation' (FMD) of the brachial artery. This non-invasive method consists of the measurement of brachial artery diameter changes caused by an increase in shear stress, mediated by local release of nitric oxide (NO) (44). Ischaemia is induced by the inflation of an arterial occlusion cuff for 5 minutes, positioned on the proximal forearm. After cuff deflation brachial artery flow increases because of downstream vessel dilation and this augmented flow increases brachial artery shear stress resulting in vasodilation of the artery itself. The mechanism of FMD is not fully understood but it is speculated to involve increased production of NO by the endothelium in response to stress-induced phosphorylation of the endothelial NO synthase (44). In arteries with impaired NO production, due to decreased endothelial function the above response is diminished. In some patients a constrictor response is seen.

Several pieces of evidence in the literature are supporting a more active role for FMD in clinical practice (45). First, decreased brachial artery FMD has been associated with the major risk factors for cardiovascular disease, including smoking, diabetes, advanced age, and hypercholesterolaemia. Moreover, FMD appears to represent coronary artery reactivity, since atherosclerosis is a systemic disease and abnormalities detected in the brachial artery reflect the mechanical properties of the patient's vessels in general. Lastly, FMD provides significant diagnostic and prognostic information in patients with coronary artery disease (CAD). Some studies have shown that FMD was almost as sensitive and more specific in detecting CAD in comparison to stress electrocardiography (45).

A meta-analysis (46), which included approximately 2500 patients with atherosclerotic coronary disease or characterized by high cardiovascular risk, demonstrated that endothelial dysfunction, evaluated by brachial artery FMD significantly predicted cardiovascular events, independently of traditional cardiovascular risk factors.

Although measurement of brachial artery FMD is a non-invasive index of endothelial dysfunction with an established relationship to CAD, it has several limitations that need to be taken into consideration for its clinical applications. The potential small vessel size makes the measurement of the brachial artery difficult, whereas another potential problem arises from the ambiguity in image timing after cuff deflation (45). Moreover, the location of the occlusion cuff, the patient's age, and size may affect FMD measurements (45). Lastly, although FMD describes one facet of endothelial dysfunction, other mechanisms also exist (45).

Measurement of carotid intima–media thickness

Another surrogate marker used to measure atherosclerosis by B-mode ultrasound burden is the measurement of carotid intima–media thickness (CIMT) (3, 47). B-mode ultrasound CIMT measurement involves a simple distance measurement between the leading edges of the lumen–intima and media–adventitia ultrasound interfaces. This measurement has been validated as an early marker of atherosclerosis progression and it can be used to quantify pathology monitoring and response to drug therapy (3).

Large follow-up studies such as the Rotterdam Study (48) and the Atherosclerosis Risk in Communities Study (ARIC) (49) provided evidence that CIMT measurements can be used to indicate the degree of existing generalized atherosclerosis and future cardiovascular disease risk. In ARIC an increase in mean CIMT of 0.2mm was associated with an increase in relative risk for myocardial infarction and stroke of 33% and 28% respectively. Several other studies have established the predictive value of CIMT for adverse cerebral, cardiac, and peripheral vascular events. Studies, such as Cholesterol Lowering Atherosclerosis Study (CLAS) (50), Asymptomatic Carotid Artery Progression Study (ACAPS) (51), Regression Growth Evaluation Statin Study (REGRESS) (52), and Atorvastatin versus Simvastatin in Atherosclerosis Progression (ASAP) (53) have shown the efficacy of CIMT in monitoring the patients' response to lipid lowering therapies.

Although observational studies have supported the use of CIMT as a surrogate marker for atherosclerosis, several randomized trials and standardization of the technique are needed before widespread clinical application. The use of B-mode ultrasound makes this technique readily available and easily applicable.

Conclusions

The vascular laboratory is pioneering in the changing technology. Virtually all peripheral arterial and venous structures may be imaged with colour DU. The identification of occlusions, the characterization of plaques, and the monitoring of vascular interventions are just a few examples. Moreover, the development of 3-D ultrasound, contrast-enhanced ultrasound, and IVUS is opening new paths in the asymptomatic diagnosis, localized treatment, and monitoring of vascular disease. The low cost and non-invasive aspect of most ultrasound methods make it the technique of choice in studying the human vasculature.

References

1. Pearce WH, Astleford P. What's new in vascular ultrasound. *Surg Clin North Am* 2004; **84**(4):1113–26.
2. Furlow B. Contrast-enhanced ultrasound. *Radiol Technol* 2009; **80**(6):547S–561S.
3. de Groot E, vuven SI, Duivenvoorden R, Meuwese MC, Akdim F, Bots ML, *et al*. Measurement of carotid intima-media thickness to assess progression and regression of atherosclerosis. *Nat Clin Pract Cardiovasc Med* 2008; **5**(5):280–8.
4. Zacharatos H, Hassan AE, Qureshi A. Intravascular ultrasound: principles and cerebrovascular applications. *AJNR Am J Neuroradiol* 2010; **31**(4):586–97.
5. Grassbaugh JA, Nelson PR, Rzucidlo EM, Schermerhorn ML, Fillinger MF, Powell RJ, *et al*. Blinded comparison of preoperative duplex ultrasound scanning and contrast arteriography for planning revascularization at the level of the tibia. *J Vasc Surg* 2003; **37**(6):1186–90.
6. Mazzariol F, Ascher E, Hingorani A, Gunduz Y, Yorkovich W, Salles-Cunha S. Lower-extremity revascularisation without preoperative contrast arteriography in 185 cases: lessons learned with duplex ultrasound arterial mapping. *Eur J Vasc Endovasc Surg* 2000; **19**(5):509–15.
7. Proia RR, Walsh DB, Nelson PR, Connors JP, Powell RJ, Zwolak RM, *et al*. Early results of infragenicular revascularization based solely on duplex arteriography. *J Vasc Surg* 2001; **33**(6):1165–70.
8. Johnson BL, Bandyk DF, Back MR, Avino AJ, Roth SM. Intraoperative duplex monitoring of infrainguinal vein bypass procedures. *J Vasc Surg* 2000; **31**(4):678–90.
9. Labropoulos N, Nandivada P, Bekelis K. Prevalence and impact of the subclavian steal syndrome. *Ann Surg* 2010; **252**(1):166–70.

10. Labropoulos N, Leon L, Kwon S, assiopoulos A, Gonzalez-Fajardo JA, Kang SS, *et al*. Study of the venous reflux progression. *J Vasc Surg* 2005; **41**(2):291–5.
11. Labropoulos N, Kokkosis AA, Spentzouris G, Gasparis AP, Tassiopoulos AK. The distribution and significance of varicosities in the saphenous trunks. *J Vasc Surg* 2010; **51**(1):96–103.
12. Labropoulos N, Jen J, Jen H, Gasparis AP, Tassiopoulos AK. Recurrent deep vein thrombosis: long-term incidence and natural history. *Ann Surg* 2010; **251**(4):749–53.
13. Labropoulos N, Bhatti AF, Amaral S, Leon L, Borge M, Rodriguez H, *et al*. Neovascularization in acute venous thrombosis. *J Vasc Surg* 2005; **42**(3):515–18.
14. Gramiak R, Shah PM, Kramer DH. Ultrasound cardiography: contrast studies in anatomy and function. *Radiology* 1969; **92**:939–48.
15. Voigt JU. Ultrasound molecular imaging. *Methods* 2009; **48**(2):92–7.
16. Cosgrove D. Ultrasound contrast agents: an overview. *Eur J Radiol* 2006; **60**(3):324–30.
17. Weyman AE. Future directions in echocardiography. *Rev Cardiovasc Med* 2009; **10**(1):4–13.
18. Seidel G, Meairs S. Ultrasound contrast agents in ischemic stroke. *Cerebrovasc Dis* 2009; **27** (Suppl. 2):25–39.
19. Wilson SR, Burns PN. Microbubble contrast for radiological imaging: 2. Applications. *Ultrasound Q* 2006; **22**(1):15–18.
20. Hölscher T, Ozgur B, Singel S, Wilkening WG, Mattrey RF, Sang H. Intraoperative ultrasound using phase inversion harmonic imaging: first experiences. *Neurosurgery* 2007; **60**(4 Suppl 2): 382–6.
21. Stieger SM, Caskey CF, Adamson RH, Qin S, Curry FR, Wisner ER, *et al*. Enhancement of vascular permeability with low-frequency contrast-enhanced ultrasound in the chorioallantoic membrane model. *Radiology* 2007; **243**(1):112–21.
22. Lindner JR Contrast ultrasound molecular imaging of inflammation in cardiovascular disease. *Cardiovasc Res* 2009; **84**(2):182–9.
23. Leong-Poi H, Christiansen J, Heppner P, Lewis CW, Klibanov AL, Kaul S, *et al*. Assessment of endogenous and therapeutic arteriogenesis by contrast ultrasound molecular imaging of integrin expression. *Circulation* 2005; **111**(24):3248–54.
24. Alonso A, Della Martina A, Stroick M, Fatar M, Griebe M, Pochon S, *et al*. Molecular imaging of human thrombus with novel abciximab immunobubbles and ultrasound. *Stroke* 2007; **38**(5):1508–14.
25. Vicenzini E, Giannoni MF, Benedetti-Valentini F, Lenzi GL. Imaging of carotid plaque angiogenesis. *Cerebrovasc Dis* 2009; **27**(Suppl 2):48–54.
26. Hernot S, Klibanov AL. Microbubbles in ultrasound-triggered drug and gene delivery. *Adv Drug Deliv Rev* 2008; **60**(10):1153–66.
27. Hynynen K. Ultrasound for drug and gene delivery to the brain. *Adv Drug Deliv Rev* 2008; **60**(10):1209–17.
28. Medel R, Crowley RW, McKisic MS, Dumont AS, Kassell NF. Sonothrombolysis: an emerging modality for the management of stroke. *Neurosurgery* 2009; **65**(5):979–93.
29. Trübestein G, Engel C, Etzel F, Sobbe A, Cremer H, Stumpff U. Thrombolysis by ultrasound. *Clin Sci Mol Med Suppl* 1976; **3**:697s–698s.
30. Alexandrov AV, Molina CA, Grotta JC, Garami Z, Ford SR, Alvarez-Sabin J, *et al*. Ultrasound-enhanced systemic thrombolysis for acute ischemic stroke. *N Engl J Med* 2004; **351**(21):2170–8.
31. Perren F, Loulidi J, Poglia D, Landis T, Sztajzel R. Microbubble potentiated transcranial duplex ultrasound enhances IV thrombolysis in acute stroke. *J Thromb Thrombolysis* 2008; **25**(2):219–23.
32. Liu JB, Goldberg BB. 2-D and 3-D endoluminal ultrasound: vascular and nonvascular applications. *Ultrasound Med Biol* 1999; **25**(2):159–73.

33. Houslay ES, Uren NG. Intravascular ultrasound: defining plaque regression. *Hosp Med* 2005; **66**(1):27–31.
34. Fayad ZA, Fuster V. Clinical imaging of the high-risk or vulnerable atherosclerotic plaque. *Circ Res* 2001; **89**(4):305–16.
35. Martin AJ, Ryan LK, Gotlieb AI, Henkelman RM, Foster FS. Arterial imaging: comparison of high-resolution US and MR imaging with histologic correlation. *Radiographics* 1997; **17**(1):189–202.
36. Potkin BN, Bartorelli AL, Gessert JM, Neville RF, Almagor Y, Roberts WC, et al. Coronary artery imaging with intravascular high-frequency ultrasound. *Circulation* 1990; **81**(5):1575–85.
37. Nissen SE, Nicholls SJ, Sipahi I, Libby P, Raichlen JS, Ballantyne CM, et al. Effect of very high-intensity statin therapy on regression of coronary atherosclerosis: the ASTEROID trial. *JAMA* 2006; **295**(13):1556–65.
38. Crouse JR, Raichlen JS, Riley WA, Evans GW, Palmer MK, O'Leary DH, et al. Effect of rosuvastatin on progression of carotid intima-media thickness in low-risk individuals with subclinical atherosclerosis: the METEOR Trial. *JAMA* 2007; **297**(12):1344–53.
39. Nissen SE. Effect of intensive lipid lowering on progression of coronary atherosclerosis: evidence for an early benefit from the Reversal of Atherosclerosis with Aggressive Lipid Lowering (REVERSAL) trial. *Am J Cardiol* 2005; **96**(5A):61F–68F.
40. Nissen SE, Nicholls SJ, Wolski K, Rodés-Cabau J, Cannon CP, Deanfield JE, et al. Effect of rimonabant on progression of atherosclerosis in patients with abdominal obesity and coronary artery disease: the STRADIVARIUS randomized controlled trial. *JAMA* 2008; **299**(13):1547–60.
41. Carlier SG, Coen VL, Sabaté M, Kay IP, Ligthart JM, Van Der Giessen WJ, et al. The role of intravascular ultrasound imaging in vascular brachytherapy. *Int J Cardiovasc Intervent* 2000; **3**(1):3–12.
42. Pearce BJ, Jordan WDJ. Using IVUS during EVAR and TEVAR: improving patient outcomes. *Semin Vasc Surg* 2009; **22**(3):172–80.
43. Fenster A, Landry A, Downey DB, Hegele RA, Spence JD. 3D ultrasound imaging of the carotid arteries. *Curr Drug Targets Cardiovasc Haematol Disord* 2004; **4**(2):161–75.
44. Ghiadoni L, Versari D, Giannarelli C, Faita F, Taddei S. Non-invasive diagnostic tools for investigating endothelial dysfunction. *Curr Pharm Des* 2008; **14**(35):3715–22.
45. Faulx MD, Wright AT, Hoit BD. Detection of endothelial dysfunction with brachial artery ultrasound scanning. *Am Heart J* 2003; **145**(6):943–51.
46. Lerman A, Zeiher AM. Endothelial function: cardiac events. *Circulation* 2005; **111**:363–8.
47. Labropoulos N, Leon LRJ, Brewster LP, Pryor L, Tiongson J, Kang SS, et al. Are your arteries older than your age? *Eur J Vasc Endovasc Surg* 2005; **30**(6):588–96.
48. Bots ML, Hoes AW, Koudstaal PJ, Hofman A, Grobbee DE. Common carotid intima-media thickness and risk of stroke and myocardial infarction: the Rotterdam Study. *Circulation* 1997; **96**(5):1432–37.
49. Chambless LE, Heiss G, Folsom AR, Rosamond W, Szklo M, Sharrett AR, et al. Association of coronary heart disease incidence with carotid arterial wall thickness and major risk factors: the Atherosclerosis Risk in Communities (ARIC) Study, 1987–1993. *Am J Epidemiol* 1997; **146**(6): 483–94.
50. Blankenhorn DH, Selzer RH, Crawford DW, Barth JD, Liu CR, Liu CH, et al. Beneficial effects of colestipol-niacin therapy on the common carotid artery. Two- and four-year reduction of intima-media thickness measured by ultrasound. *Circulation* 1993; **88** (1):20–8.
51. Furberg CD, Adams HPJ, Applegate WB, Byington RP, Espeland MA, Hartwell T, et al. Effect of lovastatin on early carotid atherosclerosis and cardiovascular events. Asymptomatic Carotid Artery Progression Study (ACAPS) Research Group. *Circulation* 1994; **90**(4):1679–87.

52. de Groot E, Jukema JW, Montauban van Swijndregt AD, Zwinderman AH, Ackerstaff RG, van der Steen AF, *et al*. B-mode ultrasound assessment of pravastatin treatment effect on carotid and femoral artery walls and its correlations with coronary arteriographic findings: a report of the Regression Growth Evaluation Statin Study (REGRESS). *J Am Coll Cardiol* 1998; **31**(7): 1561–7.
53. Smilde TJ, van Wissen S, Wollersheim H, Trip MD, Kastelein JJ, Stalenhoef AF. Effect of aggressive versus conventional lipid lowering on atherosclerosis progression in familial hypercholesterolaemia (ASAP): a prospective, randomised, double-blind trial. *Lancet* 2001; **357**(9256):577–81.

Chapter 11

The development of ultrasound in radiology in Sweden

Torbjörn Andersson

The early years

Diagnostic ultrasound in radiology started up in Sweden in the 1970s. And, as elsewhere in the world, it was a couple of enthusiasts who found out that a new and interesting technology was used in other departments and thought it could be used in radiology as well. The main inspiration came from the departments of obstetrics and gynaecology where ultrasound had been shown to be of great use in different obstetrical problem situations. Obstetrical ultrasound was initially used only in the larger university hospitals, which is why the first attempts to use ultrasound in radiology also started there. In southern Sweden, ultrasound was used extensively both for cardiac and obstetrical diagnosis, thus its use in radiology came on early at Lund and Malmö University Hospitals.

In Lund, the radiologist Wilhelm Karp introduced static ultrasound scanning in radiology. He and his co-worker Lillemor Forsberg published several papers with reference to the use of ultrasound technology in various fields (1–6) and he also defended the first Swedish thesis in radiology dealing with ultrasound. Their publications showed that this new technology was not just a flash in the pan but here to stay. In Malmö, static ultrasound within the radiology department was introduced by a group lead by Jan Hildell and Peter Aspelin. Simultaneously ultrasound became more and more popular in the larger Swedish hospitals such as Karolinska Hospital in Stockholm and Uppsala Academic Hospital. In Stockholm, several of the radiology departments were pioneering ultrasound in obstetrics and this became the incentive to also use the technology for abdominal and genitourinary diagnosis. Some of the most active radiologists in this work were Ingmar Fernström, who was responsible for both obstetric (7) and radiological ultrasound at Karolinska Hospital for several years, and Anders Törngren and Gunnar Westberg who had similar positions at Danderyd and Serafimer Hospitals.

Commercial ultrasound equipment at that time were rather complicated to use and to calibrate. The first scanners also utilized so-called bi-stable displays, which lacking in grey-scale made it rather complicated to interpret the images. Therefore ultrasound did not have the same rapid breakthrough as other later introduced radiological imaging modalities. The early users of ultrasound in radiology were all autodidacts and no organized education was available in Sweden at that time. Although the Internet was not yet invented and fax not available for the ordinary person, many of the early users found out where to go to get more information and training and some of us made odysseys to especially the United Kingdom and the United States to learn more.

One would have expected that the initiative to start up ultrasound education would come from the large university hospitals where most knowledge was acquired, but the enlightenment came from quite an unexpected quarter. A young British radiologist from Southampton, Keith Dewbury, had a summer locum tenens at the small Swedish hospital in Motala town. He informed the department chairman, Dr Göran Karner, about diagnostic use of ultrasound. This resulted in an acquisition of a Diasonograph static ultrasound scanner and subsequent introduction to the art of ultrasound for all the radiologists at Motala hospital. Karner immediately understood the potential of ultrasound in radiology and encouraged Dr Dewbury to try to find some interested colleagues in the United Kingdom and come back next year to be part of the first radiological ultrasound course in Sweden.

This course was held in May 1978 in the old monastery in Vadstena town. The course was entirely arranged by Dr Karner, but he managed to persuade the Swedish Society of Medical Radiology to be guarantor and the official organizer. Dr Karner had also arranged a technical exhibition at Motala hospital so the course participants received both theoretical and practical training. At the same occasion, a group of Swedish radiologist were for the first time introduced to dynamic ultrasound scanning with real-time equipment.

The lecturers were all non-Swedish and Keith Dewbury had found two outstanding ultrasound friends in David Cosgrove from the Royal Marsden Hospital and Hylton Meire from Kings College Hospital in London. Together with paediatric radiologist Gary W. Le Quesne from Adelaide in Australia they formed the entire faculty. This 3-day course turned out to be a great success and several of the early radiology ultrasound pioneers in Sweden attended and established close personal connections. In this way Karner's first ultrasound course became the take-off for one of the most successful annual courses in Swedish radiology.

The golden years

A successful period for ultrasound began with the second Swedish ultrasound course, held in 1980. During subsequent years the course grew into a 6-day boarding school course. Besides the three British lecturers and a growing Swedish faculty, a number of distinguished scientists and physicians were lecturing here, such as Hans-Henrik Holm, Sören Torp Pedersen, and Christian Nolsö from Denmark, William Lees and Henry Irving from the United Kingdom, Fred Lee from Ann Arbor and David Cossman from Los Angeles, United States. The high quality of the lecturers and the mix of theory and practice made this course, the Kolmården Ultrasound Course, a must for most Swedish radiologists. More than 1200 radiologists attended the course until it was phased out in 1992. This successful concept was also brought back to the United Kingdom by the British ultrasound troika when they later introduced a similar concept—the London Ultrasound Course.

During the same period the Swedish healthcare system, including radiology, expanded heavily. This expansion comprised ultrasound, which was introduced in almost every radiology department in the country. The change from static to dynamic scanning was one major factor for the spread of ultrasound since it made the technology easier to learn and master and also faster to use. The annual numbers of performed examinations grow considerably and the interest for the technology was intense in spite of the introduction of other new technologies such as computed tomography (CT) and, later, magnetic resonance imaging (MRI). The combination of the annual advanced ultrasound course with very qualified national and international teachers, and the general interest of non-invasive imaging made this period a golden era for ultrasound in Sweden. The general level of competence was high and the fast development of ultrasound in radiology also attracted a lot of junior doctors to the speciality, which created a demand for more education.

In southern Sweden this growing demand was also met by Dr Lillemor Forsberg, now working at Ängelholm General Hospital, who initiated a course in basic ultrasound for junior doctors. This was build upon the same foundation as the more advanced Kolmården Course, with both theory and practice. It is still running every year, now in Gothenburg, and still with the retired Dr Forsberg attending as an active teacher. This concept with a basic ultrasound course has later been followed by similar courses arranged by several university hospital radiology departments in Sweden.

The start of ultrasound education for Swedish radiologists came about hand-in-hand with an initiative to formalize the education and also to ensure that this new technology was firmly established as one of many radiological technologies. This was initiated by Dr Curt Lagergren at Karolinska Hospital, who as chairman of the Swedish Society of Medical Radiology, suggested that an ultrasound section of the society should be created. This was effected in 1978 at the Annual Meeting of the Society in Stockholm. This Section for Ultrasound of the Swedish Society for Medical Radiology had a very strong position for many years and became a guarantor that radiology was seen as one of the main medical specialities with a legal interest in ultrasound. The core of early Swedish ultrasound enthusiasts also fused together in the work with the Section for Ultrasound and within the board you found people like Gunnar Westberg, Göran Karner, P.G. Lindgren, Anders Törngren, Mats Aztely, Lillemor Forsberg, Lars Öberg, and myself.

The interventional years

The use of special equipment for ultrasound-guided punctures was first described in 1969 when Kratochwil presented a dedicated A-scan transducer for puncture (8). In Denmark, Professor Hans-Henrik Holm at Gentofte and Herlev Hospitals was one of the early ultrasound pioneers and he and co-workers developed a widely-used puncture technique with a special transducer for static ultrasound B-scanners (9). However, the static scanner had a number of drawbacks for puncture guidance. The most important was the lack of control of the needle position during the actual puncture moment and the technique was never widely spread and by many considered to be both complicated and dangerous.

In Sweden two technical inventions by P.G Lindgren in Uppsala, had an enormous impact on the use of ultrasound for guiding different interventional procedures. In 1980 he presented his experience of a large number of ultrasound-guided punctures performed with a dynamic mechanical sector scanner and a specially designed needle-guide unit (Fig. 11.1) fitted on the transducer head (10). The passage of the needle through the tissues could now be exactly predicted and also observed on the ultrasound monitor during puncture of both cystic lesions and solid tissues (Fig. 11.2). Two years later he presented a semiautomatic device, a 'biopsy-gun' for performing core biopsies using one hand (11). The first prototype used a 2.0mm Travenol Tru-Cut needle, originally designed for manual biopsies using two hands (Fig. 11.3, top). This made it possible to perform ultrasound-guided tissue sampling with high precision in an extremely fast way. When he later presented a modified biopsy device, Biopty-Cut® (Fig. 11.3, bottom), with the possibility to use a number of different needle diameters, this technique became extensively used, evaluated, and proven to be both highly reliable and safe (12–19).

These experiences from Uppsala Academic Hospital were soon spread internationally, initially to larger centres where interventional procedures were widely used, but also nationally and the use of interventional ultrasound was also widely adopted in small hospitals and outpatient departments. In that way the fear of using biopsies and other invasive procedures was eradicated. During these years ultrasound enjoyed a definite clinical breakthrough as a reliable and widely-used technology in Swedish radiology, and simultaneously became the preferred method for biopsies in abdomen, retroperitoneum, and superficial lesions. In parallel to the introduction of ultrasound-guided semi-automatic core biopsies other invasive procedures such as nephropyelostomy, abscess drainage,

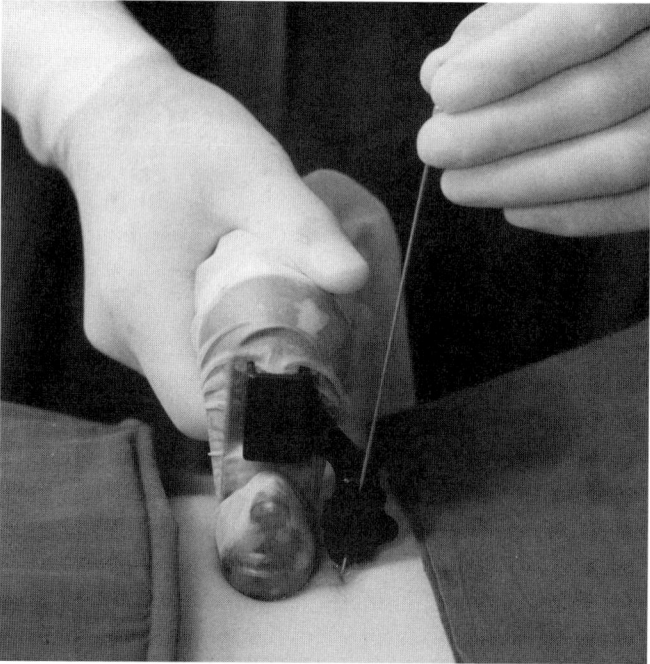

Fig. 11.1 The first needle guide unit designed by P.G. Lindgren for the ATL mechanical sector scanner. (This figure is reproduced in colour in the colour plate section.)

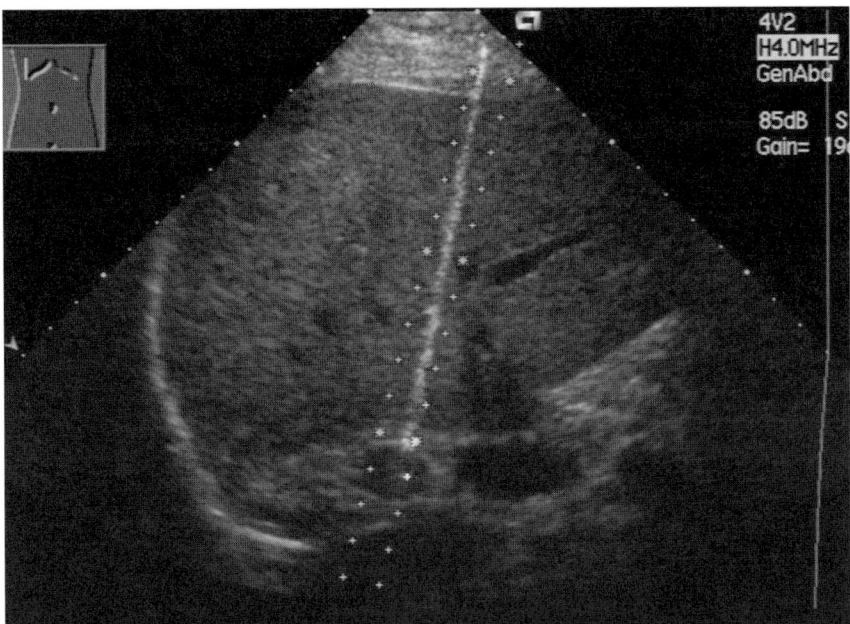

Fig. 11.2 Transhepatic biopsy of an adrenal tumour using a cutting needle. The needle path can be predicted through the electronic guide lines and the needle exactly followed in real-time during the puncture procedure.

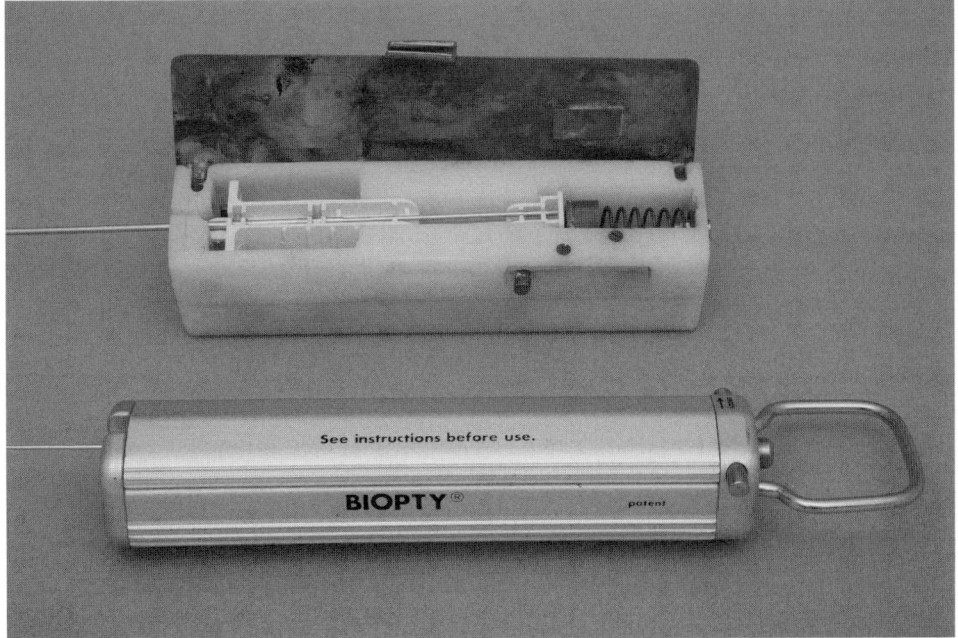

Fig. 11.3 The first semiautomatic biopsy device prototype used by Lindgren and designed for the manual Travenol TruCut® needle (top). Below is the commercial biopsy gun, Biopty® also designed by P.G. Lindgren. (This figure is reproduced in colour in the colour plate section.)

cholecystostomy, percutaneous tumour therapy, and nervous blockage were adapted for ultrasound guidance, which expanded the possibilities to perform these procedures in a simplified and safe way.

The expansion of the use of ultrasound was seen not only in radiology but also in other areas. The increasing use of endoscopic transducers, first described in the late 1960s (20), revolutionized gynaecological and early pregnancy obstetrical ultrasound and converted the procedure from a referring method to a part of an ordinary clinical gynaecological examination performed by most gynaecology physicians. This development entailed a change in the ultrasound patient spectrum in radiology departments in Sweden and within a couple of years both obstetrical and gynaecological ultrasound were completely moved away from radiology.

The re-evaluating years

This stable period—the golden years—lasted to the first half of the 1990s. At that time, the Section for Ultrasound as well as the long lasting 'Kolmården course' had been closed down. At the same time CT became more and more efficient, fast, and available. Many radiologists perceived ultrasound as a complicated technology to learn and master and therefore put more commitment into other imaging modalities. The 'old guard' of ultrasound pioneers diffused in different directions; some retired, some died, some of foreign origin went back to their home countries, and many also were promoted in the healthcare system as chairmen of radiology departments thereby abandoning the everyday work in the ultrasound laboratory.

A new and scientifically active generation of 'ultrasounders' did follow, but they were not very large in number. Some young enthusiasts in that generation revived the concept of an advanced ultrasound course. The group behind this consisted of four young radiologists from Stockholm and Uppsala—Karin von Sievers, Anna-Karin Siösten, Anders Elvin, and Anders Nilsson—and their new course was both well organized and attended. However, radiology in Sweden in many ways continued to evolve away from ultrasound, which lost its central position and more and more became an abandoned technology when younger physicians preferred more 'objective' modalities. This new advanced ultrasound course was therefore closed down after a couple of years.

One of the reasons for the decline of ultrasound in Swedish radiology departments at that time was the opinion that the technology was non-objective, too time-consuming, and also complicated to master since no objective documentation was available as in other modalities such as MRI and CT. The lack of a good and advanced education also resulted in rather large differences in diagnostic quality between examinations performed by different physicians. We could from referring clinicians see a growing scepticism towards diagnostic ultrasound and a re-evaluation of ultrasound in general and an unhealthy growth of the number of CT examinations as a result of that.

The introduction of a number of new ultrasound developments such as colour Doppler, power Doppler, harmonic imaging, ultrasound contrast examination, and elastography were expected to regain a lot of the enthusiasm and reliance in ultrasound. This has only been the case in departments with very engaged enthusiasts who have marketed the new technology aggressively and with quality. These new possibilities have, however, not routinely been introduced in a surprisingly large number of Swedish radiology departments. This is a phenomenon that stands out from the situation in many other European and North American hospitals where the new developments have been included in the clinical arsenal fast and successfully.

One controversial question in Swedish radiology is 'who should perform the examination?'. The tradition and so far the completely dominating opinion is that the radiologist should do it. Systems one can find in other countries, with sonographers and ultrasound technologists, have never been accepted in Sweden. Due to a lack of radiologists, the drive to spend a lot of time learning and performing ultrasound might have been weak and might therefore have influenced the development of ultrasound in radiology in a negative way. Few radiologists have engaged themselves in these important questions and those who have were usually met with doubts and negative reactions. Lars Thorelius, radiologist at Linköping University Hospital, has introduced a very ambitious organization at the ultrasound laboratory where sonographers perform routine ultrasound examinations according to a very well-defined scheme and with systematic dynamic documentation. The result is then jointly evaluated by the sonographer and radiologist (21, 22). Although he has raised very important questions with large impacts on the future of ultrasound in Sweden, his initiative has not been seriously discussed among Swedish radiologist but, rather, received with scepticism and silence.

What can be seen now in radiology in Sweden are, however, signs that might infuse hope for ultrasound. There are now a growing number of radiologists in Sweden, and young doctors are rather easy to recruit to the speciality. With this improved staffing more time will be available for junior doctors to train in ultrasound and to explore the unique and valuable characteristics of the technology. In that way diagnostic ultrasound might find its way back to the position in radiology it once had and also deserves.

My picture of Swedish ultrasound in radiology at the twenty-first century is therefore two-sided: partly a technology going downhill, partly a technology for which there are signs of hope and light at the horizon.

References

1. Forsberg L, Albrechtsson U, Norgren L. Acceleration ratio measurements with Doppler compared with angiography in patients with occlusive arterial disease. *Vasa* 1980; **9**(3):192–6.
2. Forsberg L, Holmin T, Lindstedt E. Quantitative Doppler and ultrasound measurements in surgically performed arteriovenous fistulas of the arm. *Acta Radiol Diagn (Stockh)* 1980; **21**(6):769–72.
3. Forsberg L, Malmfors G, Mortensson W, White T. Ultrasound examination of the kidney after Politano-Leadbetter ureteroneocystostomy. *Acta Radiol Diagn (Stockh)* 1981; **22**(3B):349–51.
4. Forsberg L, Tylen U. Ultrasound examination of lesions in the thorax. *Acta Radiol Diagn (Stockh)* 1980; **21**(3):375–8.
5. Karp W, Eklöf B. Ultrasonography and angiography in the diagnosis of abdominal aortic aneurysm. *Acta Radiol Diagn (Stockh)* 1978; **19**(6):955–60.
6. Karp W, Lunderquist A, Tylen U, Ishe I. Angiography and ultrasound examination in the evaluation of pancreatic lesions. *Acta Radiol Diagn (Stockh)* 1980; **21**(2A):169–76.

7. Belfrage P, Fernstrom I, Hallenberg G. Routine or selective ultrasound examinations in early pregnancy. *Obstet Gynecol* 1987; **69**(5):747–50.
8. Kratochwil A. Presentation. *First World Congress on Ultrasonic Diagnostics in Medicine*, June 2–7, Vienna 1969.
9. Holm HH, Kristensen JK, Rasmussen SN, Northeved A, Barlebo H. Ultrasound as a guide in percutaneous puncture technique. *Ultrasonics* 1972; **10**(2):83–6.
10. Lindgren PG. Ultrasonically guided punctures. A modified technique. *Radiology* 1980; **137** (1 Pt 1):235–7.
11. Lindgren PG. Percutaneous needle biopsy. A new technique. *Acta Radiol Diagn (Stockh)* 1982; **23**(6):653–6.
12. Andersson T, Eriksson B, Lindgren PG, Wilander E, Oberg K. Percutaneous ultrasonography-guided cutting biopsy from liver metastases of endocrine gastrointestinal tumors. *Ann Surg* 1987; **206**(6):728–32.
13. Tufveson G, Hanas E, Lindgren PG, Larsson E, Andersson T, Fellstrom B, *et al*. A review of the Uppsala experience of Biopty-Cut renal transplant biopsies. *Transplant Proc* 1989; **21**(4):3581–2.
14. Elvin A, Andersson T, Scheibenpflug L, Lindgren PG. Biopsy of the pancreas with a biopsy gun. *Radiology* 1990; **176**(3):677–9.
15. Andersson T, Lindgren PG, Elvin A. Ultrasound guided tumour biopsy in the anterior mediastinum. An alternative to thoracotomy and mediastinoscopy. *Acta Radiol* 1992; **33**(5):423–6.
16. Benediktsson H, Andersson T, Sjolander U, Hartman M, Lindgren PG. Ultrasound guided needle biopsy of brain tumors using an automatic sampling instrument. *Acta Radiol* 1992; **33**(6):512–17.
17. Hanas E, Larsson E, Fellstrom B, Lindgren PG, Andersson T, Busch C, *et al*. Safety aspects and diagnostic findings of serial renal allograft biopsies, obtained by an automatic technique with a midsize needle. *Scand J Urol Nephrol* 1992; **26**(4):413–20.
18. Kalkner M, Rehn S, Andersson T, Elvin A, Hagberg H, Lindgren PG, *et al*. Diagnostics of malignant lymphomas with ultrasound guided 1.2 mm biopsy-gun. *Acta Oncol* 1994; **33**(1):33–7.
19. Abdsaleh S, Azavedo E, Lindgren PG. Semiautomatic core biopsy. A modified biopsy technique in breast diseases. *Acta Radiol* 2003; **44**(1):47–51.
20. Kratochwil A. [A new vaginal method of ultrasonotomography]. *Geburtshilfe Frauenheilkd*. 1969; **29**(4):379–85.
21. Thorelius L. '*Sonodynamics*' website. Available at: http://www.sonodynamics.com/.
22. Thorelius L. Ultrasound in radiology – is there a future? *Ultraschall Med* 2007; **28**(3):326–7.

Chapter 12

The early development of diagnostic ultrasound in Denmark

Jørgen Jørgensen

The development of diagnostic ultrasound in medicine began in Denmark in November 1965 at the Surgical Department H at Gentofte County Hospital in Copenhagen, and a prosperous time for diagnostic ultrasound began. It was the young surgeon Hans Henrik Holm who took the initiative (Fig. 12.1), strongly supported by the head of the department Professor P.A. Gammelgaard. Hans Henrik Holm had for years studied ultrasound and earlier in 1965 he had visited Helmuth Hertz in Lund in Sweden to discuss the prospects of ultrasound.

The ultrasound laboratory

A grant from a national scientific foundation of 60 000 Danish kroner (approximately $10 000) made it possible to buy the American Physionic A-mode ultrasound machine. It was installed in a spare room at the Surgical Department H at Gentofte County Hospital in Copenhagen. An ultrasound laboratory was hereby established, and it was increasingly involved in a variety of clinical ultrasound studies and in the development and testing of new ultrasound equipment. The expenses were met by both the hospital and the University of Copenhagen, and a great deal of the research was financed by foundations.

Hans Henrik Holm became the day-to-day head of the laboratory and he kept this position for many years. The Surgical Department and the ultrasound laboratory, designated the Ultrasound Department, were relocated to the new Herlev County Hospital in 1976 where Hans Henrik Holm became consultant at the Urology Department and Professor in Ultrasound and Interventional Ultrasound affiliated with the Surgical Department. The Ultrasound Department at Herlev had an increasing number of rooms and staff members. A senior registrar (Jørgen Kvist Kristensen) was associated to the department in 1975 and Søren Torp-Pedersen was appointed consultant at the department in 1989. In 1966, 250 patients were examined annually. Thirty years later the Ultrasound Department at Herlev Hospital examined 17 000 patients annually, and ultrasound departments had been established at other hospitals in the Copenhagen area. By 1966 two papers in Danish were published and two papers in English were published in 1967 and 1968 (1, 2). The number of staff rapidly increased, and a group of enthusiastic doctors and technicians was formed, working with patients and on scientific projects. More than 400 written papers on ultrasound were published over the following 20 years.

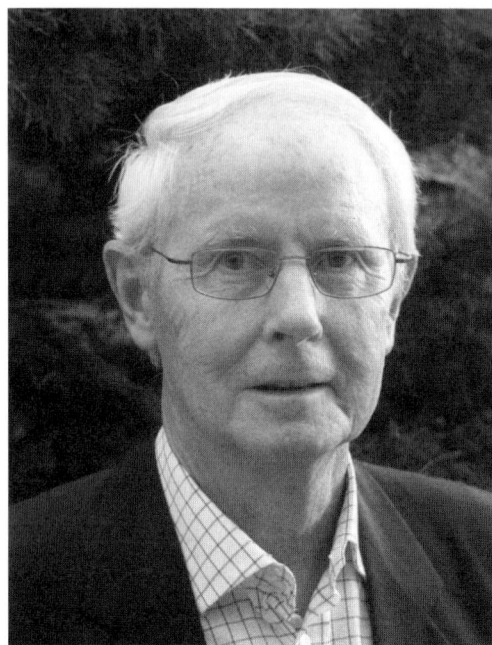

Fig. 12.1 Portrait of Professor Hans Henrik Holm, 1998. With permission from Professor Hans Henrik Holm.

Simultaneously, the members of the group acted as teachers in annual courses. Some of these members were later appointed consultants at other ultrasound departments or engaged as experts in diagnostic ultrasound at radiology departments. The group was named 'The Gentofte Group' by Goldberg and Kimmelmann in 1988 (3). The methodological approach to development of diagnostic ultrasound as well as the technical progress in ultrasound equipment in Denmark were accentuated in this monograph.

Technical developments

The Danish Welding Centre, which later became the Medico-Technical Institute and the Force Institute was experienced in ultrasound for industrial use and became interested in medico-technical collaboration with the ultrasound laboratory at Gentofte Hospital. The result was 35 years of close and fruitful collaboration with the institute and its director, the late Allan Northeved.

The Gentofte scanner was constructed in 1967 (Figs. 12.2 and 12.3) in collaboration with Allan Northeved from parts from the Welding Centre and a modified Hewlett Packard unit, and it set the standard for diagnostic ultrasound equipment up to 1980. It was purchased and used for many years and continuously improved. Grey-scale was introduced on this scanner in 1969. Many experimental instruments were tested. In 1973 a mechanical rotating transducer was constructed to be used via a cystoscope into the bladder (4), which became an international sensation. In 1980–82 a scanner with A-D converter was generated in cooperation with Brüel and Kjaer, a Danish company producing

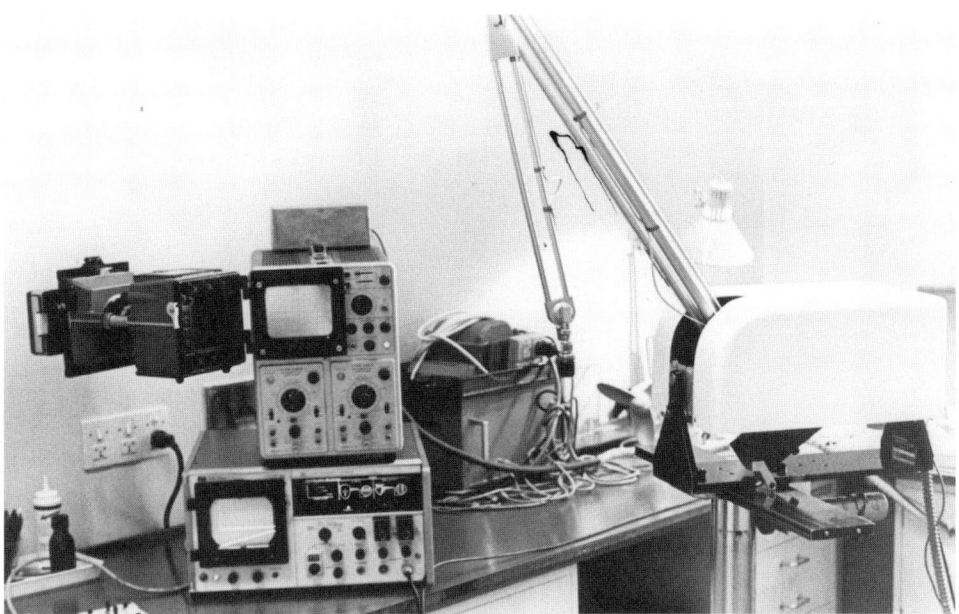

Fig. 12.2 The first Gentofte scanner 1967.
Reproduced from Jørgensen J. *Bibl Laeg* 2003; **193**:177–207, with permission.

instruments for electronic measurements (Sound and Vibration). This scanner was provided with electronic transducers of different kinds, and it had a modern design with a smooth surface. The transducers could be sterilized in liquid and the scanner was suitable for bedside examinations at the clinical wards and for scanning during operations. A mechanical real-time scanner was constrructed in 1974. Initial experiments with an electronic real-time scanner were made in cooperation with the Medico-Technical Institute, but were stopped, probably because Japanese and American products already

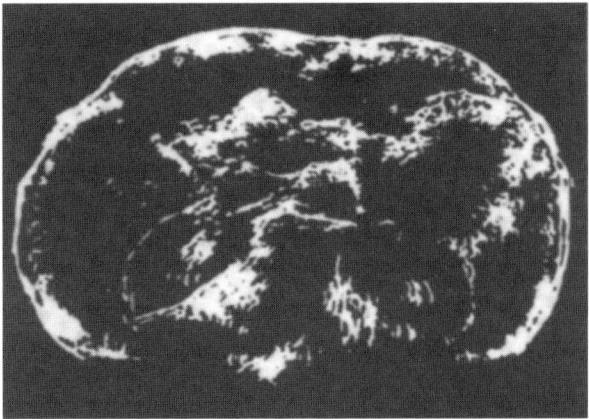

Fig. 12.3 Polaroid from the screen of the Gentofte scanner 1967.
Reproduced from Jørgensen J. *Bibl Laeg* 2003; **193**:177–207, with permission.

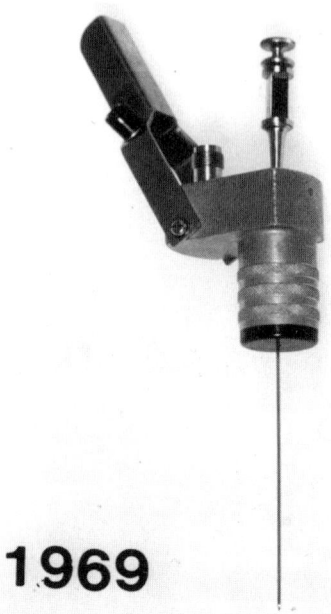

Fig. 12.4 Transducer with a central canal for a needle, to be used on the Gentofte scanner 1969. Reproduced from Jørgensen J. *Bibl Laeg* 2003; **193**:177–207, with permission.

controlled the market at that time. A paper on ultrasound examination in carotid artery disease was published in 1967, but preliminary experiments with colour Doppler were not successful. Acuson Doppler ultrasound equipment arrived in the department in 1982.

Puncture guided by ultrasound

Experiments were performed for biopsy transducers in order to ensure that the biopsy was taken accurately. A biopsy transducer with a canal for insertion of the biopsy needle was in use on the Gentofte scanner in 1972 (Fig. 12.4). Biopsy guided by ultrasound became a distinctive feature for Danish ultrasound. Liver biopsy was reported in 1972 (5) and biopsy of kidney tumours was reported in 1972. An abscess in the kidney was treated successfully in 1974, and the ultrasonic-guided percutaneous nephrostomy was described by Jan Fog Pedersen in 1975 (6). Drainage of abscesses and fluid collections guided by ultrasound became routine, as did diagnostic needle biopsy of suspected malignancies. The early experience of being able to discern between solid tumours and cysts was promising. Ultrasound failed to show a distinction between benign and malignant lesions, but cytology samples from needle puncture compensated for that.

At some ultrasound departments, puncture was performed in 15% of all ultrasound examinations. The thin needle puncture guided by ultrasound was considered to be a safe procedure and only a few complications appeared and were reported in a paper in 1990 (7). Injection of cytostatic chemicals in hepatic metastases from malignant tumours was performed early in the 1970s. Thin needle biopsy from the prostate guided by transrectal ultrasonic scanning served as a method for staging the cancer preoperatively. Steen Karstrup injected sclerosing fluid in adenomas of the parathyroid successfully. In many cases diagnostic thin needle biopsy was part of the research.

The spread of ultrasound

Early in the 1970s a few regional hospitals installed ultrasound at the same time. But, in general, the use of ultrasound examinations spread slowly to other hospitals. Ultrasound was first introduced at obstetric departments and at hospitals dealing with cardiology. In the beginning very few hospitals had access to ultrasound. A 'wait and see' attitude dominated, probably because of poor image quality and a lack of practice in this new technique. Ernst Hasch started an ultrasound laboratory at Kolding Hospital in 1971–72. It was located in the obstetric department but served other wards too. He also worked with ultrasound of children. According to a survey from 1988, all obstetric departments and most cardiologists were using ultrasound, but 34 small hospitals still had no access to ultrasound examinations. Many radiologists opposed to diagnostic ultrasound for several years. Hans Henrik Holm read a paper on abdominal ultrasound at the 348 meeting in the Danish Radiological Society in September 1967. The intention was to create interest in ultrasound as an imaging method. It was followed by a film demonstrating the technique at the 367 meeting in September 1970. However, radiologists were not interested in diagnostic ultrasound at that time. Senior radiologists expected abdominal ultrasound to be replaced by computed tomography (CT) scanning and they did not recommend any acquisition of ultrasound equipment at radiology departments. Fifteen years later a younger generation of radiologists raised the subject with the National Health Service in Denmark and the Danish Ultrasound Society in order to establish rules for specialists in diagnostic ultrasound. Instructions in ultrasound became compulsory for young radiologists, but other doctors were not required to be educated in ultrasound—any doctor was allowed to use ultrasound as a diagnostic tool. The combination of CT scanning and ultrasound scanning was supplementary and highly effective diagnostically. Strategies for CT scan versus ultrasound were described by Axel Haubek. But ultrasound examinations replaced most radiology examinations of kidneys and all radiology examinations of bile ducts and became the examination of choice of the abdomen. In 1996, 350 000 ultrasound examinations were performed in Denmark. Doctors performed the ultrasound examinations at the radiology departments and all of the invasive procedures while personnel with special training normally did the ultrasound examinations at obstetric departments.

The Gentofte Group

The Gentofte Group was not well defined. Some of the doctors in the group came from other departments working temporarily at the laboratory. Most of them were young doctors with an interest in medical research. To list all their names is impossible, but the group formed the major part of the membership of the Danish Ultrasound Society when it was founded on 1 February 1974. The initial number of members was 42. The society was immediately affiliated to the European Federation of Societies for Ultrasound in Medicine and Biology and the World Federation for Ultrasound in Medicine and Biology. The society arranged many courses, scientific meetings, and conferences in Denmark and internationally, and members of the group wrote important textbooks. Hans Henrik Holm was guest professor at Harvard Medical School in Boston, United States, in 1975–1976. He was affiliated to the University of Copenhagen as Professor in Ultrasound in 1992 and honoured in many ways for the efforts he made for ultrasound in medicine. The Gentofte Group created national and international attention by their scientific approach and intensive work with diagnostic ultrasound. It contributed to the spread of ultrasound for diagnostic imaging. The work done to improve ultrasound equipment was important and sometimes necessary for research. The laboratory at the Gentofte Hospital and the Ultrasound Department at the Herlev Hospital offered important coaching opportunities, but could not keep up with demand for many years. Surprisingly many people of different nationalities visited the laboratory every year, and some stayed for weeks or even months. The staff and former members of the staff or people with some connection to the laboratory attended as teachers in the courses held at the Gentofte Hospital or later at the Herlev Hospital. Several courses were held every year and members of the staff took part in international meetings and gave talks. The importance of this coaching to future users of ultrasound should not be undervalued. But the importance of the flow of scientific projects followed by reports might have been of even greater value, even continuing to today.

Research

A great number of articles on ultrasound from Holm or his colleagues were published in Danish and in international medical journals in the first two decades after introducing ultrasound. They put transducers in any conceivable place a transducer could be put on or in the human body! The result was a number of research projects and papers in fields of considerable importance in comparison to international research. In many cases the research project resulted in a conclusive dissertation which typically was published and defended some years later than the initial report because of delays in the academic procedure. Some projects were milestones in the development of ultrasound in medicine. A few have to be mentioned. Jørgen Kvist Kristensen was a member of the laboratory from the beginning. He wrote a number of papers on ultrasound scanning and his dissertation *Ultrasonic scanning of the kidneys* was published in 1979. Steen Nørby Rasmussen's research into organ volume took place in 1971 and 1972 (8). His dissertation *Liver volume determination by ultrasound scanning* was published in 1977. Organ volume assessment has been important in other organs as demonstrated in Lazlo Hegedüs' dissertation from 1990: *Thyroid size determined by ultrasound. Influence of physiological factors and non thyroid disease*. Søren Hancke improved the B-mode scan technique for the pancreas and combined it with needle biopsy in 1976 (9). His dissertation *Ultrasound in pancreatic cancer. Scanning and fine needle puncture* was published in 1980. In 1967 and 1970 papers were published on blood vessels. More important research with Doppler came later. A dissertation by Henrik Sillesen *Diagnosis and hemodynamic evaluation of internal carotid artery stenosis by Doppler ultrasound* was published in 1990. A dissertation by Knud Rasmussen *Non-invasive quantitative measurement of blood flow and estimation of vascular resistance by the Doppler ultrasound method* was published in 1991. Margit Mantoni published a paper on venous thrombosis of the leg with duplex sonography (10). It replaced many radiological vascular contrast examinations. Paediatric ultrasonography became important, and among others, Ernst Hasch performed important studies in 1973 and 1974 (11). In 1966, Jens Falbe Hansen began development of ultrasonography of the eye at the National Hospital in Copenhagen. Hans C. Fledelius took over in 1969 and his dissertation *Prematurity and the eye* was published in 1976 and was partly based on ultrasound studies. Dedicated eye scanners were purchased and the method had become common in all eye departments within two decades.

Obstetric ultrasound

From the early 1970s, Jens Bang performed ultrasound examinations of pregnant women at the obstetric department in Copenhagen. He had a close connection to the laboratory at the Gentofte Hospital. Hans Henrik Holm and Jens Bang published a paper on detection of movements of the fetal heart by ultrasound in 1966. Jens Bang was a pioneer in amniocentesis (12). He and his colleagues published a number of articles on amniocentesis in international journals and later became devoted to the study of fetus malformations and intrauterine intervention (13). A. Tabor published the dissertation *Genetic Amniocentesis—Indications and Risks* in 1988. As an obstetrician, Jens Bang was concerned about the effect of ultrasound on the embryo. He carried out experiments on pregnant mice to study the risk of hereditary malformations created by ultrasound radiation (14). He recommended limited maximum power values for radiation from ultrasound equipment for medical use. The result of his study was of great international importance. He became chairman of the Committee for Ultrasound Radiation and Safety under the European Federation of Societies for Ultrasound in Medicine and Biology. A study of the size of the fetus in order to determine gestational age was performed by Jan Fog Pedersen. His dissertation *Ultrasound studies of foetal crown-rump length in normal and diabetic pregnancies* was published in 1986. Margit Mantoni's dissertation *Ultrasound studies of bleeding in early pregnancy* was published in 1987. A group at the Hvidovre County Hospital (another hospital in Copenhagen) performed studies on fetal growth from 1984–87. They published schematic surveys of gestational age and weight (15).

Echocardiography

Development of ultrasound for cardiac examinations took place mainly at departments for cardiac diseases. In the beginning, the group at the Gentofte Hospital was the most prominent in that development. Hans Henrik Holm and Per Henningsen published a paper in Danish on the application of M-mode technique. Jan Fog Pedersen continued the project. He improved the technique together with Allan Northeved and published a paper on a study of endocarditis (16). Jan Fog Pedersen described a method for puncture of the pericardium guided by ultrasound in 1974. Henrik Egeblad used the scanner for a study of ischaemic disease of the heart in 1980. Echocardiography was performed at the Copenhagen National Hospital. The Cardiological Department B had a close connection to the University Hospital in Lund, Sweden. They cooperated in many fields with Inge Edler and Helmuth Hertz who had developed the M-mode. Henrik Egeblad had a dedicated scanner for echocardiography installed in 1978. This scanner became the basis for his many papers in Danish and international journals. His dissertation *Intracardiac thrombus—systemic arterial embolism. Contribution of echocardiography* was published in 1988. But he had, in the early 1970s, performed experiments with echocardiography. He also added M-mode echocardiography to electrocardiogram in uteri in 1975. Jens Berning and Henrik Egeblad from the National Hospital headed the development of echocardiography in Denmark for several years. They specified the indications for echocardiography in 1983. Echocardiography rapidly spread and became the most informative examination in the hands of the heart specialists.

Acknowledgements

The illustrations were demonstrated in Jørgensen J. *Bibl Laeg* 2003; **193**:177–207. I wish to thank the publisher for permission to use them. And I wish to thank Hans Henrik Holm for his help.

References

1. Holm HH, Kristensen JK. Ultrasonic pulse detection. *Acta Chir Scand* 1967; **133**:269–73.
2. Holm HH, Mortensen T. Ultrasonic scanning in abdominal disease. *Acta Chir Scand* 1968; **134**:339.
3. Goldberg B, Kimmelman BA. Medical diagnostic ultrasound. A retrospective on its 40th anniversary. *Kodak Health Science* 1988; **9**:88–94.
4. Holm HH, Northeved A. A transurethral ultrasonic scanner. *J Urol* 1974; **1**:183–6.
5. Rasmussen SN, Holm HH, Kristensen JK, Barlebo H. Ultrasonically guided liver biopsy. *BMJ* 1972; **2**:500–3.
6. Pedersen JF. Percutaneous nephrostomy guided by ultrasound. *J Urol* 1974; **112**:157–61.
7. Nolsø C, Nielsen L, Torp-Pedersen S, Holm HH. Major complications and deaths due to interventional ultrasonography: a review of 8000 cases. *J Clin Ultrasound* 1990; **18**:178–84.
8. Rasmussen SN. Liver volume determination by ultrasonic scanning. *Br J Radiol* 1972; **45**:579–84.
9. Hancke S. Ultrasonic scanning of the pancreas. *J Clin Ultrasound* 1976; **4**:233–9.
10. Mantoni M. Diagnosis of deep venous thrombosis by duplex sonography. *Acta Radiologica* 1989; **30**:575–9.
11. Hasch E. Ultrasound in the diagnosis of hydronephrosis in children and infants. *J Clin Ultrasound* 1974; **2**:21–5.
12. Bang J, Northeved A. A new ultrasonic method for transabdominal amniocentese. *Am J Obstet Gynecol* 1972; **114**:599–609.
13. Bang J, Bock JF, Trolle D. Ultrasound-guided fetal intravenous transfusion for severe rhesus haemolytic dsease. *BMJ* 1982; **284**:373–4.
14. Bang J, The effect of continous ultrasound in pregnant mice and measurement of intrauterine energy levels. (Proceedings of 1st World Congress on Ultrasonic Diagnosis, Vienna 1969.) *Ultrasonografia Medica* 1971; **2**:495.
15. Secher NJ, Hansen PK, Lenstrup C, Pedersen-Bjerggaard L, Eriksen PS, Thomsen BL, *et al*. Birthweight-for-gestational age charts based on ultrasound estimation of gestational age. *Br J Obstet Gynecol* 1986; **93**:128–34.
16. Pedersen JF, Berning J, Haunsø S. Single and multiple beam echocardiography in aortic valve endocarditis. Report of three cases. *Acta Med Scand* 1978; **204**: 314–19.

Chapter 13

Ultrasound in radiology—state of the art

David O. Cosgrove

The practice of ultrasound in radiology has continued to develop and shows no signs of slowing down. The changes affect the systems themselves, with important technical developments, as well as the ways they are used, and to some extent these are interlinked.

Usage of ultrasound

The earliest static scanners were so difficult to use that only dedicated personnel could find the time and make the effort required to use them. This led to a small cohort of enthusiasts offering a limited and expensive service. Strangely, they were a mixture of doctors (many of whom were not radiologists) and physicists, perhaps reflecting the complexity of the scanners. With the development of real-time systems and increasingly as they have become easier to operate, ultrasound found its place within radiology departments and, in parallel, in cardiology and obstetric units as well as in vascular labs. Here the role of physicists faded and most of the people performing the scans were medical, a situation that still obtains in many parts of the world, notably in the Far East (in China, the doctors are ultrasound specialists) and in many European countries. In others, especially in the United States, technologists or radiographers took over the actual scanning, leaving radiologists or their equivalent (cardiologists, obstetricians) to read and report the studies by analogy with other scanning modalities such as computed tomography (CT) and magnetic resonance imaging (MRI).

The driver for this major change has mainly been financial: medics are expensive and sharing the workload with technologists is cost-effective. However, this shift comes with a penalty: as ultrasound is a real-time method and the techniques required to make the studies are very interactive, simply reading a set of images on a PACS (picture archiving and communication system) workstation deprives the radiologist of dynamic information that can be critical to making the diagnosis. In some places the response to this has been to train the technicians or radiographers to interpret and report their own cases. Though often disapproved of by the regulatory authorities (1) and exposing practitioners to risks of litigation, this approach has been popular amongst radiographers only partly because their extended role is rewarded by additional pay.

Another significant trend in the practice of ultrasound has been triggered by the introduction of more affordable and portable systems, many even hand-held. Taking the scanner to the point of care, typically a clinic or general practice office, is a very practical way to improve the service a patient experiences and many general practitioners have grasped this opportunity, which also serves as a source of extra income. In addition, many specialist training programmes now include the use of ultrasound, especially by urologists, gastro-enterologists, and intensive care and emergency room doctors. In some cases the official training bodies have endorsed this practice by making ultrasound an essential requirement for specialist certification (2). While this seems a logical approach that brings many advantages and efficiencies, acquiring the necessary skills is taxing and time-consuming. The temptation to view ultrasound as an easy technique with no risks is dangerously naive: the main risk to an ultrasound examination is making a wrong diagnosis! So the training implications of moving scanners into clinics and wards is a major barrier. In an unfortunate twist, the lower end systems that are used in this way necessarily give poorer images: the less well-trained ultrasonologists are the very people who most need the best quality images. Continuing improvements in the performance of smaller machines should help improve this gap.

Scanner configuration improvements

Behind the change from the awkwardness of the early manual 'contact' scanners to the slickness and elegance of current systems lies a remarkable series of developments designed to make ultrasound more straightforward to perform. It is a tribute to the competition between manufacturers that drives the industry, but the ultrasound business sector is sometimes unusual in that a semi-hidden cooperation sometimes exists between what should be aggressive competitors: users will have noticed that innovations on one brand sometimes appear soon afterwards on another. Examples are tissue harmonic imaging and colour Doppler. Though not often openly declared, it is widely believed that many ultrasound manufacturers prefer to cross-license innovations rather than to go to the expense and delays of litigation.

A significant trend in system design has been improved ergonomics that has produced scanners with control panels whose height and angle are adjustable, together with controls that are conveniently placed for the hand. In some the control functions can be reassigned. CRT (Cathode ray tube) monitors have largely been replaced by flat screens which are lighter and easier to reposition. Though theoretically their image quality falls short of that obtainable from a high quality CRT, especially in the dynamic range achieved, in practice most users are not troubled by this and anyway many scans are interpreted on flat-screen PACS monitors.

Remaining problems that many systems suffer are noisy fans and slow switch-on and -off times—a particular handicap when the scanner must be moved between beds, as in intensive care or a ward. Some systems have developed a work-around for this problem by incorporating a rechargeable battery and a standby mode that allows instant waking and sleeping.

Transducers

Improved transducer technologies have underpinned many of the improvements in image quality that modern radiologists take for granted. Improved piezoelectric materials, including sub-dicing to suppress lateral acoustic waves, better matching layers to improve sensitivity on receive, and shaping of the probe face for improved orthogonal focussing (3) have all added to their high performance. All this has been achieved without adding to the probe weight or necessitating bulky rigid cables.

Novel transducer materials may further improve performance. Use of single crystal PZT (lead zirconate titanate) as opposed to the cheaper amorphous PZT that is currently available promises wider bandwidths and thus better range resolution. Micromachined transducers (capacitative micromachined transducers, cMUTs) which operate like microscopic drums or electrostatic loudspeaker/microphones, are constructed using the photo-etching techniques so successfully employed by semiconductor industry (4). Thus they can be inexpensive and turned out in bulk to the point that they might even become disposable, which might be useful for intraoperative or intracavitary scans. More significantly, micro-electronics could be built directly on the silicon wafer on which the cMUT is built for highly integrated transducer-amplifier systems.

B-mode imaging

Improvements in B-mode imaging have been spectacular and have leveraged the better transducers that have become available as well as the faster image processing. Compounding, in which the final image is a composite of several different images has become standard (5). The traditional way to acquire the different images is to steer the transmit beam in different directions. This means that the speckle pattern received is slightly different between the images formed from the several steerings and so are averaged out in the summing process (Fig. 13.1) Wanted echoes from tissue interfaces add and thus are emphasized so that the signal to speckle ratio is improved. Obviously, there is a loss of frame rate but this doesn't occur with the other form of compounding in which a broad-band transmitted signal is frequency filtered and the resulting several images are summed. Frequency and steered compounding are complementary ways to reduce speckle and are often used together.

Tissue harmonic imaging is another technique that has become mainstream (6). It exploits the fact that the transmitted beam becomes distorted as it travels through the tissue because of the fact that ultrasound travels faster through denser tissue. Thus the parts of the wave in the compression phase of the cycle move slightly ahead of the parts in the rarefaction part of the cycle. In this way the original sine wave acquires a saw-tooth shape and the more rapid changes this implies carry higher frequencies than the original transmitted wave. Ways to extract this part of the echo, originally developed for detecting microbubble contrast agents (see below), can be used to form the harmonic image. Advantages of this technique are a reduction in side lobes (because these are mainly formed by the higher energy parts of the transmitted beam) and less reverberation from the superficial tissue layers (because the development of harmonics is gradual so there are

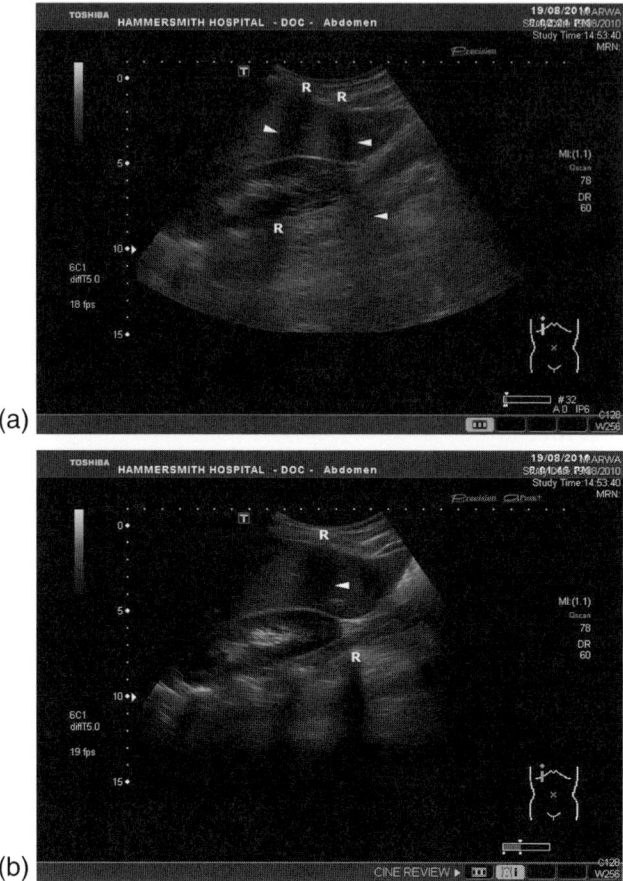

Fig. 13.1 Compounding. In the compounded scan of a normal liver and kidney (A), the parenchymal texture appears smother than in the non-compounded scan (B). In the standard scan the rib shadowing extends across the liver and right kidney (arrowheads). Because of the multi-angle scanning, the shadowing is partially removed and extends much less far (arrowheads). R = rib.

fewer in the superficial part of the beam). Overall, harmonic images are cleaner with less clutter and artefacts. The downsides are that the harmonic signal is weaker and thus harmonic images are inherently noisier, and that they are more strongly formed at higher transmit powers. Harmonic imaging is generally more effective for body and cardiac imaging than for small parts.

Image processing to smooth noise and speckle and to emphasize true structure have also made a great contribution to B-mode quality. Proprietary algorithms that adaptively smooth just the speckle in an image are used in most high-end scanners. They are processor-intensive and exploit the faster image handling that has increasingly become available. In some, computer games video cards have been hijacked for this processing. A degree of edge enhancement is often applied to ultrasound images to highlight important structure. As is often the case with such automatic systems, too much enhancement is distracting and the images are unaesthetic. Many of the algorithms suitable for ultrasound can also be used for CT and MRI.

On the other side of the coin, making use of speckle has led to speckle-tracking algorithms that can be used to form extended field of view images that are useful for communication, especially in musculoskeletal ultrasound where long spans of tissue need to be displayed. Another application is in compensating for in-slice movement, especially for contrast studies where a region of interest is placed over, for example a liver lesion; the speckle tracking can follow respiratory movement to keep the region of interest (ROI) in place (7).

Many forms of automatic image correction have been applied recently with the laudable intention of simplifying the choice of optimal settings for the scanner. A useful one is automatic optimization of the time gain compensation (TGC) and gain. The algorithms are subtle in that they do more than merely adjust the gain so that the image occupies the available dynamic range of the display. They can apply variable TGC across the image whereas in most systems the operator can only adjust the axial TGC. They also look at the noise content of the image and avoid introducing noise by over amplifying the signals.

The old topic of tissue characterization has resurfaced in the form of sonohistology in which analysis of the histograms of the distribution of signals of different intensities in a ROI can give extra information. It has been successfully applied in the prostate and for arterial plaque characterization (8, 9).

Doppler

In some respects, Doppler has been the Cinderella of ultrasound with few important advances since the introduction of power Doppler in the mid-1990s (10). One important trend that is gradually appearing on commercial systems is the attempt to remove the direction dependence of conventional Doppler while retaining the velocity quantification that is missing from power Doppler. The usual approach is to use two transducers, which could be a pair of separate transducers or, more conveniently, employ an array in which the beam is formed alternately from the left and right halves with electronic steering to form a crossed beam (11). The two Doppler signals can be combined to make the system essentially insensitive to the beam-to-vessel direction. An elegant alternative additionally modulates the system sensitivity in the lateral direction, enabling the measurement of the transverse component of blood velocity in a way that is entirely analogous to standard Doppler (12) (Fig. 13.2). By combining the two sets of information, so-called vector flow images can be obtained with no beam-to-vessels angle dependence. The information can also be displayed as vector arrows that, again, are quantitative.

B-flow imaging is also non-directional (13). Essentially a form of speckle tracking, it uses long coded pulses to achieve high sensitivity to the very weak echoes from red cells—the loss in spatial resolution caused by the long pulses is recovered by passing the echoes through an inverse code of the same type. In addition, echoes from non-moving structures are partly subtracted away. The resulting real-time images show flow patterns in complex vessels.

Tissue Doppler is important in cardiology (14). Essentially it is the colour Doppler information at low Doppler frequency and high amplitude that is rejected in vascular

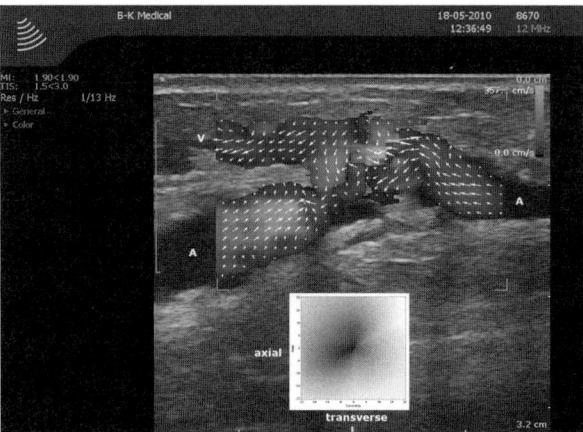

Fig. 13.2 Vector Flow Imaging. This scan of an arterio-venous shunt in a patient receiving haemodialysis shows the very complex anatomy that is readily displayed by non-directional Doppler. The arrows indicate the flow direction which goes from the afferent artery (A) to the vein (V) along a twisty fistula path. In normal colour Doppler the directional dependence would produce uninterpretable colour changes and dropouts at the 90° angles. The colour wheel indicates the coding for direction, lighter shades indicating faster flow. Image courtesy of Dr Stefen Ellebæk Pedersen. (This figure is reproduced in colour in the colour plate section.)

Doppler as wall thump. Here the movement of cardiac muscle is deliberately displayed by using the opposite filtration. It displays cardiac muscle movement. A variant of this approach is used in some elastography systems (see below).

The same kind of optimize algorithms that are used for B-mode optimization have been applied to spectral Doppler. They set the Doppler gain so that the brightness of the tracing falls in the middle of available dynamic range of the tracing and also change the pulse repetition frequency (PRF) and the baseline to avoid or minimize aliasing. These are very convenient and practical features.

Three- and four-dimensional scanning

The simplest approach to three (3-D) and four-dimensional (4-D) scanning is to house a conventional array in a hand-held water bath equipped with a motor to sweep or 'wobble' the probe so that volume data can be collected (15). Four-dimensional refers to this type of approach in which the frame rate is high enough to allow its presentation in 'real time', itself a somewhat poorly defined term that implies that significant tissue motion can be captured in an interpretable fashion. Obviously cardiac 4-D requires a higher frame rate than abdominal 4-D.

A more sophisticated approach uses a two-dimensional (2-D) array of elements, each separately connected so that the ultrasound beam can be swept through a volume of tissue (16). The technology is expensive, not least the necessary cabling, and so far has only been implemented on cardiac systems. Its attractions are the smaller size of the probe and the flexibility of steering it bestows. Silicon cMUT transducers might stimulate this development since complex arrays could prove simpler and cheaper to produce and the cabling could be simplified by the electronics that could be grown on the back of the silicon chip.

Processing the volume data entails filling in the gaps between the acquired slices and, as these are not of uniform thickness since the beam is swept in an arc, this is not a trivial task. The volume set can be re-sliced to display any plane. Since the ultrasound beam is both non-uniform and is thicker in the Z-plane, the eventual data set is not isotropic and this means that the Z-plane slices (sometimes termed the C-plane) have poorer spatial resolution than the X and Y planes. The data can also be presented as a three dimensional rendition, either as a surface or as a transparency. This is useful in obstetrics for complex anatomy, especially of the face where lip and palatal defects can be revealed. Regrettably, its main use has been to provide parents with souvenir images for the first page of the baby's photo album, a practice that various societies have condemned (17).

Ultrasound contrast agents

One of the most exciting developments that has taken ultrasound to a new level of clinical usefulness, at least in Europe and the Far East has been the development of microbubble contrast agents (18, 19). The unique behaviour of microbubbles in an ultrasound field, whereby they expand and contract in a non-linear fashion and thus generate harmonic signals that are not present in the transmitted wave, allows special imaging sequences to extract the contrast agent echoes from those of the tissue. These are usually displayed as registered side-by-side images. However, both need to be made at low transmit power to avoid destroying the microbubbles and as a result, the B-mode images are noisier than a normal B-mode image. Nevertheless they serve as a guide to the anatomy being studied which cannot be seen prior to the injection of the microbubbles because the more effective the separation of the two components, the blacker the screen in the microbubble part.

An important principle in using microbubbles is to appreciate that their detection does not depend on the flow rate of the blood that contains them. Thus they can be detected in both the macro- and the microcirculation and so much more of the circulation can be investigated than with Doppler, which fails when the velocity of tissue (from cardiorespiratory motion) approaches that of blood. Clutter from tissue motion obscures Doppler signals from such slow flowing blood so that it can only detect the macrocirculation.

The main impact of contrast-enhanced ultrasound (CEUS) has been in the heart (to improve endocardial border detection and assess myocardial perfusion) and in the liver (Fig. 13.3). Here it is used to improve the detection and the characterization of focal liver lesions, and in these applications numerous studies have shown CEUS to be the equal of contrast CT or MRI. When incorporated into diagnostic sequences, CEUS is not only cost-effective but simplifies patient flow and reduces the anxiety associated with waits for CT or MRI studies to sort out unexpected lesions that are encountered on routine ultrasound scans (20, 21).

Another important application of CEUS is in interstitial ablative therapy, especially in the liver (22). These interventions are best carried out with ultrasound guidance because of its interactive nature, but the coagulation lesions produced cannot reliably be distinguished

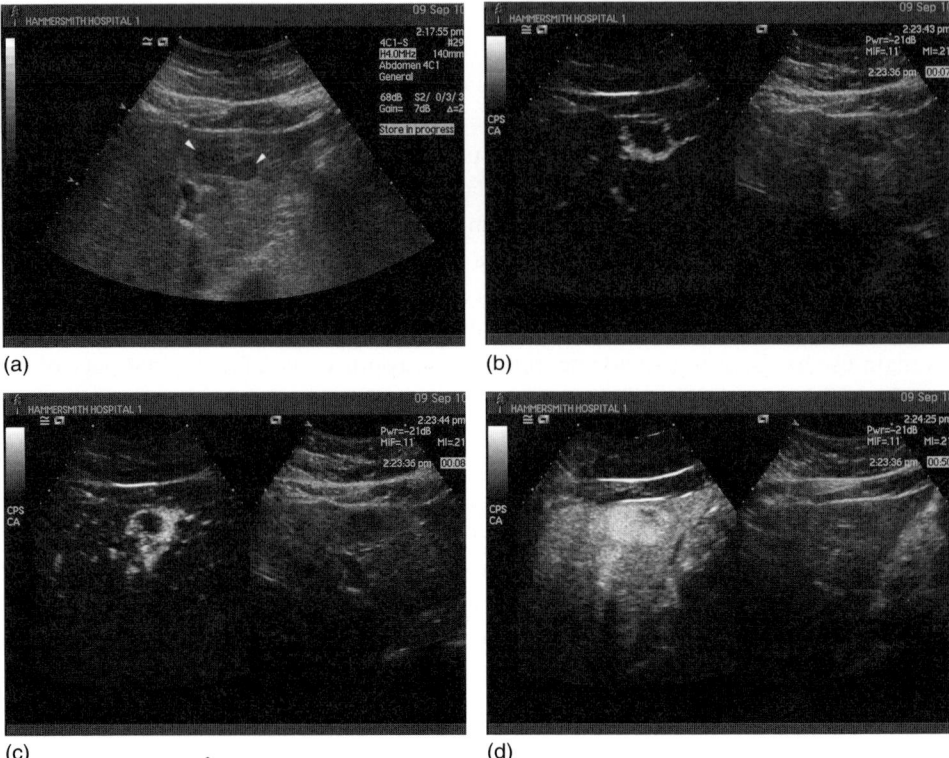

Fig. 13.3 Haemangioma of the liver. The nature of this echopoor lesion in the liver (arrowheads in (a)) is unclear, so a contrast study using SonoVue was performed. Very soon after intravenous injection (at 8s in (b)), intense enhancement is seen in the periphery of the lesion where it has a nodular appearance. This and subsequent figures are still frames extracted from the movie clip. The split screen shows the contrast image on the left with the low MI tissue image, used to keep the lesion in the field, on the right. A second later (c) there is continued filling in a centripetal pattern and by 50s (d) the lesion has filled in almost completely. The peripheral nodular enhancement and centripetal fill-in are diagnostic of a haemangioma. This example is somewhat unusual in that it is echopoor on B-mode and takes up contrast very rapidly. These are features of the high-flow variant of haemangiomas. The late enhancement is typical of benign solid lesions.

from the adjacent liver on B-mode imaging and so, historically the patient has to be sent for contrast CT—if the ablation turns out to be incomplete, the patient must be returned to ultrasound for further ablation. Because the coagulated tissue is devascularized, it shows as a filling defect on CEUS, allowing extension of the ablation to be carried out in the same session, with savings of cost and efficiency. It can truly be claimed that interstitial ablation of focal liver lesions should not be performed without CEUS.

An important advance in ablation techniques has been the development of image fusion methods that allow simultaneous display of ultrasound alongside the same slice reconstructed from a previously acquired 3-D CT or MRI data set (23). It relies on a position sensor that is attached to the ultrasound transducer and uses a radiofrequency (RF) field to track the movement of the probe in space. The benefit of such fusion imaging is the combination of the interactiveness and real time nature of ultrasound that is so useful for needle guidance with the more complete anatomical display of CT and MRI.

CEUS is used in many other parts of the body, especially in the kidneys, where it helps distinguish developmental anomalies from real masses, and in trauma where, rather as in interstitial ablation, the devitalized tissue is much more clearly seen in the liver, spleen and kidneys than on B-mode (24). It is also used for numerous small parts applications with great promise, though it has to be said that these have not become as indispensable as their use in the liver (25).

Contrast agents have opened up the new opportunity of functional imaging for ultrasound in which a bolus of microbubbles is tracked as it traverses a region of interest to produce time-intensity curves (26). These contain much haemodynamic information including even estimates of true tissue perfusion, which can be extracted mathematically. Again, the heart and the liver have been studied most intensively, in the case of the latter, mainly by measuring the time taken to cross from the hepatic artery to the hepatic veins. This 'hepatic transit time' is shortened when arteriovenous shunts form in the liver. The most striking change occurs in cirrhosis and precursor conditions, and a shortened transit time is an indicator of the severity of diffuse liver diseases. Shunts also form in response to malignancies and a shortened transit time can detect metastases (27). An important use of time-intensity curves that has entered clinical routine is in monitoring the effects of anti-angiogenesis drugs in tumours. Previously, size changes were the only measure available, but now it is possible to assess changes to these curves repeatedly and early results show that the reduction in perfusion they measure anticipates size changes, sometimes by many months, so that treatment regimens can be adapted quickly to the tumour's response (28).

In the future microbubble agents for ultrasound may well be more used as targeted agents for molecular imaging and for drug/gene delivery. Despite the simple chemistry of their shells, it is possible to attach targeted ligands to them. Since they are used as intravascular agents, the endothelium is an obvious first target using antibodies to vascular endothelial growth factor (VEGF) for new blood vessels or to activated endothelium (integrins). Studies with experimental animals have validated these approaches to molecular imaging with ultrasound.

In a second step, higher acoustic powers can be used to destroy the microbubbles and release the attached molecules, which could be chemotherapeutic drugs or nucleic acids such as small inhibitory RNAs (siRNAs). By good fortune, the interaction between the ultrasound and the microbubbles has a supra-additive effect whereby the bubbles' oscillations make pores in the cell membrane that facilitate transfer of larger molecules, a process known as sonoporation. Provided the acoustic power is not too high, these pores heal in a few minutes; at higher powers and durations of sonication, they are irreversible and cell kill occurs.

Obviously, extensive safety testing will be required before these methods can be used in the clinic but there is one application where they are already used, albeit in a relatively crude way. The combination of licensed (non-targeted) microbubbles and conventional diagnostic ultrasound has been found to accelerate the dissolution of thrombus in the intracranial arteries in stroke patients (29, 30). The ultrasound beam is directed at the middle cerebral artery and the contrast agent infused intravenously.

Elastography

It is not often that a completely new way to form images emerges but this is exactly what elastography offers (31). The principle is simple and is akin to manual palpation. A force is applied to the tissue to be interrogated and the extent to which it deforms is noted: the stiffer the tissue, the less it distorts. The attraction of elastography for diagnosis is the great range of stiffness differences between normal and pathologic tissue. Elastography has been studied for MRI with very promising results, though most work and early clinical implementation has used ultrasound.

Though the principle is straightforward, the reality is rather more subtle. This is because of the complexity of the mechanical properties of soft tissue, which displays several different types of response to a distorting force. A truly elastic tissue reverts to its original shape once the force is removed and it distorts in a linear fashion. But tissue is not only non-linear (it becomes stiffer the more force is applied) but also has viscous properties, in that, rather like treacle, it can flow and never return to its original shape. Added to that is the fact that liquids within tissue can move through it (think of pitting oedema); add this poro-elasticity to the equation and the situation become very complex. But there is yet more: tissue also supports shear waves in which the particles move across the direction of the travel of the wave, exactly as the surface of a pond responds to a pebble thrown into it. (This is the opposite to the particle movement in conventional pulse wave ultrasonography where the particles move in the same direction as the wave propagates.) All these properties can be in play during elastography measurements and keeping track of them is challenging!

Perhaps fortunately, only two approaches have been exploited clinically thus far. The older assumes that tissue is truly elastic and the force is applied by the operator moving the transducer (though in some experimental systems, a motor was used to produce reproducible movements) (32). The tissue distortion is estimated by comparing image frames before and after applying the force. The movement required is very small, amounting to less than a 1% distortion—in fact, with many more recent systems, the natural cardiorespiratory movement is sufficient, so the probe can be held still. For averaging purposes, more than just two frames are compared and many systems compare continuously so that the elastography images appear in real time on the screen. It is often called 'compression elastography' though actually the tissue is not compressed, but rather is distorted. Alternative terms are static and freehand elastography. The information that is used for the comparisons is the raw or RF data, not the images themselves, in which much of the original data has been discarded. The amount of data to be handled and the algorithms themselves make the processing computer-intensive, especially when the comparisons are performed in two dimensions, an advantage if the tissue moves across the image plane. It should be noted that these elasticity results are relative values, though comparisons with an internal reference tissue (e.g. breast fat) go a long way to correcting that limitation.

Much clinical work has been performed with static systems, especially on the breast. Elastography performs approximately as well as B-mode ultrasound in classifying breast masses using a qualitative scale devised by Itoh et al. (33). (It is often called the Ueno scale, after the breast surgeon who performed the reference clinical studies.) On this scale, stiffer tissue is colour coded as blue and softer (more deformable) tissue, e.g. fat, as red. The completeness of stiffness across the lesion and the relative sizes of the mass on B-mode and that demonstrated on the elastogram are features used in these classifications. A practical problem is the operator dependence of static elastography: much training is required to produce reliable and reproducible results. Because this system depends on the ability to move the tissues directly with the probe, it can be used for other superficial structures and it has been applied to the thyroid and to lymph nodes. It has been used for the prostate and the cervix with intracavitary probes.

A different approach is required for organs like the liver which are protected by the skeleton, so that some form of remote palpation is needed. The best established implementation, the Fibroscan (Echosens, France), was developed to measure liver stiffness based on the principle that the shear waves travel faster in stiffer tissue (34). This system uses a small vibrator to move the skin by ± 2mm to create a shear wave that travels within the liver; its speed is measured using an M-mode technique. Equipped with a quality factor analyser, as in many elastography systems, it is not an imager, but gives a quantitative readout of the stiffness of an approximately 3cm long strip of tissue in kilopascals, with a normal range from 2–10kPa increasing to 25kPa in cirrhosis. It has been widely taken up by hepatologists as a non-invasive alternative to biopsy—it also has the advantage of it sampling a much larger portion of tissue. It performs well in separating cirrhotic from normal liver but falls short in distinguishing lesser degrees of fibrosis. Since the push cannot cross fluid, ascites causes the measurement to fail.

Another form of remote palpation has been exploited more recently: this is the acoustic radiation force produced by diagnostic ultrasound (35) (Fig. 13.4). This minute force (well within the recommended upper MI of 1.9) moves tissue particles by a few microns and sets up shear waves that travel away from the line of the ultrasound beam. A problem with generating a sufficiently effective push force is that the transducer tends to overheat. In the Aixplorer (SuperSonic Imagine, Aix-en-Provence, France) system this has been overcome by sending a series of push pulses at a high PRF, so that a minute shock wave is produced without overstressing the transducer.

Though the shear waves only travel at 1–10m/s, they cross the scan's field of view in a few milliseconds, so the best way to track them is to use an ultrafast imaging method (36). This is achieved by using a completely unfocused transmit beam, with all the focusing carried out on the received information. This allows an entire image to be collected in a single pulse, so that very high frame rates can be achieved. The elastographic image is quantitative, with a read-out in cm/s or in kPa, displayed as a colour overlay on the B-mode image. Because the push is applied by the scanner itself, the method should be less operator dependant. Initially it was developed for characterizing breast masses and good results have been reported in a large multicentre trial in which adding shear wave elastography to B-mode BI-RADS scores improved the accuracy of ultrasound significantly.

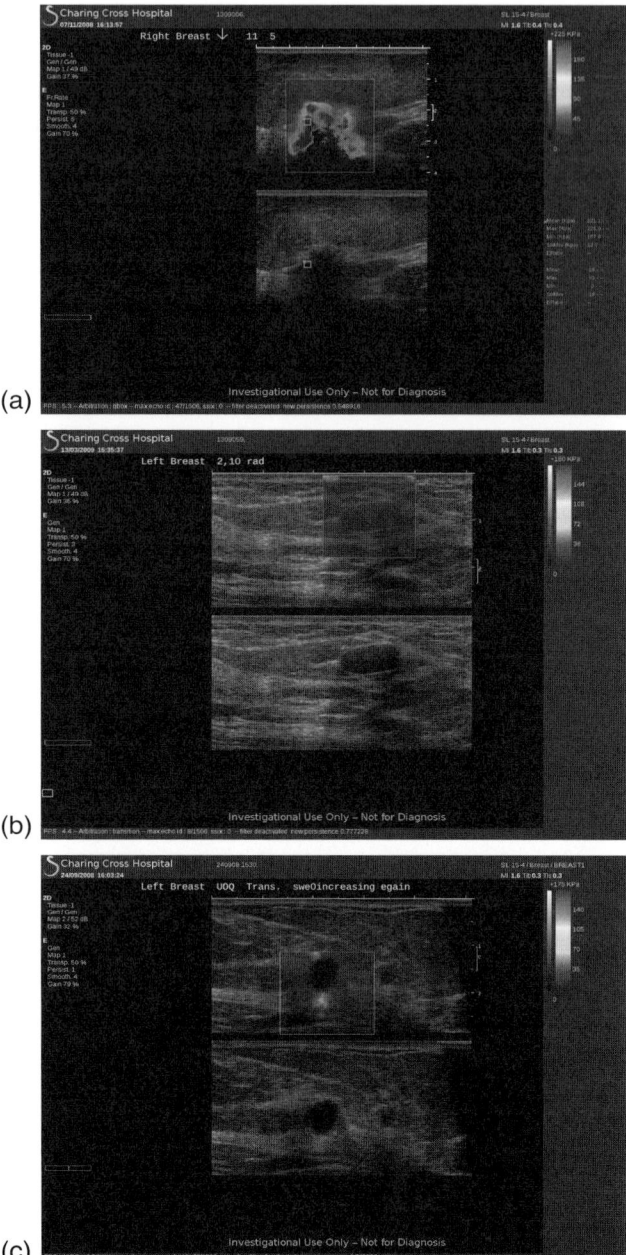

Fig. 13.4 Shear wave elastograms (SWEs) of breast lesions. In these images the SWE is shown as an overlay on the B-mode image in the upper pane; the lower pane shows the B-mode image in its original form. A carcinoma (a) shows a very stiff periphery with a maximum kPa reading of 221, corresponding to a reddish-brown colour code. The stiffness is very typically distributed around the periphery of the mass. A fibroadenoma (b) by comparison, shows low stiffness values and is depicted as a blue tint. Cysts vary in their appearance—this example (c) shows no reading at all and is depicted as a black space. If the cyst fluid is very thick, some signal may be seen. (This figure is reproduced in colour in the colour plate section.)

Studies in the liver are under way and here it shows promise for both focal and diffuse disease; for the latter, the ability to select the region of tissue to measure could be advantageous. Similar approaches have been developed by Siemens on the S-2000 system (37).

High-intensity focused ultrasound

High power ultrasound is used in industry as a means of cleaning solid objects such as jewellery and electronic circuitry. When applied to tissue, the energy is mainly deposited as heat and so this method, known as high-intensity focused ultrasound (HIFU), is part of the family of methods to achieve local heating, the most widespread of which is RF ablation using electromagnetic energy (38). HIFU has the advantage of being totally non-invasive since the transducer is merely coupled to the skin. To achieve the high power required, the transducer must be large and this also allows for the very intense focusing that is necessary. A HIFU lesion is a small (20×5mm) cigar-shaped region of coagulated tissue which is sharply demarcated from the adjacent tissue that is unaffected at a distance of only a few cells-width from the completely devitalized tissue. This is in contrast to the less well-defined margin of coagulation resulting from RF ablation and, even more so to the widespread damage resulting from radiotherapy.

In practice, the large transducer is housed in a water bath and is of fixed focus, so that it must be raised and lowered to position the lesion in the desired position. A single small lesion is rarely adequate, so the transducer is moved from side to side in a raster, delivering a series of contiguous lesions, and then repeating the raster at a more superficial level to complete the lesion. All of this requires meticulous therapy planning in the same way as for radiotherapy.

HIFU is in widespread clinical use in China, where many key developments have been made (39). It is used for ablation of fibroids and for palliative therapy of osteosarcomas. It is also used for lesions of the cervix of the uterus and for benign prostatic hyperplasia. Dedicated prostatic HIFU systems are available and their use for localized prostatic carcinoma is a topic of intensive research. An interesting use is in pancreatic carcinoma: here it has a dramatic effect on the pain that these patients often suffer. The supposition is that the HIFU damages the splanchnic nerves much as a regional local anaesthesia.

A general limitation of HIFU is that it shares the properties of ultrasound and will not penetrate bone or gas. In fact, these are regions to be avoided because the energy is selectively deposited there and produces burn injuries. Attempts to overcome this are being explored to make the method more useful for the liver, which is an important target for ablation of malignancies. One promising idea is to use an array rather than a single element transducer, and arrange for the elements overlying ribs to be switched off. This approach could also lend itself to tracking the position of a liver lesion as it moves with breathing. Another general limitation is that the HIFU lesions are slow to form so that an ablation session can take many hours. It may be possible to speed this up using sensitizers, perhaps in the form of microbubbles (40).

Another general problem is that the lesions are not well seen using conventional ultrasound, a problem shared with RF ablation. Microbubbles have greatly improved the monitoring of the eventual lesion produced by RF ablation, especially in the liver. CEUS is helpful also for HIFU, but there is an additional requirement here: it would be very useful if the temperature could be monitored throughout the HIFU session, so that the treatment could be stopped as soon as the desired temperature was reached, an approach that would likely also speed up the treatment. Temperature monitoring can be performed using routine MR sequences, but has not been satisfactorily achieved with ultrasound, which as with RF ablation, is the natural modality because of its interactivity. Coagulated tissue does conduct ultrasound more quickly and is also stiffer than normal tissue and imaging of sound speed and of stiffness (shear wave imaging is the most promising) are being developed.

Conclusions

Recent developments in ultrasound have had a hugely beneficial effect on clinical practice, not only on making important new techniques available but, by making the scanners easier to use, making it easier for less skilled operators to perform. Some might feel that this has had a negative impact in making ultrasound available to users who are not properly trained, and this is indeed a danger. Overall though, reducing operator dependence can improve consistency and thus the diagnostic power of the technique, to the benefit of our patients, surely the ultimate goal.

Acknowledgement

I am grateful to my colleague Dr Robert Eckersley PhD, for much helpful input.

References

1. Royal College of Radiologists. *Medical image interpretation by radiographers: Guidance for radiologists and healthcare providers.* London: The Royal College of Radiologists; 2010; Available at: http://www.rcr.ac.uk/publications.aspx?PageID=310&PublicationID=318.
2. The Royal College of Radiologists. *Ultrasound Training Recommendations for Medical and Surgical Specialties.* London: The Royal College of Radiologists; 2005; Available at: http://www.rcr.ac.uk/docs/radiology/pdf/ultrasound.pdf.
3. Hanafy A. Broadband phased array transducer design with frequency-controlled two-dimensional capability. In: Shung KK (ed) *Medical Imaging 1998: Ultrasonic Transducer Engineering* (Proceedings Volume 3341). Bellingham, WA: SPIE Press; 1998, pp.64–82.
4. Oralkan O, Ergun A, Johnson J, Karaman M, Demirci U, Kaviani K, *et al.* Capacitive micromachined ultrasonic transducers: next-generation arrays for acoustic imaging? *IEEE Trans Ultrason Ferroelectr Freq Control* 2002; **49**:1596–610.
5. Whatmough C, Guitian J, Baines E, Benigni L, Mahoney PN, Mantis P, *et al.* Ultrasound image compounding: effect on perceived image quality. *Vet Radiol Ultrasound* 2007; **48**(2):141–5.
6. Ortega D, Burns PN, Hope Simpson D, Wilson SR. Tissue harmonic imaging: is it a benefit for bile duct sonography? *AJR Am J Roentgenol* 2001; **176**(3):653–9.
7. Byram B, Holley G, Giannantonio D, Trahey G. 3-D phantom and *in vivo* cardiac speckle tracking using a matrix array and raw echo data. *IEEE Trans Ultrason Ferroelectr Freq Control* 2010; **57**(4):839–54.

8. Scheipers U, Konig K, Sommerfeld HJ, Garcia-Schurmann M, Senge T, Ermert H. Sonohistology – ultrasonic tissue characterization for prostate cancer diagnostics. *Cancer Biomark* 2008; **4**(4–5):227–50.
9. Abdel-Wahab M, Khattab AA, Toelg R, Geist V, Liska B, Richardt G. Plaque characteristics of nonobstructive coronary lesions in diabetic patients: an intravascular ultrasound virtual histology analysis. *J Cardiovasc Med (Hagerstown)* 2010; **11**(5):345–51.
10. Rubin JM, Bude RO, Carson PL, Bree RL, Adler RS. Power Doppler US: a potentially useful alternative to mean frequency-based color Doppler US. *Radiology* 1994; **190**(3):853–6.
11. Steel R, Ramnarine KV, Davidson F, Fish PJ, Hoskins PR. Angle-independent estimation of maximum velocity through stenoses using vector Doppler ultrasound. *Ultrasound Med Biol* 2003; **29**(4):575–84.
12. Jensen JA, Munk P. A new method for estimation of velocity vectors. *IEEE Trans Ultrason Ferroelectr Freq Control* 1998; **45**(3):837–51.
13. Chiao R, LY M, Hall A, Miller S, Thomenius K. B-mode blood flow (B-flow) imaging. *Ultrasonics Symposium, 2000 IEEE* 2002; **2**:1469–72.
14. Sutherland GR, Bijnens B, McDicken WN. Tissue Doppler echocardiography: historical perspective and technological considerations. *Echocardiography* 1999; **16**(5):445–53.
15. Merz E. [Current technical possibilities of 3D ultrasound in gynecology and obstetrics]. *Ultraschall Med* 1997; **18**(5):190–5.
16. Goncalves LF, Espinoza J, Kusanovic JP, Lee W, Nien JK, Santolaya-Forgas J, et al. Applications of 2-dimensional matrix array for 3- and 4-dimensional examination of the fetus: a pictorial essay. *J Ultrasound Med* 2006; **25**(6):745–55.
17. The problem with 'keepsake' fetal ultrasound: ECRI and other medical professionals cite potential risks. *Health Devices* 2005; **34**(11):378–80.
18. Ziskin MC, Bonakdarpour A, Weinstein DP, Lynch PR. Contrast agents for diagnostic ultrasound. *Invest Radiol* 1972; **7**(6):500–5.
19. Claudon M, Cosgrove D, Albrecht T, Bolondi L, Bosio M, Calliada F, et al. Guidelines and Good Clinical Practice Recommendations for Contrast Enhanced Ultrasound (CEUS) - Update 2008. *Ultraschall Med* 2008; **29**(1):28–44.
20. Blomley MJ, Cooke JC, Unger EC, Monaghan MJ, Cosgrove DO. Microbubble contrast agents: a new era in ultrasound. *BMJ* 2001; **322**(7296):1222–5.
21. Seitz K, Bernatik T, Strobel D, Blank W, Friedrich-Rust M, Strunk H, et al. Contrast-Enhanced Ultrasound (CEUS) for the Characterization of Focal Liver Lesions in Clinical Practice (DEGUM Multicenter Trial): CEUS vs. MRI - a prospective comparison in 269 Patients. *Ultraschall Med* 2010; **31**(5):492–9.
22. Moug SJ, Horgan PG, Leen E. Contrast-enhanced ultrasonography during liver surgery. *Br J Surg* 2004; **91**(11):1527.
23. Crocetti L, Lencioni R, Debeni S, See TC, Pina CD, Bartolozzi C. Targeting liver lesions for radiofrequency ablation: an experimental feasibility study using a CT-US fusion imaging system. *Invest Radiol* 2008; **43**(1):33–9.
24. Setola SV, Catalano O, Sandomenico F, Siani A. Contrast-enhanced sonography of the kidney. *Abdom Imaging* 2007; **32**(1):21–8.
25. Shalhoub J, Owen DR, Gauthier T, Monaco C, Leen EL, Davies AH. The use of contrast enhanced ultrasound in carotid arterial disease. *Eur J Vasc Endovasc Surg* 2010; **39**(4):381–7.
26. Kiessling F. Science to practice: The dawn of molecular US imaging for clinical cancer imaging. *Radiology* 2010; **256**: 331–3.
27. Zhou X, Liu JB, Luo Y, Yan F, Peng Y, Lin L, et al. Characterization of focal liver lesions by means of assessment of hepatic transit time with contrast-enhanced US. *Radiology* 2010; **256**(2):648–55.

28. Lassau N, Chebil M, Chami L, Bidault S, Girard E, Roche A. Dynamic contrast-enhanced ultrasonography (DCE-US): a new tool for the early evaluation of antiangiogenic treatment. *Target Oncol* 2010; **5**(1):53–8.
29. Meairs S, Culp W. Microbubbles for thrombolysis of acute ischemic stroke. *Cerebrovasc Dis* 2009; **27**(Suppl 2):55–65.
30. Alexandrov AV, Mikulik R, Ribo M, Sharma VK, Lao AY, Tsivgoulis G, et al. A pilot randomized clinical safety study of sonothrombolysis augmentation with ultrasound-activated perflutren-lipid microspheres for acute ischemic stroke. *Stroke* 2008; **39**(5):1464–9.
31. Bamber JC. Comment on new technology—ultrasound elastography. *Ultraschall Med* 2008; **29**(3):319–20.
32. Ophir J, Alam SK, Garra B, Kallel F, Konofagou E, Krouskop T, et al. Elastography: ultrasonic estimation and imaging of the elastic properties of tissues. *Proc Inst Mech Eng [H]* 1999; **213**(3):203–33.
33. Itoh A, Ueno E, Tohno E, Kamma H, Takahashi H, Shiina T, et al. Breast disease: clinical application of US elastography for diagnosis. *Radiology* 2006; **239**(2):341–50.
34. Lucidarme D, Foucher J, Le Bail B, Vergniol J, Castera L, Duburque C, et al. Factors of accuracy of transient elastography (fibroscan) for the diagnosis of liver fibrosis in chronic hepatitis C. *Hepatology* 2009; **49**(4):1083–9.
35. Montaldo G, Tanter M, Bercoff J, Benech N, Fink M. Coherent plane-wave compounding for very high frame rate ultrasonography and transient elastography. *IEEE Trans Ultrason Ferroelectr Freq Control* 2009; **56**(3):489–506.
36. Tanter M, Bercoff J, Sandrin L, Fink M. Ultrafast compound imaging for 2-D motion vector estimation: application to transient elastography. *IEEE Trans Ultrason Ferroelectr Freq Control* 2002; **49**(10):1363–74.
37. Clevert DA, Stock K, Klein B, Slotta-Huspenina J, Prantl L, Heemann U, et al. Evaluation of Acoustic Radiation Force Impulse (ARFI) imaging and contrast-enhanced ultrasound in renal tumors of unknown etiology in comparison to histological findings. *Clin Hemorheol Microcirc* 2009; **43**(1):95–107.
38. ter Haar G. Therapeutic applications of ultrasound. *Prog Biophys Mol Biol* 2007; **93**(1–3):111–29.
39. Lu J, Hu W, Wang W. Sonablate-500 transrectal high-intensity focused ultrasound (HIFU) for benign prostatic hyperplasia patients. *J Huazhong Univ Sci Technolog Med Sci* 2007; **27**(6):671–4.
40. Yue Y, Chen W, Wang Z. [The impact of microbubbles-mediated intermitten HIFU on bloodflow in femoral artery of rabbit]. *Sheng Wu Yi Xue Gong Cheng Xue Za Zhi* 2010; **27**(1):58–61.

Chapter 14

Use of contrast in ultrasound

Tomas Jansson and Anders Nilsson

In 1968, Drs Pravin M. Shah and Raymond Gramiak at the University of Rochester, New York, were conducting a study with the ultimate goal to investigate whether heart stroke volume could be estimated from the extent and duration of cusp separation of the aortic valve, as measured with M-mode ultrasound (1). Simultaneously, as the reference, they also measured cardiac output with the indicator dilution technique. Here, a bolus of a dye (indocyanine green) is injected and blood is sampled downstream to determine the rate at which the indicator has been transported from the injection site. In Dr Shah's own account of the experiments, he explains that the routine at his university then was to place a catheter in the left atrium with the trans-septal technique, i.e. inserting the catheter in a vein and penetrating into the left atrium via the right atrium (2). During the injections of the dye, somewhat to their surprise, they observed a striking echo enhancement across the aorta. The enhancement also appeared when saline and dextrose in water was flushed through the catheter. Dr Gramiak reminded himself of a comment from Dr Claude Joyner, that a temporary echo-enhancement could be observed during saline injections, and they speculated that miniature bubbles produced by gaseous cavitation upon rapid injection of the fluid gave rise to the enhancement, and raised the idea that this could be used as a contrast agent. An *in vitro* study by Frederick Kremkau provided strong evidence that gas bubbles were actually responsible for the echo enhancement (3).

It is interesting to note how discoveries are made independently around the world, when the time is ripe. At the same time in Lund, Drs Inge Edler and Kjell Lindström performed studies to measure blood flow in the heart (4). At this point no ultrasound Doppler signals had been recorded from the inside of the heart, and they used a calf heart in an *in vitro* model to verify that signals could be obtained when water and blood was led through the model. They saw that a louder Doppler signal was obtained when fluids were changed from water to blood, or vice versa, and noted that 'this effect can eventually be used for ultrasonic "contrast injections"'. Thus a different approach, but the same discovery. Edler and Lindström however did not pursue the contrast application.

The fundamental idea of a contrast agent is that it enhances (or diminishes) the signal that makes up the image, thereby accentuating the areas where the contrast agent is present, i.e. the blood pool or specific blood vessels. In the case of ultrasound contrast agents, a substance that has dramatically different acoustical properties compared to tissue will give this effect. Ultrasound imaging relies on sound reflection from various tissue interfaces, and the larger the difference in density and compressibility between two media, the larger the reflection will be. Gas is a good example, but metal particles could also theoretically be used. The governing parameter is, however, compressibility, and thus gas has a much larger contrast effect than does metallic objects, even though metal nanoparticles are being developed as contrast agents for ultrasound—usually, however, with a different mode of detection than pure reflection (5, 6).

Modern contrast agents are, however, not of the kind where catheterization is necessary, nor are they based on the production of free bubbles. There are several reasons for this, apart from the obvious practical complications with catheterization. First and foremost, free bubbles that are produced by injection are much too large to pass the pulmonary bed, and thus would need a catheter to be used anyway. Second, micrometer-sized bubbles collapse due to surface tension within milliseconds, or coalesce to dissolve somewhat more slowly.

To realize a contrast agent that permits intravenous injection, bubbles need to be stabilized with a surface film, or shell. This can be, for instance, non-ionic surfactants (which reduce surface tension) or be with proteins or phospholipids, that also hinder diffusion. Moreover, modern agents also contain gases that have minimal driving force for diffusion and dissolution in the blood, such as perfluorocarbons or sulfur hexafluoride (7).

Intuitively it could be argued that a smaller bubble would serve as a smaller target, and thus be less effective as a contrast agent (actually, the scattered energy scales as the radius to the sixth power, which makes it a very plausible proposition indeed). But there is a factor that helps micrometre-sized bubbles in blood to be very effective scatterers—resonance. The crucial point is namely that gas bubbles in a liquid can be considered as a mechanical oscillating system where the gas pressure acts as a spring, and the surrounding liquid as a mass. As in all mechanical systems it possess a resonance frequency which can be derived to be (given some assumptions):

$$f_{res} = \frac{1}{2\pi R_0} \sqrt{\frac{3\gamma p}{\rho}}$$

where f_{res} is the resonance frequency, R_0 is the equilibrium radius of the bubble, γ is the ratio of specific heat of the gas at constant pressure and at constant volume, p is the hydrostatic pressure outside the bubble, and ρ is the density of the surrounding fluid (8). For air bubbles in water under one atmosphere, this means that $f_{res} R_0 \approx 3.26$MHz, and consequently that a 2μm air bubble will resonate at 3.26MHz, in perfect range for diagnostic ultrasound. Thus there is the fortunate coincidence that bubbles that are small enough to pass into the pulmonary circulation, are in resonance at employed ultrasound frequencies, and thereby appear as bubbles that are 10–100 times larger.

In the 1990s, ultrasound contrast agents began to be introduced commercially to a larger market. The first applications of modern-type contrast agents were simply as an echo enhancer, for instance to improve delineation of the endocardial border of the left ventricle to evaluate heart function. Another area was as Doppler signal enhancers but that application never really took off, at least partly because the problems with separating slow flow from tissue movement remained, regardless of the Doppler signal strength.

However, as these microbubble-based agents were designed to be of a size that would allow an intravenous injection and passage through capillary beds it was soon noticed that the bubbles accumulated in organs such as the liver, some due to Kupffer cell uptake, some merely because of slow flow in the liver sinusoids. Methods designed to detect the contrast, apart from Doppler, were soon developed. Stimulated acoustic emission (SAE) was one such method where the agent was injected and allowed to accumulate in the liver parenchyma for 3–5min. After that the Doppler mode was switched on (usually power Doppler), the high mechanical index (MI) Doppler bursting the contrast bubbles which then emitted a signal detected by the ultrasound machine as a Doppler signal. Thus normal liver parenchyma would appear as completely filled with Doppler colour but lesions consisting of other tissues, i.e. tumours, would not. SAE somewhat lacked the spatial resolution to be incorporated into day-to-day clinical practice and as the bubbles were destroyed, only allowed for a single pass of the ultrasound beam. It was possible to do such a single scan, store on a cine loop, and review it afterwards but this was cumbersome and took away the real time ability that is one of ultrasound's major advantages.

The proper incorporation of ultrasound contrast into daily routine practice only happened when research had developed contrast agents where the bubbles were more stable, and detection schemes that could effectively differentiate the contrast signal from tissue. In cardiac ultrasound for instance, to achieve more precise diagnosis it is desirable to determine not only the resulting wall movement deficiency, but also the blood flow, or perfusion, in the myocardium. For this purpose the ultrasound contrast agents did not suffice: enhancement of blood in larger blood vessels is fine, as blood normally is not very echogenic. For smaller vessels that cannot be resolved, the tissue signal will overwhelm the contrast signal making the presence of contrast in the tissue very difficult to determine unless the tissue signal can be suppressed and the contrast agent enhanced. To achieve this next clinical useful step, other strategies were called for. It had long been known that bubbles in an acoustic field will undergo asymmetric radial pulsations provided the driving pressure is large enough. The asymmetry comes from the fact that when the pressure in the acoustic wave is high, the bubble is compressed, and expanded when the pressure is low. When the bubble is compressed it becomes stiffer, and resists further compression. In the rarefaction phase, the bubble can readily expand to several times the diameter it has in the equilibrium state, even with a shell. The scattered pressure waveform will thus also be asymmetric, and if so it will also contain harmonics, i.e. multiples of the fundamental frequency.

The first detection strategy that utilized the non-linear effect was what is known as harmonic imaging (9). In this mode, pulses with a given (centre) frequency are transmitted, and the receiver is tuned so that only frequencies that correspond to the band around the second harmonic are detected. In this way the image is made up only from echoes that have twice the transmitted frequency. This may at first glace seem like a simple proposition, but the technique requires broadband transducer arrays and digital beamformers. These developments were underway at this time because broadband transducers also significantly improve image resolution (as shorter pulses can be generated).

Eventually, with a variant of harmonic imaging (harmonic power Doppler) it was possible to successfully detect deficiencies in myocardial perfusion (10).

The drawback with harmonic imaging is that relatively long pulses are needed, and this will reduce the spatial resolution. The reason is that long pulses are needed to separate the fundamental and second harmonic frequency bands. Short pulses correspond to wide-frequency bands, with harmonics equally wide. This means that fundamental and harmonic bands will interfere for short pulses, counteracting the purpose of harmonic imaging. This is especially troublesome when the harmonic signals are weak compared to the fundamental tissue signal.

To overcome this, an entirely new class of contrast-specific imaging schemes have been developed. The key idea is to not only base the detection on the result of one transmitted pulse, but two (or a whole sequence). That is, each image line is made up from two transmissions, and not one, as usually is the case. These two pulses can differ in phase, as was first suggested ((11), see Fig. 14.1), or amplitude, or a combination thereof. Any target that behaves linearly, such as tissue interfaces, will produce an echo that is a mirror image of the transmitted pulse (left panels, Fig. 14.1). Thus the registered echoes of that target will also be identical, apart from the phase difference. In the case of phase inversion between two successive pulses, simple addition of the resulting echo lines will yield zero amplitude from linear echoes. On the other hand, if a bubble is present, the response will be asymmetric as explained above, and the resulting sum of the echo-lines will produce a contribution at the location of the bubble (right panels, Fig. 14.1). It can be shown that this corresponds to a time domain cancellation of odd harmonics (including the fundamental).

In this way the spatial resolution can be improved without sacrificing the sensitivity to the harmonic response. The pulse inversion technique does require twice the data collection time, and tissue movements will also cause the two echo lines to not perfectly line up. The latter can be alleviated by transmitting not only two pulses, but a whole sequence of pulses, named power pulse inversion (12). The resulting echo lines can be combined in a way that eliminates the effect of moving tissue. For example, three transmitted pulses can be considered, where the first and third are identical, and the second inverted. If the tissue has moved

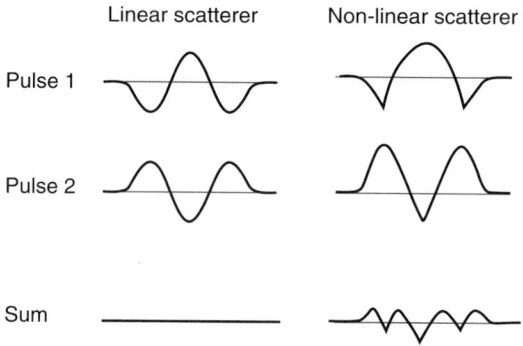

Fig. 14.1 The principle of pulse inversion imaging. The sum of two phase-inverted echoes from a target that produce linear reflection cancels (left), while the sum of echoes from a target with non-linear effects is detectable (right).

during the time between pulse one and three, the technique can be thought of as forming an average of pulse one and three, which will line up with line two, and the subtraction can be performed successfully. This method can be generalized onto a train of pulses.

Using power pulse inversion, myocardial areas with no perfusion can be localized, but those where perfusion is impaired only, careful consideration needs to be taken on how the first part of the contrast bolus enters the area, i.e. the dynamics. Wei et al. (13) introduced a standardized way to achieve this by utilizing that the contrast bubbles break if exposed to a high-amplitude ultrasound wave. The strategy is to apply a constant infusion of contrast agent, so that a constant level of contrast is achieved in the bloodstream. A short burst of high energy ultrasound can then be applied to the image plane that will be investigated. All bubbles within the plane will be destroyed, akin to SAE, but here subsequent images acquired at a low power level, allows the reperfusion of contrast agent into the image plane to be studied. Areas with impaired perfusion will have a marked slower reperfusion rate, and possibly also lower total contrast intensity (vascular volume) in that area. This technique is especially useful in investigations of myocardial perfusion, whereas a bolus technique usually is sufficient for radiological studies (see below).

Having thus improved the detection strategies and thereby the sensitivity, only more stable agents were needed. The bubbles of earlier agents were destroyed even by low MI signals making also pulse or phase inversion techniques one-pass scans. However, the development of agents such as Sonovue and Sonazoid, coinciding with the new millennium, restored the real-time ability of contrast-enhanced ultrasound (CEUS) and it has now become an established clinical tool. The most widely accepted clinical use to date is in the detection and characterization of focal lesions, mainly in the liver (14), where it is as good as contrast-enhanced computed tomography (CT) or magnetic resonance imaging (MRI) (Fig. 14.2). Equally importantly is that even though no modality can detect all lesions, they

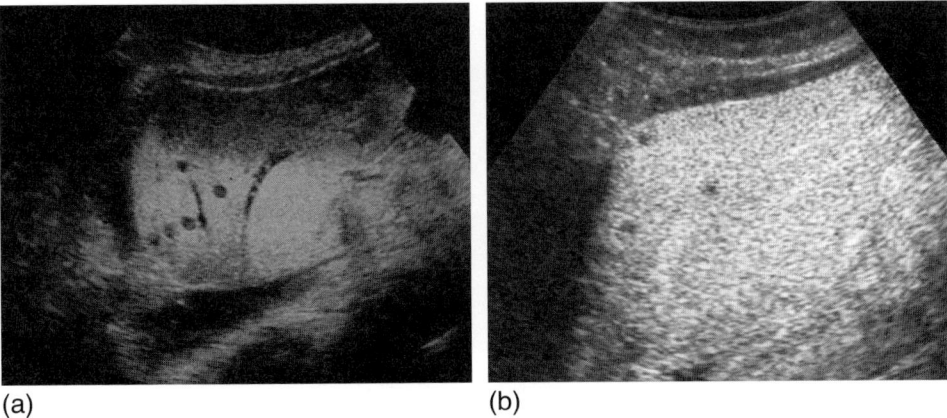

Fig. 14.2 Small metastatic liver lesions (a) detected with a 'single scan' pulse inversion technique before the time of stable contrast agent and (b) real-time contrast-enhanced ultrasound image of three small liver metastases from a breast cancer, seen as dark 'holes' in the otherwise enhancing liver parenchyma. Their size of <3mm makes them, at least in this patient, impossible to detect on CT or MRI.

seem to detect different lesions, i.e. any work-up of a patient really should include more than one modality, CEUS often being one of them due to the availability, low cost, lack of side effects, etc.

Ultrasound contrast agents are blood pool agents, i.e. they do not leave the blood vessels, as they are particles rather than chemical compounds. It therefore follows that the presence of contrast agent means the presence of blood vessels, i.e. we are looking at solid, viable tissue. Conversely, the excellent sensitivity to even small amounts of contrast in most modern, high-end, ultrasound machines means that the opposite often also can be assumed, i.e. no contrast equals no blood vessels. Though this seems a very simple fact it has many uses in everyday ultrasound. Lesion characterization in other parts of the body than the liver is such an application. The spatial resolution of CEUS can be used to distinguish small cysts or cystic masses from solid lesions when this is not possible on CT or MRI due to the small size of the lesion, lack of contrast resolution, etc. Likewise, tissue coagulated by modern ablation therapy can be distinguished from residual perfused tumour, echogenic fluid collections like abscesses separated from surrounding tissue, small solid portions in otherwise cystic tumours detected, etc. (15). In virtually every situation where an unknown lesion is detected, CEUS has a role in the work-up. A specific field that should expand is in the examination after trauma. Blunt abdominal trauma almost without exception now leads to a trauma CT regardless of the power and position of the impact. When trauma is light to moderate and localized to either flank, a CEUS exam can do the same job without the radiation. CEUS may even turn out to be better than CT as it is possible to distinguish between an organ contusion and a proper rupture (Fig. 14.3).

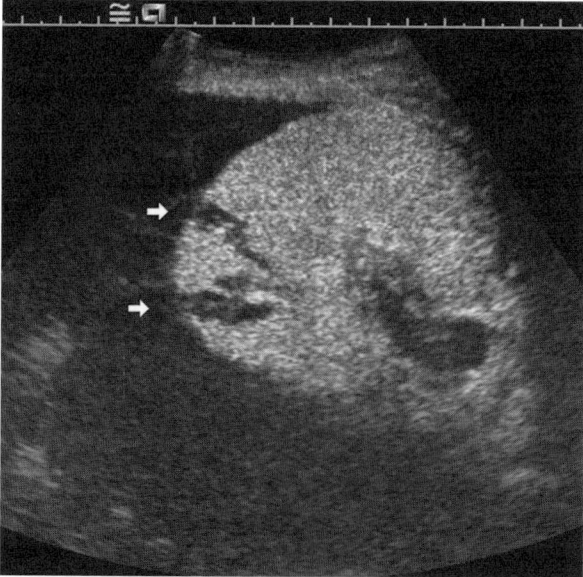

Fig. 14.3 Rupture of the left kidney after blunt trauma. Note the sharp delineation of the lesions and non-contrast-enhancing haematoma (no blood vessels, e.g. no contrast) surrounding the upper pole of the kidney.

Another emerging application, made all the more feasible by the contrast agents being blood pool agents, is the quantification of tissue perfusion, i.e. not just perfusion or no perfusion assessment but the ability to detect and numerically quantify differences in perfusion between different tissues, same tissue before or after treatment, or simply perfusion in an organ compared to a normal variation. Such applications have been surprisingly slow to reach clinical practice, even though they were already devised by 1998 (13), partly due to lack of adequate software in the ultrasound machines. But quantification of tumour perfusion before and after treatment is very promising (16) and this may pave the way for other areas such as transplant perfusion, stenosis detection, and hyperaemia quantification. As contrast can be given both as a bolus or an infusion, a wash-in/wash-out curve can be obtained and many parameters calculated, eventually giving perfusion in ml/min/cm^2 or such.

At a recent ultrasound meeting, Peter Burns, one of ultrasounds pioneers, pointed out that ultrasound really came into clinical practice in the 1970s. Then over the next decades came CT, MRI, positron emission tomography (PET), PET-CT, etc. and every time such an improvement is made we think that ultrasound is out for the count. Ultrasound, however, has always come back with improvements of its own, like Doppler, colour and power Doppler, and now contrast with ever increasing novel applications. In the future, more stable bubbles may improve image quality ever further and agents with a pronounced Kupffer cell uptake will add another dimension both to lesion detection, characterization, and image resolution. Other exciting emerging applications include molecular imaging and targeted drug delivery, assuring ultrasound to continue to be one of the cornerstones of modern medicine.

References

1. Gramiak R, Shah PM. Echocardiography of the aortic root. *Invest Radiol* 1968; **3**:356–66.
2. Nanda NC, Schleif R, Goldberg BB. *Advances in Echo Imaging using Contrast Enhancement.* Dordrecht: Kluwer Academic Publishers; 1997.
3. Kremkau FW, Gramiak R, Carstensen EL, Shah PM, Kramer DH. Ultrasonic detection of cavitation at catheter tips. *Am J Roentgenol Radium Ther Nucl Med* 1970; **110**(1):177–83.
4. Lindström K, Edler I. Ultrasonic Doppler technique used in heart disease. An experimental study. In: Bock J and Ossoinig K (eds) *Ultrason Graphia Medica Separatum 1st World Congress on Ultrasonic Diagnosis in Medicine, Vienna, Austria, June 1969*. Vienna: Verlag Wiener Medizinischen Akademic; 1969, pp.447–54.
5. Wang LV (ed). *Photoacoustic Imaging and Spectroscopy.* Boca Raton, FL: CRC Press; 2009.
6. Oh J, Feldman MD, Kim J, Condit C, Emelianov S, Milner TE. Detection of magnetic nanoparticles in tissue using magneto-motive ultrasound. *Nanotechnology* 2006; **17**:4183–90.
7. Goldberg BB, Raichlen JS, Forsberg F. *Ultrasound Contrast Agents, Basic principles and Clinical Applications*, 2nd edn. London: Martin Dunitz Ltd; 2001.
8. Leighton TG. *The Acoustic Bubble.* San Diego, CA: Academic Press; 1994.
9. Burns PN, Powers JE, Fritzsch T. Harmonic imaging—new imaging and Doppler method for contrast-enhanced ultrasound. *Radiology* 1992; **185**:142.
10. Burns PN, Becher H. *Handbook of contrast echocardiography.* Frankfurt: Springer-Verlag; 2000.
11. Simpson DH, Burns PN. Pulse inversion Doppler: a new method for detecting nonlinear echoes from microbubble contrast agents. *Proc IEEE Ultrasonics Symp* 1997; **2**:1597–600.

12. Simpson DH, Chin CT, Burns PN. Pulse inversion Doppler: a new method for detecting nonlinear echoes from microbubble contrast agents. *IEEE Trans Ultrason Ferroelectr Freq Control* 1999; **46**(2):372–38.
13. Wei K, Jayaweera AR, Firoozan S, Linka A, Skyba DM, Kaul S. Quantification of myocardial blood flow with ultrasound-induced destruction of microbubbles administered as a constant venous infusion. *Circulation* 1998; **97**:473–9.
14. Bryant TH, Blomley MJ, Albrecht T, Sidhu PS, Leen EL, Basilico R, *et al*. Improved characterisation of liver lesions with liver-phase uptake of liver-specific microbubbles: prospective multicentre study. *Radiology* 2004; **232**:799–809.
15. Ding H, Kudo M, Onda H, Suetomi Y, Minami Y, Chung H, *et al*. Evaluation of posttreatment response of hepatocellular carcinoma with contrast-enhanced coded phase inversion harmonic US. Comparison with dynamic CT. *Radiology* 2001; **221**:712–30.
16. Krix M. Quantification of enhancement in contrast ultrasound: a tool for monitoring of therapies in liver metastases. *Eur Radiol* 2005; **15**(Suppl.):E104–E108.

Chapter 15

The development of ultrasound in ophthalmology

Karl C. Ossoinig

Introduction

The clinical applications of diagnostic ultrasound in ophthalmology were initiated by G.H. Mundt and W.F. Hughes (1) (1956) as well as A. Oksala and A. Lehtinen (2) (1957) introducing A-scan, and by G. Baum (3) (1958) introducing and pioneering B-scan. The first medical society for diagnostic ultrasound was founded in 1964 (Societas Internationalis de Diagnostica Ultrasonica in Ophthalmologia) with subsequent biennial congresses. Ophthalmic diagnostic ultrasound is the only ultrasonographic method heavily relying on A-scans besides the B-scans. Today, four distinct echographic methods (utilizing different types of instrumentation) are being used in ophthalmology:

1) *Biometric A-scans* for measuring the axial eye length.
2) *Low-frequency B-scans* for the examination of the posterior eye segment and the anterior orbit utilizing 10–20MHz.
3) *High-frequency B-scans* for the evaluation of the anterior eye segment applying 25–50MHz.
4) *Standardized Echography*, a combination of diagnostic as well as biometric A-scan (8MHz) and B-scan echography (10–50MHz) for a comprehensive ultrasonographic examination of the eye (anterior and posterior segments) and of the entire orbit and periorbital region.

Biometric A-scans

A-scan (8–12MHz) is used for measurements of the axial eye length, today an important contribution to the calculation of intraocular lens power in cataract surgery. F. Jansson (4) (1963) proposed biometric A-scan as an immersion (non-touch) technique and also measured the involved sound velocities of the anterior chamber, the lens, and the vitreous cavity which since then have been the accepted standard values.

At first, axial eye length measurements were mostly used in studies regarding glaucoma and myopia. When, in the early 1970s, the implantation of artificial lenses during cataract surgery spread quickly, the much more precise but more time-consuming and demanding immersion method temporarily gave way to an easier and quicker contact method. Lately, however, advances in cataract surgery, especially the use of multifocal lenses as well as the competition from laser technology, resulted in a return of Jansson's immersion method.

Low-frequency B-scans

Ever since the introduction of real-time B-scanning by N. Bronson (8), low-frequency B-scans (10–20MHz) evolved into a popular screening tool used to detect or rule out posterior segment lesions in eyes with opaque media (e.g. opaque corneas, dense cataracts, anterior chamber and vitreous haemorrhages). Since then diagnostic B-scan instrumentation has been remarkably improved, particularly in terms of their resolution and grey-scale quality.

Low-frequency B-scan echography (5–7, 9) is an accepted and widespread tool for screening the posterior eye segment and for accomplishing a number of diagnoses based either on a lesion's location and distribution, its specific configuration or movement pattern, or an acoustic shadowing. In many instances, however, B-scan findings alone represent only probabilities, possibilities, or suggestions of ocular lesions or remain altogether inconclusive as to the underlying pathology. This is, for instance, the case in the clinically very important early diagnosis of endophthalmitis, in the diagnosis and differentiation of tumours, and the differentiation between retinal detachments and dense fibrovascular membranes (severe diabetic vitreoretinopathies, trauma). In addition, measurements with the low-frequency B-scan method are neither precise nor reliable (falsified by refraction, erroneous because of 'blooming' artefacts).

Since in many ophthalmic practices low-frequency B-scan echography is still the only echographic tool available, being frequently overtaxed rather than used according to its limited capacity, it has, as a consequence, given diagnostic ophthalmic ultrasound in general a totally unjustified poor clinical reputation.

High-frequency B-scans

High-frequency B-scan echography (50MHz), so-called ultrasonic biomicroscopy (UBM), is a very different matter. Introduced and pioneered by Pavlin and Foster (13) (1994), it has revolutionized the echographic evaluation of the anterior eye segment (in particular that of the cornea, chamber angles, and iris). Markedly improved software in newer instrumentation (e.g. the Aviso series by Quantel Medical) has made available a wide range of diagnostic data competitive with, and at times, superior to similar evaluations with laser technology. UBM usage in the evaluation of the anterior eye segment is rapidly spreading and advancing (Fig. 15.1).

Standardized echography

Standardized echography combines diagnostic A-scan (8MHz), diagnostic B-scan (10–50MHz), and biometric A-scan (8MHz) techniques. It was introduced and pioneered by K. Ossoinig (5–7, 10–12, 15) in the 1960s. Today it is a widely used ultrasonic method in ophthalmology. Based on extensive experimental and clinical studies it evolved into the most efficient and reliable ultrasonic method in ophthalmology, surpassing by far the low-frequency B-scan method and ordinary A-scan biometry in terms of its applicability, and its diagnostic and differential capabilities for lesions of the eye and orbit, as well as in

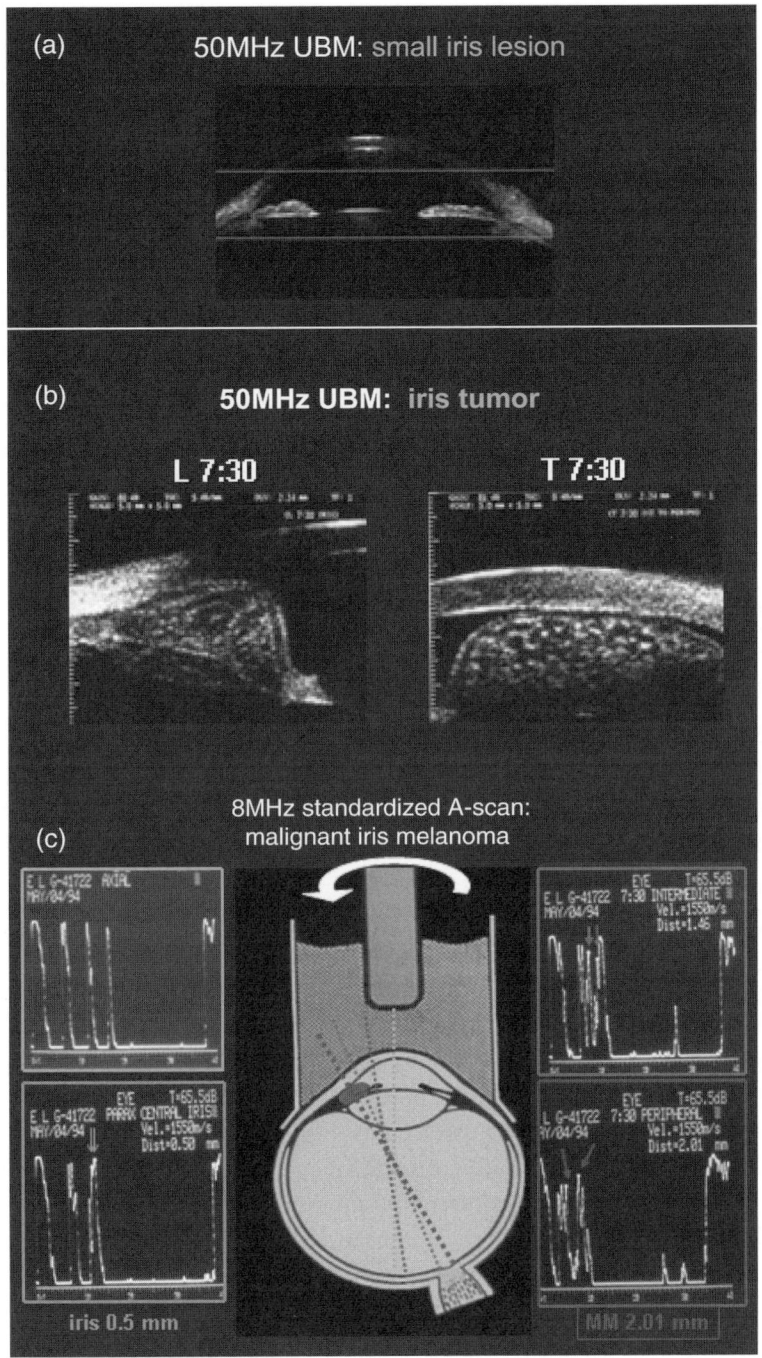

Fig. 15.1 (a) Iris tumour (benign nevus by A-scan). (b) Longitudinal (L), transverse (T) high-frequency ultrasonic biomicroscopy sections of a larger solid iris tumour. (c) Standardized A-scan (immersion technique) proves this iris tumour to be a malignant melanoma. (This figure is reproduced in colour in the colour plate section.)

its accuracy and precision of measurements of normal and abnormal ocular structures. Each of the available echographic techniques (i.e. diagnostic A-scan, diagnostic low-frequency and high-frequency B-scan, and biometric A-scan) is applied in the course of an echographic examination according to each one's optimal suitability and capability.

A multitude of ophthalmic echographers worldwide have contributed immensely to the development and consolidation of standardized echography. Their names are listed in the *Comprehensive Literature* available from the website on Standardized Echography (14).

What is standardized echography? (10, 15)
Optimal design
All internal instrument parameters of signal reception, amplification, and processing, which affect the A-scan display, including the A-scan probes, are specifically designed to allow a wide range of tissue diagnoses at a single gain setting, called tissue sensitivity (T). In addition, both B-scan and A-scan examination techniques are organized to fully support this instrument design and result in optimal sensitivities and specificities of tissue diagnoses as well as in a clear documentation of tissue locations and topographies.

Standardization
This optimal design of the A-scan instrumentation and of the A-scan and B-scan examination techniques is standardized, which gives the method its name, leading to the following effects:

- Standardized echography is *one* optimal echographic language.
- It produces unique, accurate, and safe differential diagnoses, localization, and measurements.
- Its results are reliable, understandable, comparable, and repeatable.
- All users of standardized echography can pool together and build on each other's experience.

B-scan
B-scan (5–7, 10–12, 14, 15) is utilized for topographic evaluations of a lesion (of its location, shape, insertion, and its relationship to normal structures), for estimations of a lesion's dimensions, and for some kinetic assessments of a lesion's mobility and consistency. B-scan of 10–20MHz is used for the posterior eye segment and anterior orbit; B-scan of 25–50MHz is preferred for evaluations of the anterior eye segment.

The 50MHz UBM presents one exception: its (B-scan) measurements are so precise that they replace A-scan biometry in the evaluation of the anterior eye segment. Fifty MHz B-scan techniques are standardized just like the low-frequency B-scan techniques are, in order to deliver understandable and unmistakable localizations. In the differentiation of tumours of the anterior eye segment (iris and ciliary body) the UBM clearly differentiates between cysts and solid tumours, but fails to further differentiate the solid ones; solid iris (and ciliary body) tumours are differentiated with standardized A-scan in the very same fashion as the posterior eye segment lesions are; but as is the case in axial eye length measurements with A-scan biometry, for the standardized A-scan diagnosis of anterior eye segment lesions an immersion procedure is required (Fig. 15.1).

A-scan

A-scan (5–7, 10–12, 14, 15) is used to diagnose and differentiate lesions—mainly through quantitative measurement of their internal structure, reflectivity, and sound absorption, and through kinetically determining their consistency, motion, motility, and vascularity. These kinetic evaluations are not duplicating those available with B-scan, but deliver different kinds of information.

For diagnosis and differentiation, A-scans are displayed at 'Tissue Sensitivity', an absolute, high, standardized gain setting obtained with the help of a 'Tissue Model'. Tissue structure is derived from the height, length, and width of the spikes and their distribution within the tissue echogram and is assessed as regular or irregular. Tissue reflectivity is indicated by the average height of all tissue spikes (excluding surface signals) as a percentage of the display height. Tissue absorption is measured from the decline of spike height within the tissue echogram from left to right (expressed by the angle 'kappa' and indicated in dB/mm tissue).

For precise peak-to-peak measurements 'Measuring Sensitivity', a relative, usually much reduced gain setting is applied. A perpendicular sound beam is aimed at both large surfaces whose distance is to be measured. Thus the height or thickness of tumours, the thickness of tissue sheets (e.g. cornea, lens, retina, choroid, sclera, optic nerve, extra-ocular muscles, peri-orbita), and the width or depth of fluid-filled spaces such as the anterior chamber, vitreous cavity, subarachnoidal fluid surrounding the optic nerve, etc. are measured.

Progress in hard- and software achieved since the 1990s has turned the originally time-consuming and difficult method of standardized echography into a quick, much less demanding, and more accurate method. The diagnosis of retinal detachment and its differentiation from dense fibrovascular membranes is, for instance, established and documented automatically within a few seconds of using a special software program (called 'A1') (15). All the echographer needs to do in this time-frame is to slightly angle and shift the probe (ultrasonic beam) in an attempt to aim a perpendicular sound beam at the surface in question (see Fig. 15.2).

Posterior eye segment

A host of posterior eye segment lesions and conditions (more than 75 different ones) ranging from vitreous detachments and haemorrhages to endogenous endophthalmitis, from synchysis nivea to posterior hyphemas, from macular oedema to retinal holes, from choroidal exudative detachments to expulsive haemorrhages, can be diagnosed and differentiated with standardized echography. Particularly important indications for this method are: the diagnosis and differentiation of tumours, retinal detachments, and the detection and localization of intra- or periocular foreign bodies.

Tumours in adult eyes

The diagnosis of intraocular tumours of the adult eye focuses primarily on their differentiation from *malignant melanoma*; many intraocular tumours clinically mimic that particular

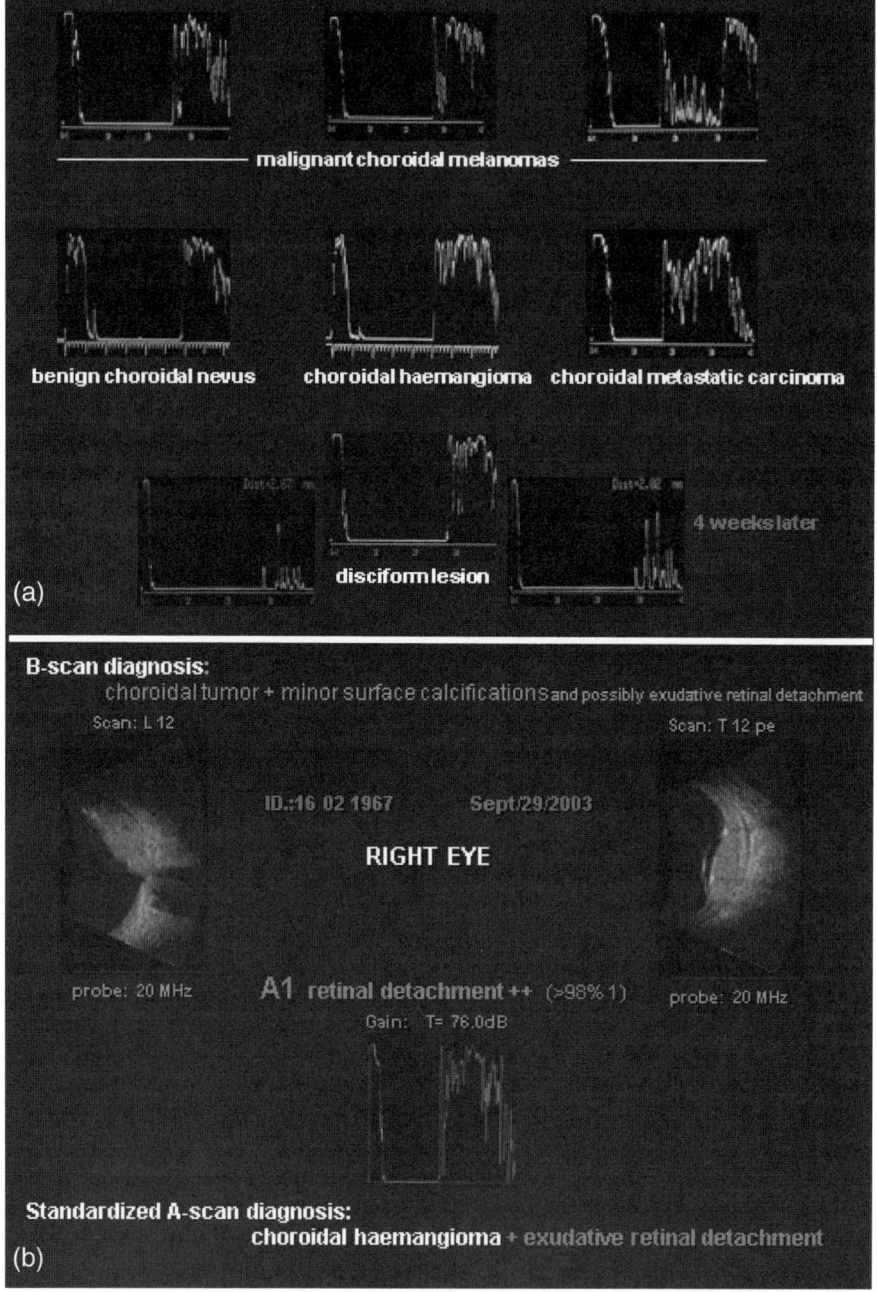

Fig. 15.2 (a) Acoustic patterns typical for different intraocular tumours. (b) Longitudinal (L) and transverse (T) 20MHz B-scans from intraocular tumour with small superficial calcifications producing shadows and overlying the tumour what probably is an exudative retinal detachment. Standardized A-scan confirmed choroidal haemangioma and proved (through an A_1 procedure) the overlying large surface to be retina; this diagnosis was automatically displayed and in parenthesis the reason for retina ++ is given: (reflectivity >98% + great smoothness of surface). (This figure is reproduced in colour in the colour plate section.)

Table 15.1 International melanoma study using standardized echography

# Cases of suspected melanomas*	1629
# Examiners	92
Sensitivity	99.0%
Specificity	97.9%

*All histopathologically verified.
Presented at San Francisco International Ophthalmology Congress 1980 (11).

malignant tumour. The following are the most important tumour types and their key A-scan differential criteria (Fig. 15.2):

- **Malignant melanoma:** in an International Study (11) (led by the ophthalmic echography service at the University of Iowa) of 1629 histologically proven ocular malignant melanomas, examined by 92 echographers in 13 different countries the unique value of standardized echography in the diagnosis and differential diagnosis of malignant ocular melanomas became obvious; the results were obtained at a time, when enucleation and thus histopathological examinations were still the standard management (Table 15.1).
  - Structure: regular
  - Reflectivity: 2–50%
  - Blood flow: + to +++.
- **Benign (elevated) nevus:** this rather frequent tumour clinically resembles a small malignant melanoma. It does not require treatment which would unnecessarily cause damage to the surrounding retina and its function.
  - Structure: slightly irregular
  - Reflectivity: very high (90–100%)
  - Blood flow: –.
- **Choroidal haemangioma:**
  - Structure: regular
  - Reflectivity: 85–95%
  - Blood flow: – (Doppler +).
- **Metastatic carcinoma:**
  - Structure: irregular
  - Reflectivity: 65–98%
  - Blood flow: –
  - Tumour spike height increases toward sclera.
- **Disciform macula degeneration (Kuhnt–Junius):**
  - Structure: regularly layered—3–4 long spikes
  - Reflectivity: 85–98%

- Blood flow: –
- Follow-up: elevation decreases.

Tumours in infants and children

The malignant retinoblastoma forms another important diagnostic task for standardized echography. Retinoblastomas are not easily recognized ophthalmoscopically when present and on the other hand often suspected when actually benign lesions ('pseudogliomas') occur.

Retinoblastomas are frequently calcified and then easily diagnosed with both B-scan and A-scan. Non-calcified (diffuse) retinoblastomas are diagnosed with standardized A-scan on the basis of their vascularity.

- **Calcified retinoblastoma:**
  - Irregular tumour mass
  - Partially calcified (dust-like): very high reflectivity
  - Shadowing.
- **Non-calcified (diffuse) retinoblastoma:**
  - Irregular structure
  - Low to medium high reflectivity
  - Vascularity.

Similarly to the malignant melanoma study, an International Collaborative Study (11) involving 319 consecutive cases of histologically proven retinoblastomas, examined by 56 different echographers in 13 different countries resulted in a sensitivity of 98.1% and a specificity of 97.8% (Table 15.2).

Orbit and periorbital region

The echographic diagnosis and differential diagnosis of orbital tumours (5–7, 10–12, 14) was developed by the author together with the echography of intraocular tumours and reached its peak popularity in the late 1980s. With the spread of advanced computed tomography (CT) and magnetic resonance imaging (MRI) technology orbital echography lost some of its leading status in the field of orbital diagnostics. Here again, the echography centres that used primarily or exclusively B-scan technology (which, for orbital examinations, is further limited by poor or insufficient sound penetration) caused the poor reputation of

Table 15.2 International retinoblastoma study using standardized echography

# Total cases of retinoblastomas*	319
# Examiners	56
Sensitivity	98.1%
Specificity	97.8%

*All histopathologically verified.
Presented at San Francisco International Ophthalmology Congress 1980 (11).

ophthalmic ultrasound in orbital diagnostics as compared to the improving radiological imaging procedures.

Standardized echography, however, remains clearly superior to the radiological imaging procedures in a number of areas, mostly because of greater resolution, real-time display, and safety in multiple re-examinations:

Reliable preoperative tissue differentiation

With standardized echography more than 60 different neoplasms and other space-occupying lesions can be detected and differentiated with a high degree of sensitivity and specificity. In orbital echography, A-scan is the primary method to detect and differentiate orbital and periorbital tumours including those within the posterior orbit and orbital apex. The differentiation is based on nine acoustic differential criteria evaluated with *quantitative echography* (structure, reflectivity, sound absorption), *topographic echography* (location, outline, shape), and *kinetic echography* (vascularity, mobility, consistency). Figure 15.3 illustrates some of the more frequent orbital tumours and their differences in structure, reflectivity, sound absorption and delineation.

Preoperative tissue diagnoses are very important for optimal patient treatment; they reveal whether partial or total biopsies or drainage are indicated and what surgical approach to the tumour will be appropriate. For instance, partial biopsies are standard in the presence of a lymphomatous neoplasm, whereas they are contraindicated in benign encapsulated tumours such as haemangiomas of the adult type, polymorphic adenomas, schwannomas, to mention a few. While small lacrimal gland tumours are best approached from anterior incisions at the brow region, larger tumours may require a lateral Kroenlein's approach with temporary resection of the lateral bone. When a malignant lacrimal gland tumour such as an adenoid cystic carcinoma is present, however, such an invasive procedure involving the peri-orbita and bony wall should be avoided.

Precise repeatable measurements

Precise measurements of the thicknesses of all six extraocular muscles at up to five well-defined and reproducible measuring points (Fig. 15.3) provide diagnoses of frequent orbital conditions such as *endocrine orbitopathy* and *orbital myositis* with a sensitivity and specificity of almost 100%. Unlike CT and MRI, echographic measurements include muscle sheaths, thus allowing an early diagnosis of optic nerve compression, a blinding condition.

Exact measurements of optic nerve thickness and optic nerve sheath distension are an important aid for early diagnosing optic nerve lesions and differentiating papilloedema from other causes of disc swelling (12).

Other advantages of standardized echography

Echographic evaluation of inflammatory and vascular lesions, unlimited follow-up examinations, easy examination of infants and children, intraoperative use (e.g. in localizing organic foreign bodies), and, last not least, relatively minimal costs of equipment and usage, all are beneficial advantages of standardized echography.

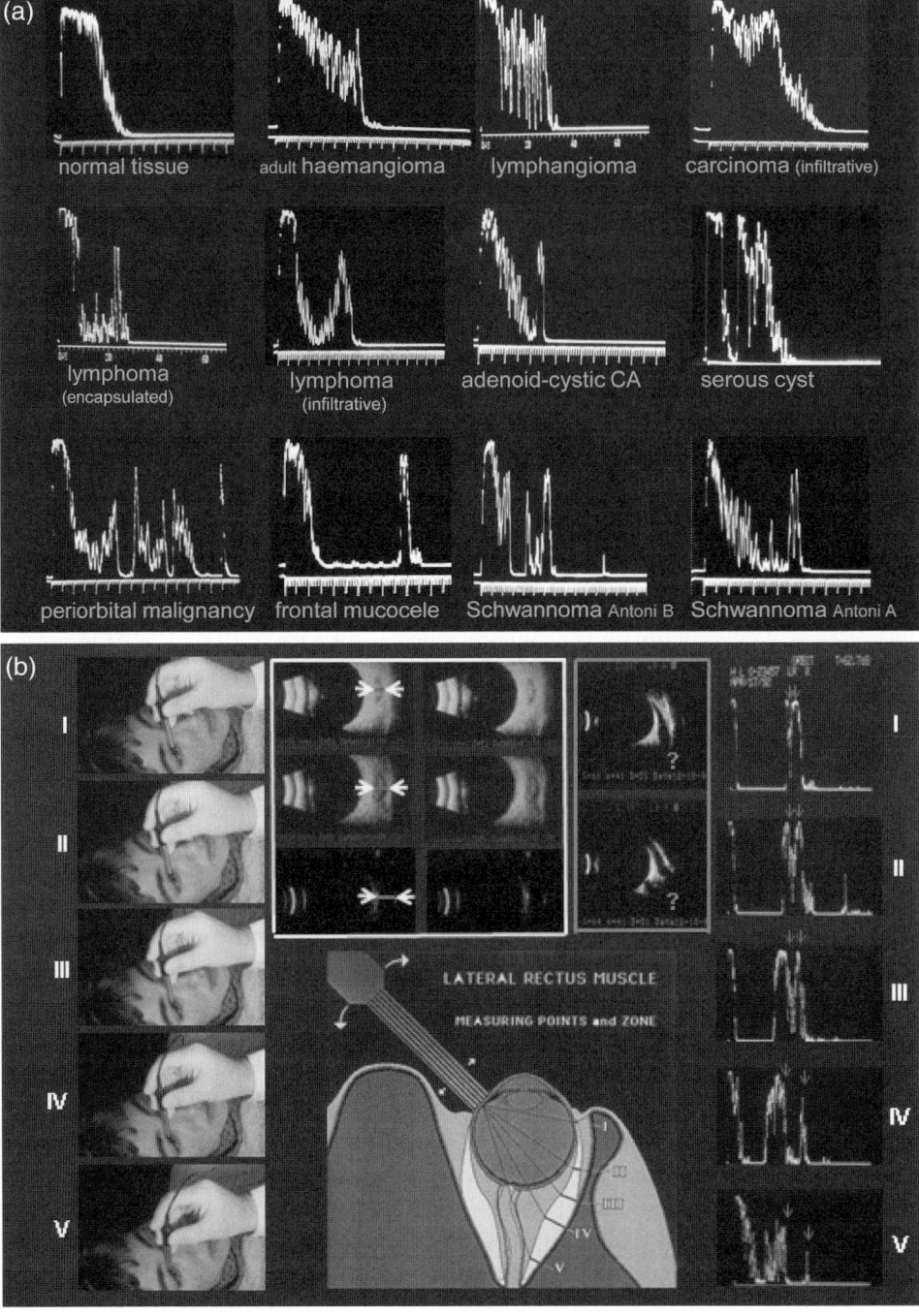

Fig. 15.3 (a) Acoustic patterns typical for different orbit tissues. (b) Illustration of the measurement of the thickness of an extraocular muscle in five different well-defined measuring points. (This figure is reproduced in colour in the colour plate section.)

References

1. Mundt GH, Hughes WF. Ultrasonics in ocular diagnosis. *Am J Ophth* 1956; **41**:488–98.
2. Oksala A, Lehtinen A. About the diagnostic use of ultrasound in ophthalmology (German). *Ophthalmologica (Basel)* 1957: **134**:387–95.
3. Baum G, Greenwood I. The application of ultrasonic locating techniques to ophthalmology. *Am J Ophth* 1958; **46**:319–29.
4. Jansson F. Measurements of intraocular distances by ultrasound. *Acta Ophthal Kbh* 1963; Suppl. 74.
5. Ossoinig KC. Echographic diagnosis of ocular tumors – clinical and experimental examinations (German). *Klin Monatsbl Augenheilkd* 1965; **146**:321–37.
6. Ossoinig KC. Routine ultrasonography of the orbit. *Int Ophthalmol Clin* 1969; **9**(3):613–42.
7. Ossoinig KC. Basics, methods, and results of ultrasonography used in the diagnosis of intraocular tumors. In: Gitter KA, Keeney AH, Sarin LK, Meyer D (eds) *Ophthalmic Ultrasound* (Proceedings of International Symposium in Philadelphia 1968). St Louis, MO: CV Mosby Company; 1969, pp.282–93.
8. Bronson NR. Development of a simple B-scan ultrasonoscope. *Trans Am Ophthal Soc* 1972; **70**:365–40.
9. Coleman DJ, Lizzi FL, Jack RL. *Ultrasonography of the eye and orbit*. Philadelphia, PA: Lea & Febiger, 1977.
10. Ossoinig KC. Standardized echography: Basic principles, clinical applications and results. *Int Ophthalmology Clinics* 1979; **19**(4):127–210.
11. Ossoinig KC. Advances in diagnostic ultrasound. In: Henkind P (ed) *ACTA XXIV, International Congress of Ophthalmology, Vol 1*. New York: J.B. Lippincott; 1982, pp.89–114.
12. Ossoinig KC. Standardized echography of the optic nerve (Jules Francois Memorial Lecture). In: Till P (ed) *Ophthalmic Echography 13 (Documenta Ophthalmologica Proceedings Series 55)*. New York: Kluwer Academic Publishers, 1993, pp.3–99.
13. Pavlin CJ, Foster FS. *Ultrasound biomicroscopy of the eye*. New York: Springer-Verlag, 1994.
14. Comprehensive literature on standardized echography available at http://www.echography.com under 'History'.
15. Ossoinig KC. *Diagnostic ultrasound in ophthalmology, Vol 1: Basics of Standardized Echography* [CD]. Echographic Teaching Services, 2009. Available at: www.echography.com.

Chapter 16

The development of ultrasound in otorhinolaryngology

Pernilla Sahlstrand Johnson and Magnus Jannert

Summary

The use of ultrasound in the field of otorhinolaryngology goes back almost 40 years. Ultrasonography with simple A-mode has proved to be successful for identifying diseased maxillary and frontal sinuses. It is generally accepted that ultrasonography is of value in diagnosing acute rhinosinusitis; in cases of chronic rhinosinusitis both A- and B-mode ultrasound have limited value. B-mode ultrasound is mainly used for soft tissue examination of the neck and has not developed to the extent that was expected for the paranasal sinuses. Computed tomography (CT) is still the gold standard for investigation in chronic rhinosinusitis when grading the severity of the disease and when the patient will be subject to surgical intervention. Ultrasound-guided fine-needle biopsy of the neck and Doppler ultrasound for evaluation of the blood vessels of the neck will also be of great value in the future. Doppler ultrasound of the paranasal sinus shows promising results in identifying the characteristics of sinus secretion, and there is ongoing research on this application. The first clinical evaluation in patients with sinusitis, examined with ultrasound Doppler, will be performed in 2011.

Ultrasound in the field of otorhinolaryngology

Ultrasound examination of the neck and ultrasound-guided fine-needle biopsy are well established methods in the field of otorhinolaryngology (1). The ultrasound technique is of great value when identifying lymph nodes, cysts, and abscesses of the neck. Furthermore, ultrasound can be used to differentiate diffuse changes in the thyroid and salivary glands from solitary lumps and cysts. Ultrasound is also of importance when examining the parathyroid glands (2). Additionally, Doppler ultrasound is a very successful method to diagnose stenosis of the arteries of the neck (3). However, these examinations are mainly executed by physicians skilled in ultrasound outside the departments of otorhinolaryngology.

Another field of application is the development of user-friendly ultrasound equipment, which can be used by physicians in primary care or by otolaryngologists in order to improve the diagnostics of rhinosinusitis (4, 5). This is an important diagnostic tool, since it has been known for more than 40 years that diagnoses of acute rhinosinusitis (ARS) based on clinical examination alone, is correct in only 50% of cases (6).

Ultrasound of the paranasal sinuses

The idea of using ultrasound in order to separate healthy air-containing sinuses from diseased ones goes back to Keidel in 1947 (7). Essential experiments and development were performed in Germany by Mann, in Finland by Revonta, and in Sweden by Jannert and Holmer, in the 1970s and 1980s (4, 8, 9). In a productive cooperation with the industry, simple inexpensive ultrasound equipment for use in the outpatient clinics was produced in all three countries. The method has now been used, mainly in Europe, in clinical practice for more than 30 years, and the method is available around the world.

Two separate ultrasonic methods are employed for examination of the paranasal sinuses, the A-mode and B-mode. From a technical point of view the A-mode is the least advanced and the least expensive method. In cases of healthy air-containing sinuses the ultrasound beam penetrates the anterior wall of the frontal or maxillary sinus but is totally reflected by the air in the sinus. On the display unit only the transducer pulse and the air–mucosa echo (AME) are seen (Fig. 16.1). The distance between the transducer pulse and the AME can be used to estimate the thickness of the mucosa of the anterior wall. If the AME is within a distance of 1.5–3.0cm from the transducer pulse it indicates mucosal swelling of the anterior sinus wall. If the sinus is filled with fluid, e.g. secretion, the ultrasound beam passes through the secretion and is reflected in the back wall of the sinus cavity. The corresponding echogram shows a distinct back-wall echo (BWE), indicating a pathological process in the sinus (Fig. 16.2). In 1986 the capture-mode was added to the A-mode equipment (11). This application implies that all reflected echoes are collected on the screen and the risk of missing information can hereby be reduced. The capture-mode can be used for screening, but every examination must be repeated with ordinary A-mode before any conclusion can be drawn. The A-mode can be used for the maxillary sinus as well as for the frontal sinus, but not for the ethmoidal or sphenoid sinuses.

The B-mode employs the same principle as the A-mode, but in the B-mode the transducer consist of many piezoelectric crystal elements used in combination creating a

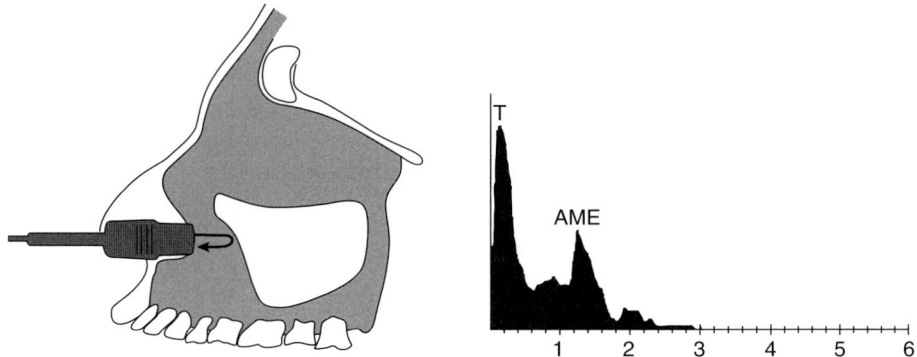

Fig. 16.1 Normal air-containing sinus and the corresponding normal echogram. An air–mucosa echo (AME) found at a distance of 1.5–3.0cm from the transducer pulse (T) indicates mucosal swelling of the anterior wall. Reproduced from Stierna P, Karlsson G, Melén I, Jannert M (eds). *Aspects on Sinusitis. Diagnosis and treatment in Adults*. Sweden: Eli Lilly Sweden AB; 1996, with permission.

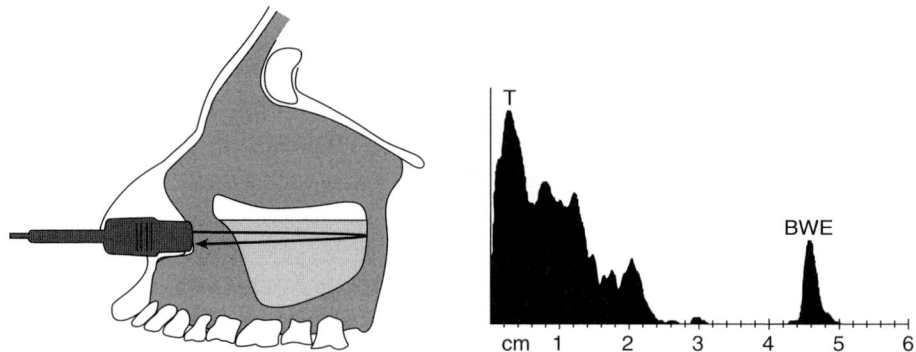

Fig. 16.2 Maxillary sinusitis with secretion and the corresponding echogram showing a back-wall echo at a distance of 4.6 cm. BWE, back-wall echo; T, transducer pulse. Reproduced from Stierna P, Karlsson G, Melén I, Jannert M (eds). *Aspects on Sinusitis. Diagnosis and treatment in Adults*. Sweden: Eli Lilly Sweden AB; 1996, with permission.

two-dimensional image. The B-mode requires a much more sophisticated technique and therefore makes it more expensive than the A-mode device.

Clinical relevance for ultrasonic examination of the paranasal sinuses

Acute rhinosinusitis is one of the most common reasons for seeking medical advice today. It was found in 1999 that an average of 8.4% of the Dutch population had at least one episode of ARS per year and according to National Ambulatory Medical Care Survey data in the United States, rhinosinusitis is the fifth most common diagnosis for which an antibiotic is prescribed. In 2002, rhinosinusitis accounted for 9% of all paediatric and 21% of all adult antibiotic prescriptions in the United States. The diagnosis of ARS is often based on clinical examination alone, which leads to high rates of false positive results. Consequently, the risk of unnecessary prescription of antibiotics for ARS is large, with the effect of increased antimicrobial resistance which is a serious public health problem in the world today. Sinus radiography, CT and ultrasound are useful tools in improving the diagnostic of ARS. However, both plain radiography and CT imply that the patient is exposed to radiation, which might be harmful, while ultrasound for medical purposes is proven to be harmless. Conventional A-mode ultrasound is successful for diagnosing ARS and detecting fluid of the maxillary sinuses with a sensitivity of 90–97% (5, 8, 12).

Non-invasive staging of a sinus infection with Doppler ultrasound

Ultrasound and CT determines the presence of fluid in the paranasal sinuses, but it says nothing of the property of the sinus fluid. In antibiotics-demanding ARS the paranasal sinuses contain purulent secretions. The only way to identify mucopurulent sinus fluid, and thereby determine if antibiotics are needed, is by performing a sinus puncture. Sinus puncture and irrigation involves penetrating the maxillary sinus cavity with a needle via the nose through a bony wall, which is an uncomfortable procedure for the patient. From mucopurulent secretions (with a high grade of viscosity) it has generally been possible to isolate bacteria, whereas bacteria have only rarely been isolated from serous type of sinus secretions (fluid with low viscosity). The hypothesis is that the viscosity of the sinus secretions is related to the need of treatment with antibiotics in ARS. If the consistency of the sinus fluid could be determined non-invasively, it would indicate if the fluid contains bacteria or not and consequently if antibiotics, and possibly sinus irrigations, are needed to treat the rhinosinusitis. With such a method it would also be possible to follow the recovery of a patient with serous rhinosinusitis and prescribe antibiotics only if the sinus fluid becomes mucous. A more specific diagnostic method would reduce the discomfort for patients with ARS, and in addition mean a significant reduction of cost in terms of reduced number of irrigations, antibiotic treatments, antimicrobial resistance, and patients in need of an extended sick-leave.

The Doppler technique

Acoustic streaming is the term applied to unidirectional flow currents in a fluid, caused by sound waves. It is generated by the absorption of energy from acoustic oscillations of the sound wave (13). The technique of using acoustic streaming to non-invasively measure the viscous properties of an enclosed fluid is not new. In the early 1990s, Dymling et al. used the method to observe a difference in acoustic streaming from fresh and sour milk (14). More recently there has also been a growing interest in utilizing acoustic streaming for medical purposes. Nightingale et al. showed that acoustic streaming could be induced and detected in breast cysts *in vivo*. Later Clarke et al. used acoustic streaming to estimate the viscosity of ovarian cyst content. In both these works acoustic streaming was induced in a fluid volume with dimensions close to 15ml, which is a typical size of a maxillary sinus. However, there is at least one crucial difference; the maxillary sinus is surrounded by bone. Bone is highly sound attenuating and therefore a large part of the sound will be lost to the bone before it arrives at the sinus cavity. However, by restricting the incoming sound beam to a region in front of the maxillary sinus called the fossa canina, where the bone is thin and compact, the influence of bone attenuation is minimized. When testing Doppler ultrasound equipment developed for this purpose, a measurable acoustic streaming can be generated in serous sinus fluid with low viscosity, but not in mucopurulent secretions with high viscosity *in vitro*. The attenuation of the mucopurulent sinus fluid is shown to be 10 times higher than that of serous cyst fluid, whereas the viscosity of the mucopurulent secretion was 1000-fold times higher than that of the cyst fluid. As the acoustic streaming is proportional to the attenuation of a fluid, but inversely proportional to the viscosity the results indicate that the method seems to be applicable in clinical practice to separate non-purulent secretions from purulent (15). Clinical studies on the Doppler technique in rhinosinusitis are now in progress.

Safety of the ultrasound technique

Ultrasound examination of the sinus is a safe method and can, for example, be used without risk on pregnant women. There are no reports of biological side effects of medical ultrasound for examining body tissue. For the examination of the paranasal sinuses an intensity of maximum 10mW/cm^2 is used. This is one-tenth of the intensity which, according to a very early World Health Organization recommendation, can be used without any time limit.

When using Doppler for examination of the maxillary sinus there is a risk of increased heat within the bone of the frontal wall. However, tests performed at the Department of Electrical Measurements, Lund University, Sweden, shows that the temperature increase of the bone is within a safe limit. The safety experiments gave a temperature increase of the bone of less than 1.5°C, which is below the temperature increase considered to be harmful according to the World Federation for Ultrasound in Medicine and Biology (15).

Future clinical applications

Another application of the Doppler ultrasound in the future might be examination of children with otitis media with effusion, in order to obtain a non-invasive guidance of the necessity for myringotomy, evacuation of middle ear effusion, and tubulation of the middle ear. Additionally, from a theoretical point of view, ultrasound may also be useful, for example, to eliminate stones in the submandibular glands, but clinical experiments in patients are still missing.

Studies from recent years have proposed the use of therapeutic pulsed ultrasound to relieve symptoms of chronic rhinosinusitis (CRS) (16). Rhinosinusitis is said to be 'chronic' when there have been symptoms and signs of disease for 3 months or more, despite adequate therapy. The background to this ultrasound application is the possible role for bacterial biofilms in the pathophysiology of CRS. Bacterial biofilms have been defined as a 'structured community of bacterial cells enclosed in a self-produced polymeric matrix and adherent to an inert or living surface' (17) and there is ongoing research in this field. Ultrasound appears to improve the antibiotic effect, but the exact mechanism is still unknown. The intensity used in published studies was up to 1500mW/cm^2 (16), significantly above the levels reported in diagnostic Doppler ultrasound of the paranasal sinuses. Disregarding the safety issues with the proximity of the eye, those results have suggested that a positive effect may be achieved from the ultrasound. Finding an acceptable power level may lead to an instrument, which can serve both as a diagnostic tool as well as a therapeutic device, and thereby offer simultaneous diagnosis and therapy.

Acknowledgement

We thank Professor N.-G. Holmer for factual examination of the text.

References

1. Baatenburg de Jong RJ, Rongen RJ, Verwoerd CD, van Overhagen H, Laméris JS, Knegt P. Ultrasound-guided fine-needle aspiration biopsy of neck nodes. *Arch Otolaryngol Head Neck Surg* 1991; **117**:402–4.
2. Solbiati L, Osti V, Cova L, Tonolini M. Ultrasound of thyroid, parathyroid glands and neck lymph nodes. *Eur Radiol* 2001; **11**(12):2411–24.

3. Grant EG, Benson CB, Moneta GL, Alexandrov AV, Baker JD, Bluth EI, et al. Carotid artery stenosis: gray-scale and Doppler US diagnosis. Society of Radiologists in Ultrasound Consensus Conference. *Radiology* 2003; **229**(2):340–6.
4. Revonta M. Ultrasound in the diagnosis of maxillary and frontal sinusitis. *Acta Otolaryngol.* 1980; **370**(Suppl.):1–55.
5. Jannert M. *Maxillary Ostial Function Tests and Diagnostic Ultrasonography of Paranasal Sinuses–An Experimental and Clinical Study.* (Thesis.) Skurup, Sweden: Lindbergs Blankett AB; 1982.
6. Axelsson A, Grebelius N, Chidekel N, Jensen C. The correlation between the radiological examination and the irrigation findings in maxillary sinusitis. *Acta Otolaryngol* 1970; **69**(4):302–6.
7. Keidel WD. Über die Verwendung des Ultraschalls in der klinischen Diagnostik. *Ärtzliche Forschung* 1947; **1**:349.
8. Mann W, Beck C, Apostolidis T. Liability of ultrasound in maxillary sinus disease. *Arch Otorhinolaryngol* 1977; **215**(1):67–74.
9. Jannert M, Andreasson L, Holmer NG, Lorinc P. Ultrasonic examination of the paranasal sinuses. *Acta Otolaryngol* 1982; **389**(Suppl.):1–52.
10. Stierna P, Karlsson G, Melén I, Jannert M (eds). *Aspects on Sinusitis. Diagnosis and treatment in Adults.* Sweden: Eli Lilly Sweden AB; 1996.
11. Jannert M, Andréasson L, Benthin M, Dahl P. Ultrasonography of the paranasal sinuses. A new computerized equipment using LCD-display and capture mode. *Rhinology* 1987; **25**(2):133–7.
12. Varonen H, Makela M, Savolainen S, Laara E, Hilden J. Comparison of ultrasound, radiography, and clinical examination in the diagnosis of acute maxillary sinusitis: a systematic review. *J Clin Epidemiol* 2000; **53**:940–8.
13. Wu J, Du G. Acoustic streaming generated by a focused Gaussian beam and finite amplitude tonebursts. *Radiology* 2003; **229**(2):340–6.
14. Dymling SO, Persson HW, Hertz TG, Lindström K. A new ultrasonic method for fluid property measurements. *Ultrasound Med Biol* 1991; **17**(5):497–500.
15. Sahlstrand-Johnson P, Jönsson P, Persson H W, Holmer N-G, Jannert M, Jansson T. In vitro-studies and safety assessment of Doppler ultrasound as a diagnostic tool in rhinosinusitis. *Ultrasound Med Biol* 2010; **36**(12):2123–31.
16. Young D, Morton R, Bartley J. Therapeutic ultrasound as treatment for chronic rhino-sinusitis: preliminary observations. *J Laryngol Otol* 2010; **124**(5):495–9.
17. Costerton JW, Stewart PS, Greenberg EP. Bacterial biofilms: a common cause of persistent infections. *Science* 1999; **284**:1318–22.

Chapter 17

The industrial development of ultrasound—a Swedish perspective

Gunnar Arveheim

My first contact with diagnostic ultrasound was in 1969, when I attended a demonstration of a Siemens Vidoson at Falun hospital, Sweden. A few Vidoson systems were installed in Sweden by the end of the 1960s. I was at that time sales engineer at the Medical Electronics Department at LIC, supplier of products to the public Swedish healthcare system.

I joined Roche Bio-Electronics in 1971. There were some early ultrasound products—Fetasonde continuous wave (CW) Doppler and Arteriosonde blood pressure units made in Cranbury, United States, and a French echoencephaloscope. I visited Lund several times in 1972 and became fascinated by the pioneering ultrasound work performed by Dr Inge Edler.

Roche Bio-Electronics was transferred to Kontron, Zürich in 1973. I was entrusted to start up the Swedish subsidiary Kontron AB in February 1973. Bio-Electronics service engineer, Åke Larsén, also accepted the Kontron offer.

I decided to focus on ultrasound in 1974, left Kontron, and joined a small trading company, Wabloprodukter, as a third part-owner, starting an electromedical department, without salary but 10% commission on sales. Wablo became distributor for Parks Medical Electronics, Oregon, one of the early Doppler manufacturers.

Doptone, the first fetal pulsedetector, was released in 1965 by Smith Kline Instruments (SKI), after a technology transfer agreement with Professor Rushmer's team, headed by Don Baker, Bioengineering Department, University of Washington, Seattle. Later, in 1965, Loren Parks released Parks first fetal and vascular CW Doppler instruments.

The two first Wablo years became economically tough. I was close to giving up, but made a final week sales trip in southern Sweden in May 1975. On Friday of that week, visiting Allmänna Sjukhuset, Malmö (part of Lund University), Professor Lindell, of the Clinical Physiology Department said: 'We have tried to find a Parks distributor, so far without success, we need to order two 806 Dopplers'. That became the turning point, and I decided to continue. During the coming years Wablo delivered thousands of Parks Dopplers in the Nordic countries. Most of them are still today, 30+ years later, in daily clinical use!

At the 2nd European Ultrasound Congress, Munich 1975, the Advanced Diagnostic Research (ADR) booth was crammed. Finally, on the 3rd day, I managed to see what was creating such huge interest. An ADR representative dressed as an American cowboy was scanning an aquarium with the new ADR 2130 linear array scanner and you could see swimming fishes on the monitor! I wanted to negotiate Nordic distribution, but was asked to talk to Marty Wilcox, ADR founder/President, who, however, already had left. Later I found out that ADR had appointed Kranzbühler, Solingen, Germany, as European distributor.

Attending the 1st World Federation of Ultrasound in Medicine and Biology (WFUMB), San Francisco August 1976, I met several ultrasound pioneers: Feigenbaum, Goldberg, Strandness, Birnholz, Kossoff, Cosgrove, Holm, and Jouppila.

In October 1976, Wablo signed a Nordic contract with Advanced Technology Laboratories (ATL), Seattle, as their second distributor. ATL was founded in 1969 and after a technology transfer agreement with the University of Washington started developing ultrasound equipment. ATL exhibited the first pulsed wave (PW) Doppler at the American Institute of Ultrasound in Medicine meeting (AIUM), Seattle, 1974. Their PW-Doppler 500A was released in 1975. Their 600B M-mode scanner (1976) became a big success, replacing the SKI Ekoline20 as the 'gold standard'.

In 1976 I became majority owner of Wabloprodukter, when the founder/President decided to concentrate his business into another company he owned.

ATL introduced MarkV, the first Duplex scanner 1977, by adding a module for real-time sector scanning to the M-mode and PW Doppler modules. Wablo bought an ATL MarkV demo system on a 6-month sales or return basis. Despite intense demo activities no order was received before the 6-month deadline. That became the most difficult decision in my business career. I convinced my bank, borrowed the required money, paid, and kept the system. Åke Larsén joined Wablo that year as Service Manager.

In April 1978, Wablo got the first MarkV order outside the United States from Dr Sivertsson, Östra Sjukhuset, Gothenburg, followed by another from Professor Areskog, Linköping. Four more ATL orders were received in 1978—one from Sweden and one each from Norway, Finland, and Denmark.

State-of-the-art general imaging ultrasound at that time was the huge, expensive static compound B-scanners. I found that the cardiac ATL produced more diagnostic information and better images in real time, compared to those B-scanners. Doctors and decision-makers claimed that you couldn't use a cardiac system in general imaging. However, I was not convinced.

Professor Curt Lagergren, Karolinska University Hospital, arranged an ultrasound symposium at Riksstämman in 1977 (Swedish Doctors Annual Meeting), attended mostly by interested surgeons. Dr Göran Karner, Motala argued, however, that ultrasound should stay within radiology. He convinced Lagergren he could arrange a radiology ultrasound course in 1978. At this Vadstena/Motala course in August, UK ultrasound doctors Keith Dewbury, David Cosgrove, and Hylton Meire were lecturers and instructors. I invited sonographer Sandra Hagen, then working for Dr Goldberg, Thomas Jefferson University Hospital, Philadelphia for hands-on instruction. (Sandra Hagen-Ansert later became President of the American Sonographer's Society.)

Monday morning started with an ultrasound system overview. It was said you needed a compound B-scanner to get optimum structure information, but some B-scanners have an optional dynamic sector module, which may be valuable as guide deciding the best scanning plane, although insufficient for diagnoses because of poor resolution.

After lunch, groups of seven or eight doctors were organized and allocated 30 minutes in each examination room. Sandra was scanning—no comments in the first group. Then the second group entered the room. Suddenly one doctor said: 'I think these images are better than the compound B-scanner images we saw in the first room.' Another doctor agreed and everybody started talking. Somebody suggested finding Cosgrove to have him see this system. He replaced Sandra scanning and agreed this was the best dynamic images he ever had seen, but added that the penetration needed improvement.

The following week a demonstration was booked at a hospital with a budget for a B-scanner twice the ATL price. When asked if the doctor might recommend buying an ATL, he answered they were doing many biopsies, which was why they needed a compound B-scanner—but they wanted to budget an ATL within 2–3 years. Unfamiliar with biopsy procedures, I accepted this explanation.

The next demonstration was for Dr PG Lindgren at Akademiska University Hospital, Uppsala, and this also went well, especially after Lindgren insisted that the monitor settings should be changed.

I told Lindgren that another hospital couldn't consider ATL, as they were doing many biopsies and therefore needed a compound B-scanner. Dr Lindgren turned around saying: 'That's exactly what we should use this scanner for. Biopsies should be done in real-time, not by static ultrasound guidance!' That night he built at home a biopsy adaptor to the ATL scanhead and the next morning started the first real-time ultrasound guided biopsies globally! He had a budget for a B-scanner, but convinced the hospital to also invest in the ATL. Dr Lindgren thus became, in 1978, the first ATL radiology customer globally.

First-wave ultrasound market consolidation started in 1979. Technicare was acquired by Johnson&Johnson for US$87 million. Squibb bought ATL for US$60 million and Spacelabs, a manufacturer of Intensive Care Unit/Critical Care Unit patient monitoring, for US$34.4 million. Squibb formed Squibb Medical Systems (SMS) in 1980 bought ADR in 1982 for US$37 million, and finally also Kranzbühler, ADR's European distributor.

In 1981, as distributor for Ausonics, Australia, commercializing the ultrasound pioneer research by George Kossoff, Wablo installed Ausonics Octoson water-based breast scanners in Linköping and at Karolinska.

Wablo was extremely successful but seriously undercapitalized, which is why I sold Wablo in 1980 to Finnish Kone Corporation, but continued as employed President. Kone also had acquired Olli Elektromedicin. Wablo and Olli were merged to Kone Instrument AB with me as President. Kone sales in 1983 continued growing, although that summer I began questioning the future.

After Squibb acquired ATL in 1979, the research and development (R&D) budget was reduced, and ATL started losing their technology leadership. The brightest ATL engineers joined Quantum, Issaquah to continue colour Doppler imaging (CDI) development. The ADR move from Arizona to Seattle 1983–84 also created problems, as new SMS/ATL managers were hired, with limited ultrasound and/or international knowledge/experience.

During the ECR (European Congress of Radiology), Bordeaux, 1983 it became obvious that competition had increased in all market segments. I asked for a meeting with my boss in Helsinki and handed over my resignation. He read it, looked at me, and demonstratively tore it to pieces and threw it in the waste basket saying he could not accept this. I received several promises and accepted to stay. As nothing changed, I sent my final resignation letter some months later, but agreed to stay until year end. Kone received 37 ATL orders in 1983, over 50% of the Nordic cardiac and radiology ultrasound market.

In January 1984, I founded Amedic AB. The business idea was to commercialize Swedish biomedical inventions. As the Swedish market of 9 million people is quite small—compared to the United States (265 million), Germany (82 million), or California (36 million)—my focus was to address at least the Nordic market (25 million), but preferably the global market.

The major products became ultrasound biopsy systems based on cooperation with Dr Lindgren. In 1984–85 Amedic signed OEM contracts with ATL, Kranzbühler, CGR, Acuson, and Philips.

Several Kone suppliers including SMS/ATL offered Amedic Nordic dealerships. My response to ATL was no, mainly because I didn't have enough capital. However, Amedic signed a Nordic distribution agreement with Parks.

Meeting John Larsson, owner/founder of Medata AB, Stockholm and ATL distributor in USSR Communist countries, I told him about the ATL offer. He suggested a joint venture, a new company Medata Nordic AB; he could invest needed capital as a 'sleeping partner' if I ran the day-to-day business. Thus Medata Nordic was founded in May 1984. John Larsson and family paid 69%, my family and some key officers 31% of the share capital. An office near Stockholm-Arlanda airport was rented and staff hired, including several from Kone Instrument. Medata Nordic/ATL recaptured the Nordic market leadership with about 60% market share in 1985.

John Larsson was one of very few Westerners who personally knew influential Communist leaders having free access to Kremlin. He owned a magnificent apartment on the classy, expensive Strandvägen, downtown Stockholm and had a Rolls Royce Silver Shadow limousine in the garage. He allowed Communist leaders to stay in that apartment and use the Rolls-Royce whenever they visited Stockholm. As Lenin had three Rolls Royces in Moscow, the Communist leaders during the 1970s and 1980s had difficulty resisting this offer.

At the 1st WFUMB Congress, San Francisco, 1976 I saw the first phased array systems by Grumman and Varian. Both were huge, expensive, and had mediocre image quality and never became successful in the market. Hewlett-Packard (HP) became, in 1981, the first to successfully market a phased array, the 77020 Echocardiography system. The first international installation was at Akademiska University Hospital, Uppsala, under Dr Johan Landelius.

HP 77020 was developed by a team headed by Sam Maslak. He wanted to continue ultrasound development, but HP instead offered him other development projects, as HP considered diagnostic ultrasound was now close to perfection. Maslak left HP, forming a general partnership with Robert Younge, a HP colleague. Another HP engineer,

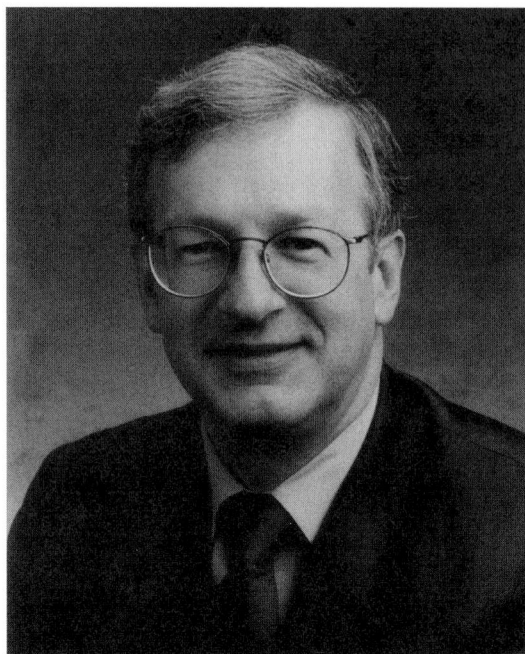

Fig. 17.1 Sam Maslak, founder, President, and Chief Executive Officer, Acuson Corporation 1979–2000. (This figure is reproduced in colour in the colour plate section.)

Amin Hanafy, joined in 1981. They continued ultrasound development and managed to raise US$2.5 million in venture capital, starting Acuson in 1981 (Fig. 17.1).

In an American financial journal in 1983 I saw a notice that a start-up company, Acuson, had presented a new general imaging ultrasound system, the Acuson128 system, at the Leading Edge Ultrasound Conference, Atlantic City. As Åke Larsén, Wablo/Kone service manager was soon to visit ATL together with Dr PG Lindgren, to discuss and explain ultrasound-guided biopsy, I told Larsén to continue to San Francisco to find Acuson, before returning home. Lindgren joined him. They found Acuson in Mountain View, south of San Francisco, and went there offering Acuson the Lindgren biopsy guide solution, and also to gain information about Acuson and their technology and to suggest Kone as the Nordic distributor.

Dr Lindgren was in the process of buying a premium ultrasound system 1984 and so wanted to evaluate the Acuson128. Together we flew to California. Dr Lindgren insisted on visiting clinics which used Acuson and listened to their experience. The closest references were around Los Angeles, which is why we visited two different Los Angeles hospitals.

Dr Lindgren became convinced; Amedic signed an Acuson Nordic distribution contract and received the first order outside the United States in October 1984. Amedic agreed with Akademiska to exhibit this system during Riksstämman in Stockholm, before installation in the beginning of December. I believed then in a possible Nordic market of a maximum of three to five systems/year because of the price (twice that of the ATL UltraMark 8), which is why I focused on ultrasound luminaries passing the booth.

Dr Adiels, from Oskarshamn countryside hospital, became extremely interested; I politely answered his questions, while I noticed several luminaries passing by. He called 10 months later in October 1985 telling me he had approval to buy an Acuson. Originally, he had asked unsuccessfully for a computed tomography (CT) scanner, then instead requested an advanced ultrasound system, which was accepted. Now I understood—although Acuson was twice the price of premium ultrasound systems, it still was cheap compared to other diagnostic modalities like CT. I also realized that the purchase price only was a part of an investment, more important was diagnostic capability (Acuson had two to three times higher detail and contrast resolution), offering quicker diagnosis and reduced need of other examinations, with total time and cost reduction potential.

In 1985 Acuson and Parks distribution were transferred from Amedic to Medata Nordic, in order to establish a complete Nordic ultrasound supplier.

Acuson's United States market success in 1985 made SMS/ATL nervous. The general imaging ultrasound market in the United States in 1985 showed a new market leader. Acuson captured 27%, Diasonics 20%, ATL 13%, Johnson & Johnson (J&J) (Technicare) 11%, Philips 7%, Picker 7%, General Electric (GE) 4%, and Toshiba 4% in $ order value. In a SMS letter in December 1985, Medata Nordic was told to cancel Acuson distribution or SMS would cancel Medata Nordic dealership. We explained, as the Acuson price was twice the most expensive ATL, we did not see those systems competing and our vision was to become established as the number one Nordic ultrasound supplier.

SMS/ATL did not listen and instead increased their threat to also cancel the Medata AB CSSR distribution agreement—blackmailing, as Medata/ATL was the largest ultrasound supplier in the USSR. Larsson got worried and we discussed several possible solutions in spring 1986.

Acuson Vice President Bob Gallagher, suggested an urgent meeting, but my calendar was completely full. I suggested that he flew to Helsinki, as I was booked on the Helsinki-Stockholm ferry on Friday, April 26, and we could meet and have dinner onboard. In the restaurant, Bob explained that Acuson was establishing more subsidiaries and wanted me as Country Manager of a Swedish Acuson subsidiary. He wanted to fax an employment contract proposal, for my consideration.

I had to fulfil a few criteria before accepting this offer: find a new Medata Nordic President; make sure that no Medata Nordic or Amedic employees or suppliers were negatively affected; and that Medata got fairly compensated for Acuson market introduction expenses.

I contacted first the deputy managing director at Technicare AB. J&J had sold Technicare in 1986 to GE, who decided to wind up Technicare and its global subsidiaries, which was why he had been given notice. We met at a roadside restaurant. I asked if he might be interested in succeeding me as Medata Nordic President and he accepted to succeed me in August 1986.

On 27 June 1986, Medata Nordic sent the famous telex, 187cm long, starting with: 'WE HAVE THE PLEASURE TO ORDER ONE DOZEN ACUSON 128.'

This was globally the largest order Acuson so far had received, with a total customer end price of more than SEK13 million (US$2 million+).

John Larsson accepted a fair compensation for the 12-system order stock in July 1986. My wife and I sold our shares in Amedic and Medata Nordic at nominal value. I then became Acuson AB Managing Director. Also the pioneer Nordic FAS (Field Application Specialist) Monica Schedin was allowed to change employment to Acuson. We moved out Acuson equipment and ourselves from Medata Nordic during July. Marianne Jönsson was contracted as office manager; Larsén joined as Service Manager in August 1986.

At RSNA (Radiology Society of North America congress) in 1984, Quantum, Issaquah, showed the first colour Doppler images. Dr Merritt, New Orleans, presented the first clinical paper at RSNA 1985. Quantum started shipping their first CDI system in 1986.

Aloka became the Japanese CDI pioneer. Their first cardiac SSD-880CW in the Nordic countries (second in Europe) was installed 1985 in Turku, Finland, under Dr Markku Saraste.

Toshiba introduced the SSH-65A cardiac CDI system in 1986.

Vingmed, Norway released CFM700 CDI and HP their Colour Flow Option at AHA (American Heart Association Congress) in 1986. ATL surprisingly launched the UM6 CDI system by Fujitsu, Japan at AHA. UM9CDI replacing UM8, and was first released in 1988. Acuson exhibited the 128CDI option at RSNA 1986 as works-in-progress. In August 1987, the Acuson 128CDI option/system started shipping.

The global ultrasound market in 1988 was dominated by Japanese manufacturers—Toshiba (19%), Hitachi (16%), Aloka (12%) followed by HP (7%), ATL (6%), and Acuson (4%).

At Riksstämman in 1984, Dr Ingemar Wallentin, Sahlgrenska University Hospital, Gothenburg attended an Acuson demonstration. He was impressed with the high resolution and asked for a formal quotation. I told him the system had no cardiology functions, but he explained that he needed the high image resolution. A Cardiac Option was developed for release in the summer of 1986, and I sent him the requested quotation, resulting in one of the 12 orders received in June 1986.

Globally he was the first to buy an Acuson cardiovascular system. First at ACC (American Congress of Cardiology) Atlanta in March 1988 Acuson market introduced the dedicated 128CV Cardiovascular System.

By the end of the 1980s, the diagnostic performance gap decreased, when ATL and Diasonics/Vingmed began using mechanical Annual Array technology. 128XP introduction in 1990 again increased that performance gap and also proved the Acuson upgradability statement—installed bases were offered affordable upgrades to 128XP performance.

Vingmed was acquired by Interspec (1988), Diasonics-Sonotron (1990) for US$17 million, Elbit, Israel (1994) for US$80 million, and finally by GE (1998) for US$228 million. Those frequent owner changes created customer uncertainty, and Acuson became the cardiovascular market leader in Norway, Vingmed's home market, during the early 1990s.

ATL acquired Interspec in 1984; Philips acquired ATL in 1998 for US$800 million and Agilent HSG (former HP ultrasound) in 2000 for US$1700 million.

Siemens acquired Quantum in 1990 and introduced a new premium system Elegra in 1995.

In 1989, the European ultrasound pioneer Kretztechnik, Zipf, Austria, introduced the Combison 330, the world's first three-dimensional ultrasound, and was acquired by

Medison, Korea in 1996. In 1998, Kretztechnik/Medison released Voluson730, the first four-dimensional ultrasound. In 2001 GE acquired Kretztechnik from Medison for US$83.9 million.

At RSNA 1992, Acuson released the Aegis ultrasound miniPACS, providing an open gateway to the emerging ACR/NEMA standard for picture archiving and communications system (PACS) and hospital information systems. At RSNA 1993 the DICOM 3.0 Standard (Digital Imaging and Communication in Medicine) was introduced, allowing imaging devices of different types/brands to connect with servers, review stations, and printers.

Early PACS systems were developed for filmless radiology and black/white static images. Sectra-Imtec AB, Linköping, Sweden was an early pioneer. Professor Torbjörn Andersson at the University Hospital in Örebro initiated in 1994 the Pax Vobiscum project that became one of the first and then biggest PACS installations in Europe.

PACS systems could, however, not handle dynamic clips and colour images. That need was first addressed by Acuson when releasing the KinetDx in 1999. The first Nordic (second in Europe) installation was performed at Södersjukhuset, Bildcentrum in Stockholm.

So far, all ultrasound systems were beamformer based and used only the amplitude information in returning echoes. Acuson introduced the Sequoia in 1996, using coherent image formation to acquire and encode both amplitude and phase data. This major technology step offered twice the information in half the time. Acuson invited global luminaries in 1995–96 to preview Sequoia in MView. During a cardiac scanning demonstration, coronary flow was seen by ultrasound for the first time ever, by a group of Nordic doctors.

Dr Lindgren at Akademiska, Uppsala, placed the first global Sequoia512 order in April 1996.

Sequoia was market released in May 1996 and quickly became the global market premium system leader, despite being almost twice the price of conventional systems. Twenty-three Nordic Sequoia orders were received in 1996. In the first 5 years, 237 Sequoia of a total of 351 Acuson systems were sold in the Nordic countries (Fig. 17.2).

Siemens acquired Acuson in 1999 for US$700 million. Siemens Ultrasound worldwide headquarters in Issaquah, WA was moved to Mountain View and outside the United States all Acuson subsidiaries were integrated into Siemens subsidiaries during 2000–2001. Acuson Nordic sales were then more than three times Siemens ultrasound sales. Acuson had installed more than 750 systems in the Nordic countries. After successful integration I asked in the summer of 2001 for an early retirement and Siemens granted a generous 4-year retirement package as of that October.

In the twenty-first century a new market segment emerged; Hand Carried Ultrasound (HCU).

In 1979, Organon Teknika, Holland released MiniVisor, an ultrasound stethoscope formed as a mushroom, battery operated with 2-inch display, but mediocre image quality. It never became a market success.

Start-up Ecton introduced a cardiac HCU system 1998. Ecton was acquired by Acuson 1999 for US$40 million and became Acuson Small Systems Division and the system was named Cypress. The first five Nordic systems were installed in late 2000.

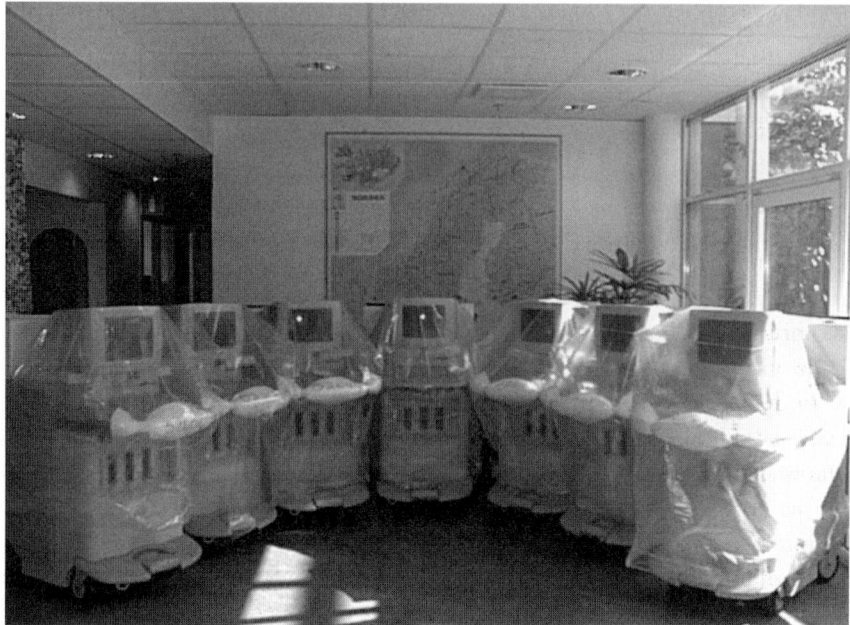

Fig. 17.2 Acuson Sequoia systems waiting for delivery to different Swedish hospitals at Eurostop Arlandastad office in June 1999. (This figure is reproduced in colour in the colour plate section.)

Sonosite was spun-off from ATL in 1998 and released their first HCU system 1999. GE introduced their cardiac HCU system, Vivid I, in 2005, followed by a family laptop systems in 2006.

Several ultrasound companies offered me consultancy contracts in 2005, when my Siemens non-competitive agreement ceased. I did some consulting for Sonosite's Danish distributor, introducing the MicroMaxx lap-top sized HCU in Sweden.

I was then contacted by start-up company, Zonare, Mountain View, which introduced their z.one system in 2004. After Siemens acquired Acuson, the R&D budget was reduced, and Siemens-Acuson started losing the technology leadership. Several of the brightest engineers instead joined Zonare.

At RSNA 2005 I met Zonare management and was invited to California to meet the brain behind Zonare technology, Glen McLaughlin, VP Engineering/CTO. He convinced me that Zonare was the fifth-generation ultrasound—the second-generation being the ATL Dynamic sectorscanner (1979), third-generation Acuson Computed Sonography (1983), and fourth-generation Acuson Sequoia (1996). I signed a 2-year consultancy agreement to help Zonare establish a Swedish subsidiary in March 2006.

Zonare AB (ZAB) was founded, an office rented (in the same building Acuson AB had been located), Marianne Jönsson and Monica Axberg from Siemens recruited, and Åke Larsén contracted as technical support consultant. The z.one rev.2 was introduced at Swedish Annual Radiology meeting in Örebro, September 2006, creating a lot of interest.

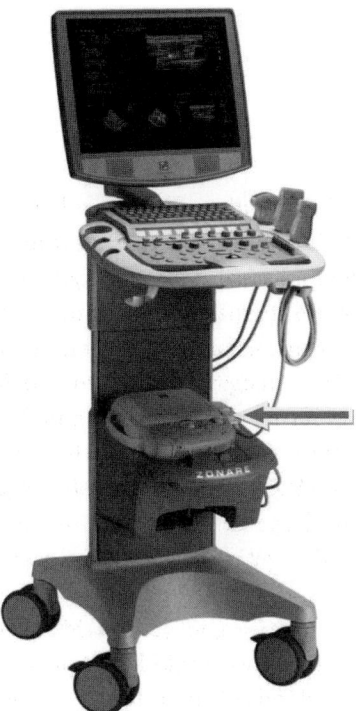

Fig. 17.3 Zonare 2.5kg Hand Carried System (HCU). Reproduced with permission from ZONARE. (This figure is reproduced in colour in the colour plate section.)

The revolutionary technology was Zone Sonography—instead of conventional line-by-line acquisition echo information is acquired more quickly by interrogating zones of anatomy, resulting in equal or more diagnostic information than competitive superpremium big systems of 150–200kg weight. Zonare design is software-based and implemented on a digital signal processor (DSP) and inherently compact, 2.5kg light, and convertible/hybrid as it can be docked to different carts (docking-stations) (Fig. 17.3).

In July 2008 Zonare filed for an IPO (Initial Public Offering) of US$86.25 million, which however, was withdrawn in December due to the global financial crisis.

Zonare decided at the end of 2007 to close down ZAB and instead appoint distributors in the Nordic countries. ZAB was already negotiating with Fujifilm, Stockholm a subdealer contract for the veterinary market, which was why those discussions were expanded to a Nordic dealership, and this was signed in March 2008. All four ZAB 'Zone Sonography ambassadors' were offered continued contracts at Fujifilm.

The results of ZAB's intense sales and marketing efforts began to be realized in spring 2008. We had focused on leading Swedish ultrasound centres and had received several orders from, e.g. Lund (Professor Maršál), Uppsala (Professor Lindgren), and Karolinska during the first quarter of 2008.

The first pocket-sized unit, the Siemens P10 weighting 0.7kg, was released in 2007, followed by the Sonosite NanoMaxx (2009), and GE Vscan (2010).

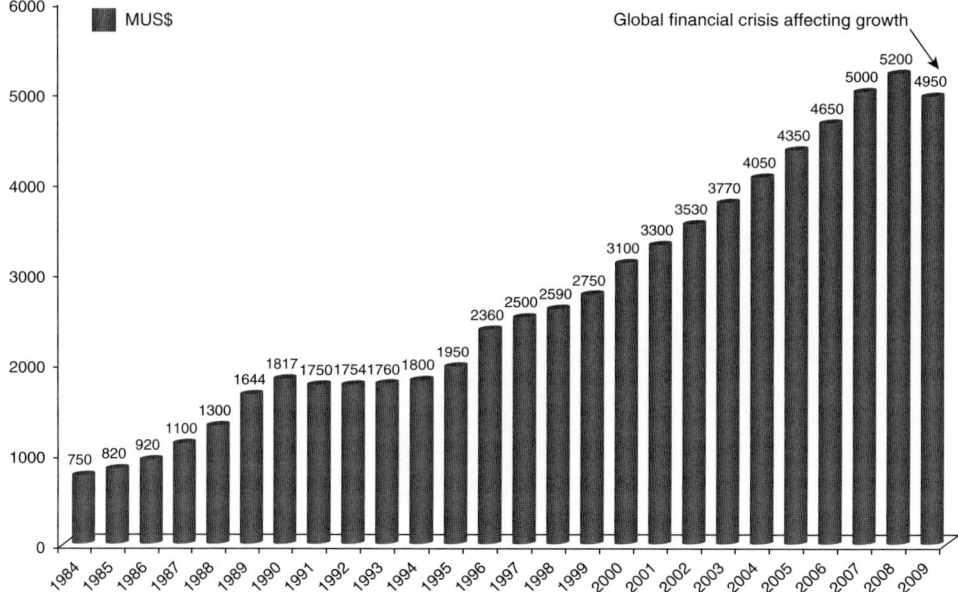

Fig. 17.4 Worldwide diagnostic ultrasound market 1984–2009 (million US$). Swedish market 0.5–0.6% of worldwide sales; Nordic market 1.0–1.1%.

In summer 2008, Fujifilm, hit by the global financial crisis, wanted to renegotiate my consultancy agreement, and I decided to finally retire at 68 years of age.

Fifty years of ultrasound development has been truly spectacular. From the early pioneers in Lund, encountering strong scepticism, to the present as a major diagnostic tool with a global market worth more than US$6000 million (Fig. 17.4), with development to continue in the years ahead. It has indeed been a privilege to closely follow.

Appendix

KUNGL. FYSIOGRAFISKA SÄLLSKAPETS I LUND FÖRHANDLINGAR
Bd 24. Nr 5. 1954.

The Use of Ultrasonic Reflectoscope for the Continuous Recording of the Movements of Heart Walls.

By

I. Edler[1] and C. H. Hertz[2].

Communicated by Prof. B. Edlén, March 10, 1954.

Introduction.

The effectivity of the pumping action of the heart is essentially dependent on cyclic variations in the volume of the heart chambers and the function of the valves. Increased difference between the diastolic and systolic volume in a heart chamber implies greater amplitude in the movements of the walls. In patients with valvular stenosis or insufficiency the curve for the variation in the volume of heart chambers will deviate from normal (1). Therefore, methods showing the variation in the volume of the heart chambers or the movements of the walls of the heart during the cardiac cycle should be useful in the investigation of cardiac function. Roentgenkymography and electrokymography are methods applied in the investigation of changes in the outline of the heart during the cardiac cycle. Rushmer et al. (2) made continuous measurements of left ventricular dimensions in intact, unanesthetized dogs. The method they used is based on the introduction of a variable inductance gauge in the ventricle, but their method can only be used in animal experiments. In recent years serial angiocardiography with several exposures per second has become an important method for the study of the variation in the volume of the heart chambers during systole and diastole. This method has been used in the clinic, among other things, for the investigation of mitral valvular disease, but it must be performed under anesthesia, it is time-consuming and by no means free of risks.

Many other methods for registering periodic movements caused by the

---

[1] Medical Clinic, University of Lund.
[2] Dept. of Physics, University of Lund.

heart are under investigation, but only one of these uses ultrasonic sound (3). But that method differs fundamentally from that presented here, since it uses continuous sound waves of 60 kc that pass through the body from the praecordium to the posterior of thorax. On its way, the sound passes the heart and other parts of the body, whereby the sound intensity is decreased by absorption, reflection and refraction. By measuring the sound intensity at the back of thorax it was found that it varied in phase with the heart frequency, but no relation between these intensity variations and the heart volume could be shown.

None of the methods mentioned above give the actual movements of the inner walls of the heart, the knowledge of which would be of importance both for studying the movements of the heart in the body and for clinical diagnosis of heart diseases. It was therefore thought that a technique already well known for some years in industry for the non-destructive testing of materials with respect to flaws might be used (4, 5).

Experimental Method.

The method, known as supersonic reflectoscope, uses short supersonic sound pulses, which are generated by an electrically excited quartz crystal and delivered to the material under investigation. This is done by pressing the disk-shaped quartz crystal directly against the surface of the material under investigation. A good acoustical contact should be secured by using a thin oil film between the quartz and the surface of the material.

If there are any boundaries in the material which are impinged by the sound pulse and which reflect part of the sound back in a direction opposite to its original direction, this reflected sound pulse (echo) will reach the quartz crystal, which then acts as a microphone. If the velocity of the sound in the material under examination is known and constant, the time elapsed between the emission of the sound pulse and the reception of the echo is a measure of the distance between the quartz crystal and the reflecting boundary. This time difference (or distance) can be read directly on a cathode-ray-tube (CRT). This CRT forms part of an apparatus which also contains the electrical equipment for the generation of the electrical signal for the excitation of the quartz crystal, etc. The quartz crystal is connected with this apparatus by a coaxial cable about 3 m. long.

On the left side of the CRT screen, the outgoing sound pulse is represented by a vertical signal 0 (see Fig. 2), while each returning echo pulse shows up as a vertical signal to the right of this outgoing sound pulse. The distance between the outgoing signal and the echo signal along the x-axis on the CRT screen is directly proportional to the distance between the crystal and the reflecting boundary. Further, the height of the echo signal shown on the CRT screen is a measure of the echo intensity.

The apparatus used in the investigations described here was the Ultraschall-Impulsgerät manufactured by the Siemens Reiniger Werke (Erlangen, Germany). In this apparatus the pulse length and intensity could be varied, the pulse length used was usually about $2-5 \times 10^{-6}$ sec., the maximum pulse intensity about 2 W/cm^2. The pulse repetition rate was 200 per second. Sound frequencies of 0.5, 1, 2.5 and 5 Mc could be chosen at will.

In nearly all of the experiments described below a frequency of 2.5 Mc was used. When selecting the frequency, different factors have to be observed, the most important of which are the sound absorption in the material under examination and the divergence of the sound beam due to diffraction. Since the absorption of the sound waves increases with increasing sound frequency in both tissue (6, 7, 8) and blood (9), it would be advantageous to use as low a frequency as possible. On the other hand, the necessity of sharp echoes requires both short pulse length and, to reduce diffraction, small wave length of the sound in tissue or blood. With a crystal shaped like a disk, 12 mm. in diameter, as used in these experiments, a frequency of 2.5 Mc was usually found to be the best compromise, except for children below 12 years, when better results were often obtained with 5 Mc.

The apparatus used in these experiments was equipped further with an electronically controlled "lens" device to enlarge and thereby facilitate observation of echo signals on the CRT screen along the x-axis. This device proved to be valuable in the investigations. Finally, a time scale was incorporated in the apparatus, which appeared as a broken line along the x-axis on the CRT screen. This scale could be adjusted so that the breaks in the line between the outgoing and the echo pulse on the CRT screen give the distance directly in centimeters between the quartz crystal and the reflecting boundary for a certain homogeneous medium. In this work the scale was adjusted in such a way that the distances between the quartz crystal and the reflecting boundary could be read directly in centimeters on the CRT screen if the medium between was blood or muscle tissue, the velocity of sound in both being nearly the same.

Preliminary Experiments on Isolated Hearts.

It has been pointed out above that only sound reflecting boundaries can be detected by this method. Thus for the present purpose it was ne-

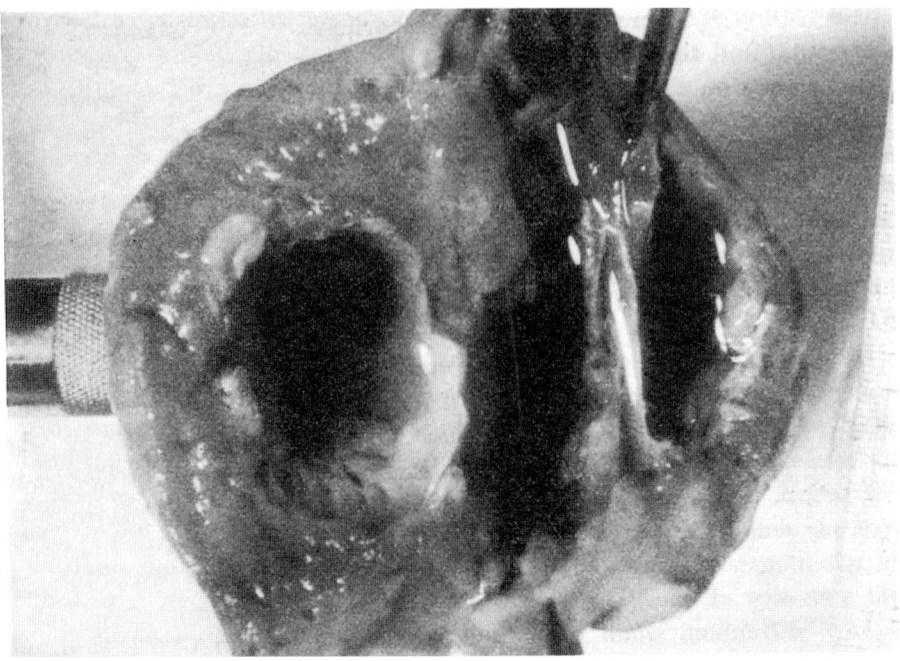

Fig. 1. Quartz — crystal applied to isolated human heart. Crystal frequency 2,5 Mc.

cessary to check that the boundary blood-heart wall fills this condition. This was not to be expected for certain, since the acoustic impedances (10, 11) for blood and muscle tissue are nearly the same. Therefore experiments with isolated hearts were made before starting the investigations on human hearts *in vivo*. The most informative of these experiments is shown by Fig. 1. It shows a human heart from above, which is cut transversely. From left to right we see the left ventricle, the right ventricle and the right atrium. All the chambers are filled with water, and the quartz crystal of the supersonic reflectoscope is applied to the outer heart wall in such a way that the sound beam traverses the heart just under the water surface. The echogram seen on the CRT screen is shown in Fig. 2. According to the figure, many echoes arise, but the co-ordination of the echoes to the different heart walls cannot be seen at a glance. But this is evident at once if both pictures are cut in halves and put together at the line along which the ultrasonic beam is traversing the heart, as is shown by Fig. 3. Each boundary of the type water-heart tissue that is traversed by the sound shows up as an echo signal on the CRT screen, even the thin wall between the right atrium and the right ventricle. The

The Use of Ultrasonic Reflectoscope

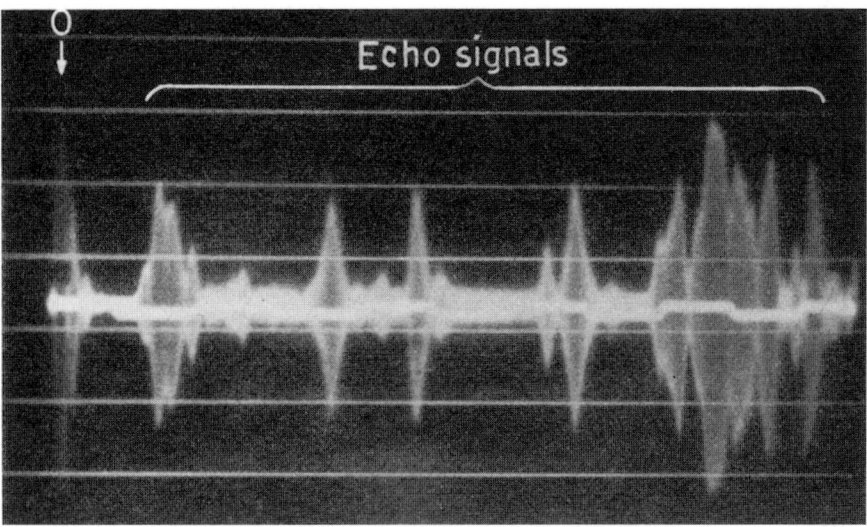

Fig. 2. Echogram obtained on the CRT screen by the arrangement shown in Fig. 1. 0 = outgoing pulse signal.

places at which the heart wall is curved or irregular give rise to diffuse echo signals, since the distance quartz crystal — reflecting boundary at these spots is not constant for different parts of the 12 mm. wide ultrasonic beam. On the other hand, the wall between the right atrium and right ventricle, which has been artificially stretched so as to lie precisely perpendicular to the ultrasonic beam, gives rise to sharp echo signals. The complex echo signal seen at the place where the sound beam, after traversing the heart, strikes the outer heart wall is probably due to the highly convex form of the heart at this place. Naturally, the height and the width of the echo signals vary very much if the direction of the sound beam is changed. The experiments described here were done with water so that the shape of the heart chambers under the water surface can be seen on the photographs. In later experiments the heart chambers were filled with blood instead of water but the results obtained were exactly the same as those found with water.

To check that the co-ordination between the heart walls and the echo signals on the CRT screen given above was correct, the following experiment was performed. An injection needle ca. 0.5 mm. thick was dipped from above into one of the heart chambers shown in Fig. 1 in such a way that it crossed the axis of the ultrasonic beam. This resulted in an additional echo signal on the CRT screen from reflection at the needle.

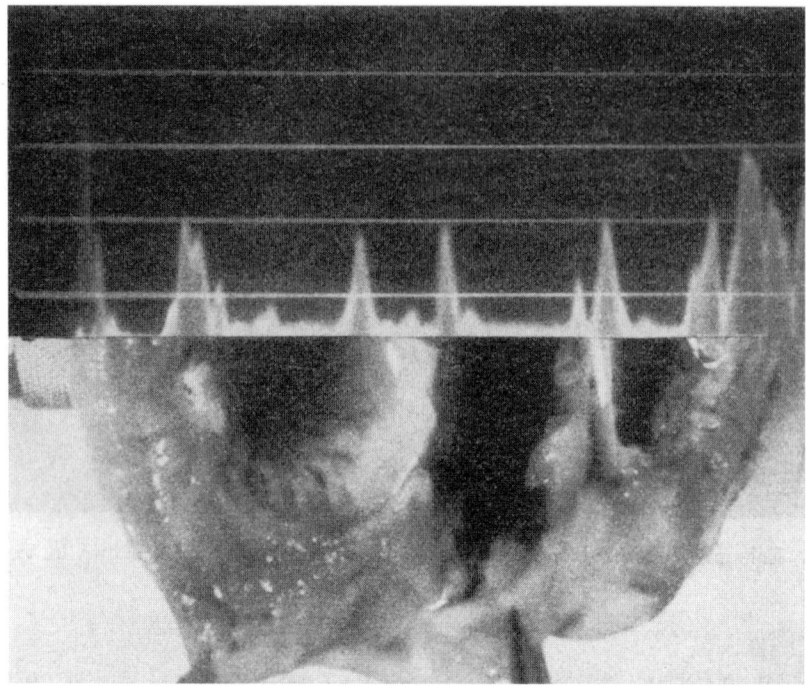

Fig. 3. (For explanation, see text).

The lower half of the Figs. 4 a–c shows the echogram without the needle in one of the heart chambers, as already shown by Fig. 2. In Fig. 4 a the needle was placed in the right atrium and in Fig. 4 b it was placed in the right ventricle and in Fig. 4 c it was placed in the left ventricle. As can be seen from the echograms, the echo signal due to the needle always shows up between the echo signals from the walls of the heart chamber into which the needle was dipped in each case. By moving the needle along the axis of the ultrasonic beam from one wall to the other in the heart chamber, the needle echo signal could be seen moving between the echo signals of the respective walls.

In other experiments, the authors examined echograms from the right atrium of the isolated calf heart. With the aid of a heart catheter passed into the atrium, the volume of the latter was varied, with a resultant corresponding shift of the echo signal from the medial wall of the atrium.

Fig. 4. Needle echo signal (N) appeared on the echogram when the needle was dipped into the right atrium (4 a), right ventricle (4 b) and left ventricle (4 c).

The Use of Ultrasonic Reflectoscope

APPENDIX | 195

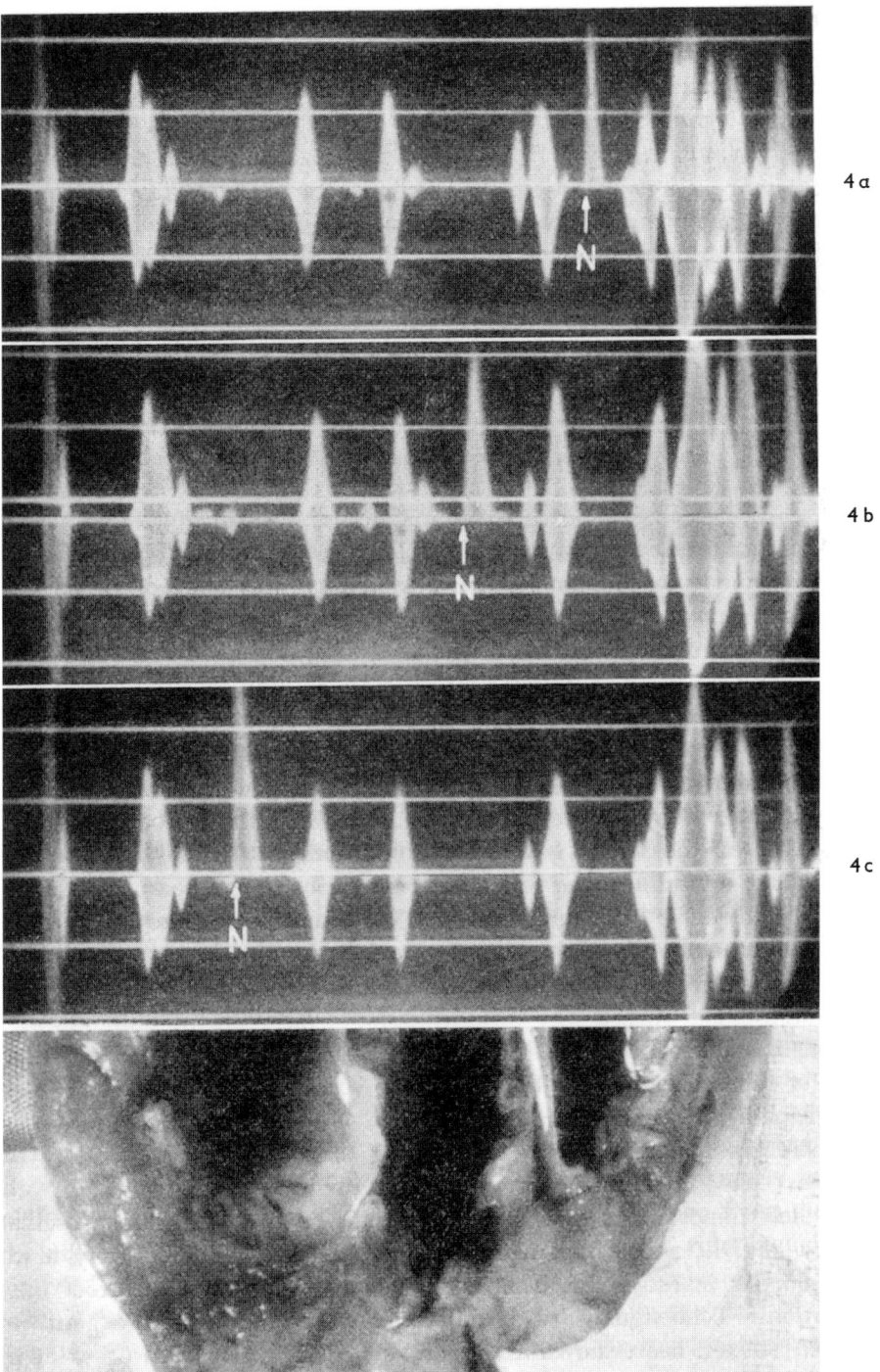

4 a

4 b

4 c

During the experiments it was felt that the reason for the unexpected large reflection coefficient encountered at the inner heart walls were due to the endocardium, since the removal of the latter seemed to diminish the reflection coefficient appreciably. This would be in agreement with the results obtained by J. J. Wild & J. M. Reid (12) with the supersonic reflectoscope on muscle tissue. As yet, no convincing evidence has been produced in support of this assumption.

Short experiments showed, further, that auricular thrombosis may also be located by this method. This should be of interest in the diagnosis of such cases. Even here, more detailed experiments are required.

Experiments on Human Beings.

After the preliminary experiments stated above, an investigation as to the applicability of the supersonic reflectoscope method for the study of the movements of human heart walls *in vivo* was started. In all cases described below a 12 mm. disk shaped quartz crystal was directly applied to the praecordium. Paraffin oil was used to ensure good acoustic contact. The quartz crystal was brought into such a position that the sound beam could pass through an intercostal space and was directed into the heart regions under investigation. A typical echogram obtained on the CRT screen is shown in Fig. 5. It was taken on a patient with enlarged heart. The distance between the outgoing signal 0 and the echo signals along the x-axis on the screen is directly proportional to the distance between the quartz crystal and the reflecting boundaries in the heart. This is true with a fair degree of accuracy, even if the sound passes muscle tissue and blood alternately, since the sound velocities in muscle tissue and blood are nearly the same. Thus, the time scale incorporated in the apparatus was adjusted in such a way that the distance between the outgoing pulse signal and the echo signals could be read directly in centimetres. Each part of the broken line of the time scale seen in Fig. 5 represents 1 cm. sound path in muscle tissue or blood.

There are two reasons for interpreting the echo signals found in this way as echoes resulting from reflections on inner or outer heart walls. The most important is that the echo signals on the CRT screen oscillate both along the x-axis and in their magnitude with the frequency of the heart under investigation. This is very convenient for the correct interpretation of echo signals arising on the CRT screen. Since the experiments on the isolated heart shown above prove that reflections can occur at the

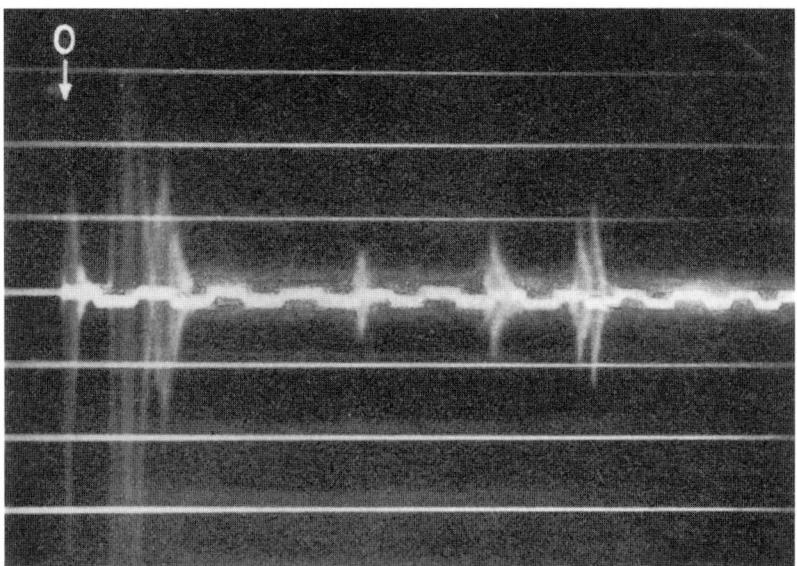

Fig. 5. Echogram obtained on the CRT-screen when quartz crystal was applied to the praecordium of a patient with cardiac enlargement.

boundary blood — heart tissue, this assumption is not contradicted. Further, no such echo signals can be found when the crystal is placed elsewhere on the thorax of a person except on the praecordium. This is due to the large absorption coefficient of the aerated lung tissue for high frequency sound.

On account of this large absorption of high frequency sound in lung tissue and pronounced reflection in skeletal parts (13), the sound beam should be delivered in such a manner as to avoid these media as far as possible. It was found that, when the quartz crystal was placed against the skin of the praecordium and in the intercostal space and when the ultrasonic beam was directed against the heart, one or more echoes ranging from 4 cm. to 11 cm. were recorded in persons with a heart of normal size. The echo signals were best obtained when the crystal was placed in the left I: 4 and I: 3. In the investigation of apparently normal adults, the ultrasonic beam is directed in sagittal direction from the left I: 4 adjacent the sternal border, whereby the posterior echo signal was recorded at a distance of 9—11 cm. from the outgoing pulse signal. If the heart is enlarged, this posterior reflecting surface will lie at greater distance from the anterior wall of the chest. Table 1 shows the relationship between

Table 1.

	Distance in centimeters of the echo signals from the outgoing signal.	Distance in centimeters from the anterior thoracic wall to the posterior of the heart, as measured on the roentgen film.	Total heart volume in millilitres.
E. L.	16	17	2440
A. L.	9,7	10,5	
B. N.	8,8	9,5	510
M. L.	12	13	
E. B.	11,3	13	1185
G. M.	12,2	13,5	1090

the distance to the posterior wall, as measured by the echo signal, and the distance from the anterior thoracic wall to the posterior part of the heart shadow, as measured by the roentgen film at the same level, in persons with varying heart volume. It is in this plane which passes through the left sternal border that the sagittal diameter of the heart is greatest, for which reason the distance measured on the roentgen film corresponds to the plane passed by the ultrasonic beam. It is apparent from the table that the posterior echo signal lies within the structure of the heart and thus represents a partition in the heart. The difference between the distance to this partition and the distance to the posterior part of the heart shadow corresponds to the thickness of the posterior wall of the heart and therefore the echo signal may correspond to the inner surface of this wall.

If the sound passes a rib, the results obtained are less accurate, and sometimes no reflection is obtained from the heart walls. If the crystal is placed against the chest outside the praecordium and where the sound waves will meet lung tissue as soon as the thoracic wall has been passed, no echo from the heart walls will be obtained. As mentioned above, this was expected.

In patients with cardiac enlargement, reflections are obtained over the major part of the praecordium which is explained by the fact that the lung tissue between the wall of the chest and the heart has been pushed aside. On the other hand, patients with emphysema and those of pyknic body build have more lung tissue between the anterior wall of the chest and the heart, which explains that it is much more difficult to obtain satisfactory echo signals in such persons.

Continuous Recording of the Echo Signals.

Since mere visual observation of the motion of the echo signals seen on the CRT screen does not yield much more information than the

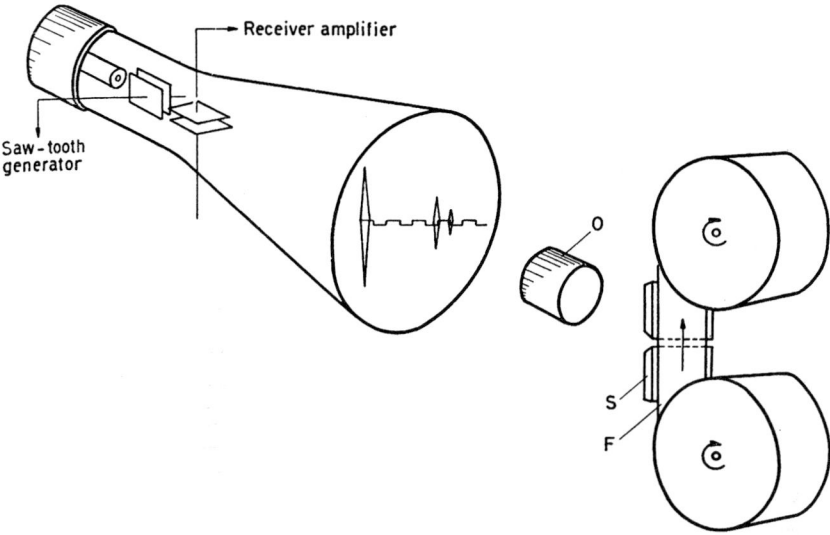

Fig. 6. Apparatus for recording UCG-curves.

distance of the reflecting heart walls from the crystal surface, a continuous photographic recording of this motion was required. To this end a horizontal slit S (see Fig. 6) was mounted in the image plane of the camera objective O, otherwise used for photographing the CRT screen, the slit width being 0.5 mm. Directly behind this slit, a 24 mm. Ilford HP3 film F was continuously moved at right angles to the slit at a rate of 1 cm/sec. The slit should be placed parallel to, but a little above, the image of the x-axis of the CRT, so that no light coming from the x-axis and the time scale visible on the CRT screen reaches the film. If no echo signal appears on the CRT screen, nothing will be marked on the film except the outgoing pulse signal which will be recorded as a straight line parallel to the direction in which the film is moved. If a constant, non-pulsating echo signal appears on the screen, even this will produce a straight line on the film parallel to the outgoing pulse line. The distance between these two lines is then proportional to the distance crystal-reflecting boundary. If the echo signal pulsates along the x-axis (which is the case in these investigations) a curve will be recorded on the film. The distance of this curve to the outgoing pulse line will correspond at any moment to the distance crystal-reflecting boundary. In this way, the variations of the distance crystal-reflecting boundary can be recorded with respect to time.

Because of the relatively large slit width relative to the film velocity, the resolving power of the present apparatus is not too good. Using higher

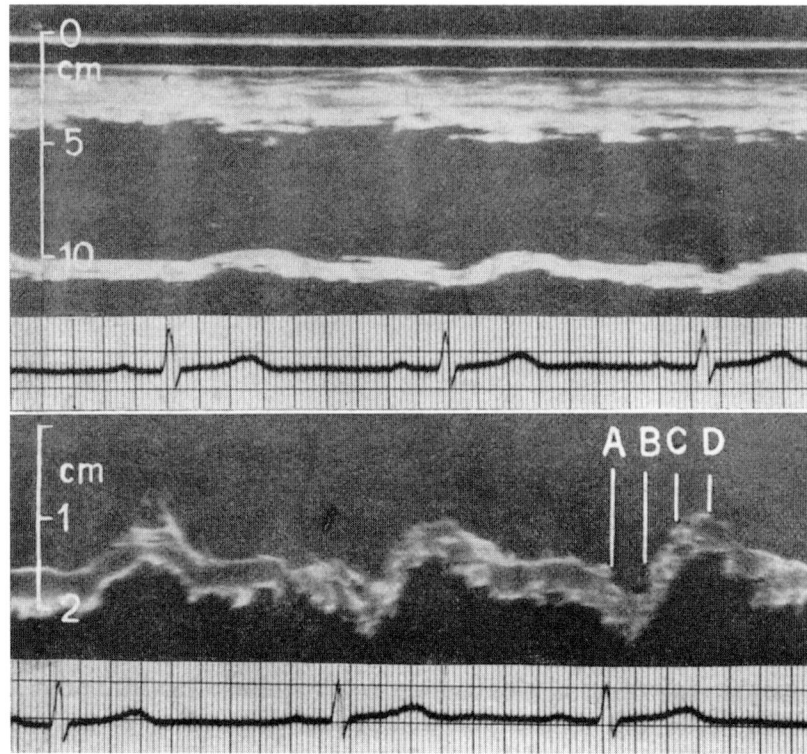

Fig. 7. Top: General view. Bottom: Enlargement of the movements of the posterior wall of the heart. A—B indicates the isometric contraction when the wall moves 2—3 mm. in dorsal direction. B—C denotes the first part of the emptying phase, maximum ejection, when the wall rapidly moves in ventral direction. C—D denotes the final phase of emptying, reduced ejection, when the wall moves slowly in ventral direction.

light intensities on the CRT screen, it will be possible without much difficulty to increase the resolving power to the same degree as is achieved in commercial ECG apparatus.

Typical curves obtained in this way from heart walls are shown in Fig. 7 to Fig. 11. Since the method uses supersonic sound to gain information about the function of the heart, in the following these curves will be referred to as UCG (Ultrasonic Cardiogram). In the lower figures the electronically controlled "lens" device mentioned above has been used. In these cases the movements of the echo signals are magnified about 4 times, whereby a more detailed study of these movements is possible. Using the scale given on the side of each figure, the actual size of the movements

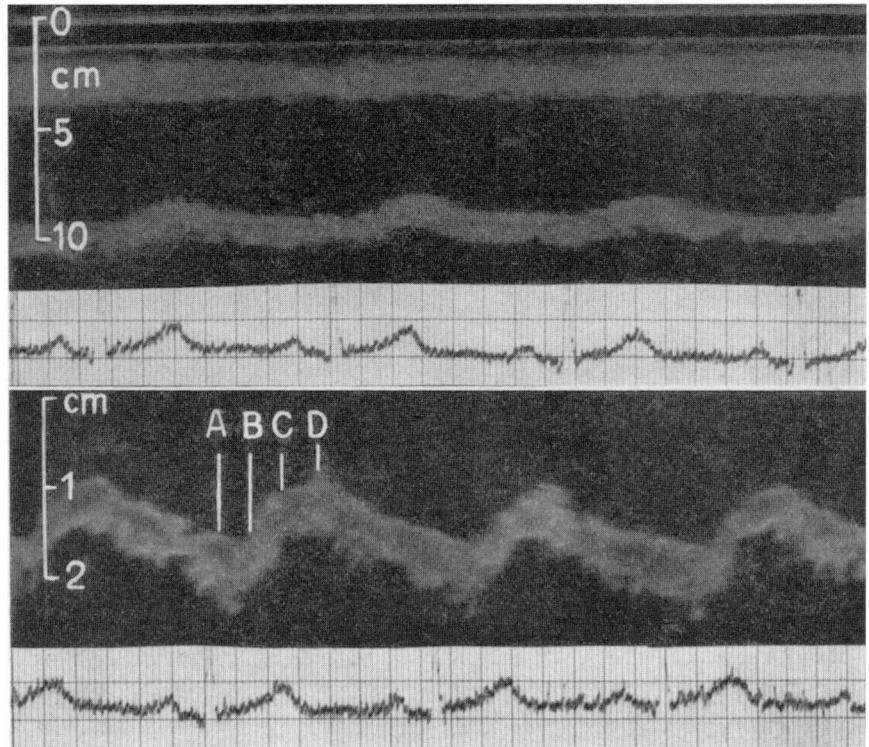

Fig. 8. UCG from a normal case. Top: General view. Bottom: Enlargement of the movements of the posterior wall of the heart.

of the heart wall under observation can be measured directly. The film velocity is the same both for the normal and for the enlarged recordings.

As can be seen from the figures, the echo signal width on the CRT screen also varies periodically. There are two reasons for this behaviour. If the reflecting boundary is not a plane or is not placed exactly at right angles to the sound beam, the echo signal will broaden, since the distance crystal-reflecting boundary is different at different places on the crystal surface. Further, in the apparatus used in these experiments, not even an echo signal reflected from an ideal plane placed at right angles to the beam direction will show up as a thin vertical line on the CRT screen, but more like an isosceles triangle with a very narrow base along the x-axis. This base width increases with the strength of the returning echo signal. Thus the base width of the echo signal pulse on the CRT screen increases with the height of the pulse, thereby making both the base width and the

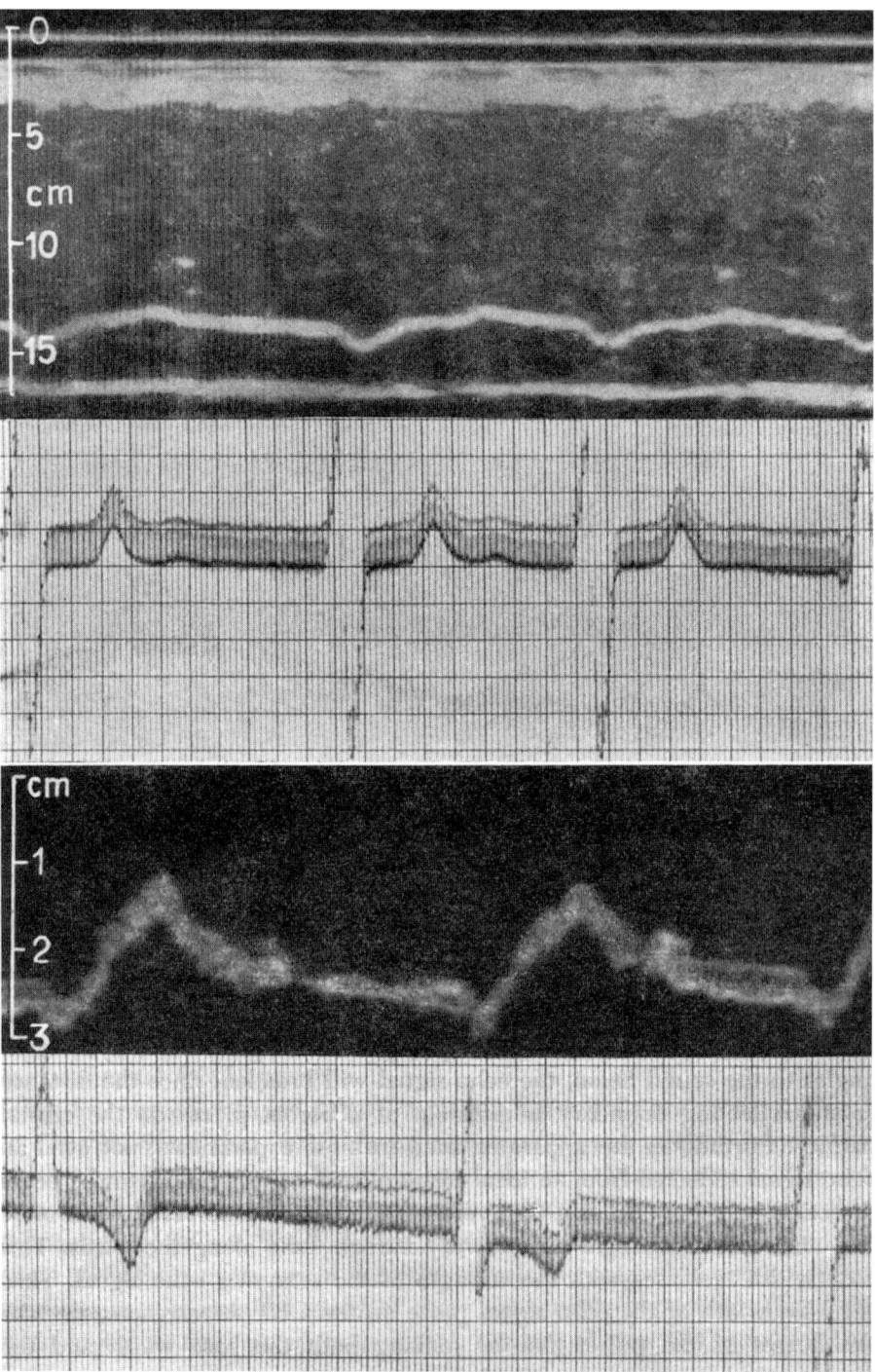

Fig. 9. UCG from a patient with aortic regurgitation. Top: General view. Bottom: Enlargement of the movements of the posterior wall of the heart.

height of the echo signal a measure of the strength of the reflected sound pulse. Thus the cause of a broad track in the UCG's may have been that the reflecting boundary was curved or not situated at right angles to the sound beam or that the echo signal was very strong. A thin track indicates a sharp but faint echo.

Since it was felt that the information about the movements of different parts of the heart gained by this method would be much easier to interpret if a simultaneous recorded and synchronized ECG were available, a synchronization device was applied to the UCG and ECG apparatus. After developing the 24 mm. UCG-film, the negative was enlarged just so much that the synchronization marks on the UCG film and ECG paper coincided. In this way a synchronization of UCG and ECG was achieved.

Preliminary Results.

The factors influencing the distance crystal-reflecting boundary are respiratory excursions of the chest and the movements of the heart. The influence of respiratory movements in the experiments hitherto performed appear to be of minor importance, so that it was not necessary for the patient to hold his breath during the examination. The movements of the heart during the cardiac cycle are complex. They are determined partly by the movements of the individual walls in association with the variation in the volume of the respective heart chambers and, second, by movements of the heart as a whole. The latter movements are due to changes in the shape of the heart during isometric contraction and relaxation.

Figs. 7 and 8 show curves for two normal persons. The crystal was placed in the left I:4 immediately lateral to the sternal border and the ultrasonic waves were delivered in sagittal direction. The maximum distance to the reflecting wall of the heart was 10.0 respectively 9.3 cm. The curves thus represent the dorsal part of the heart. In the enlargement of Fig. 7 the various phases of the movements occurring during the cardiac cycle are marked.

Fig. 9 shows the curve for the posterior wall of the left ventricle in a patient with aortic regurgitation and hypertrophy of the left ventricle. The curve deviates from normal by showing much greater amplitude during ejection systole and a much more abrupt return in dorsal direction during the beginning of diastole. This latter movement coincides in time with the rapid regurgitation in the beginning of diastole in advanced aortic insufficiency (1).

UCG's taken from the left I:3 about 3—5 cm. lateral to the sternal border over the region of the left atrium showed very rapid movements

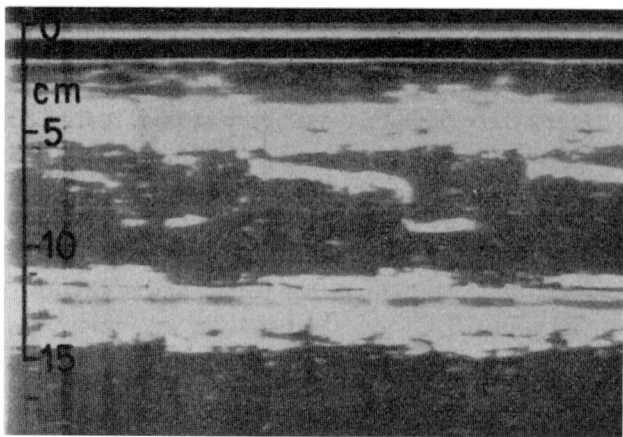

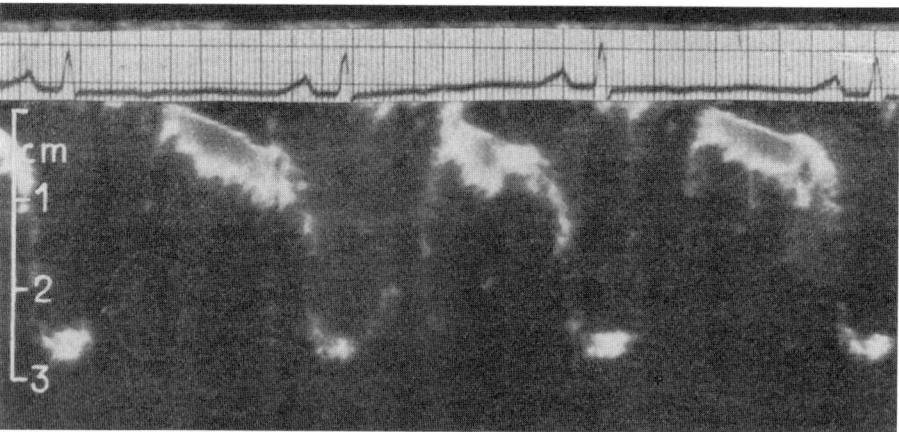

Fig. 10. UCG-curve showing the movements of left auricular wall in a case of mitral stenosis. Top: The curve shows a reflecting surface about almost 6 cm. from the anterior thoracic wall in the beginning of diastole. Bottom: Enlargement of the reflecting surface. From the beginning of ventricular diastole, when the atrio-ventricular valves open, the reflecting surface moves 6—7 mm. in dorsal direction. Immediately after the beginning of the P-wave in the electrocardiogram the sound reflecting surface makes a rapid movement in dorsal direction. This movement has an amplitud of about 2 cm.
During ventricular systole the wall returns to its original position.

at a depht of 5—7 cm. in some cases. In normals such movements were recorded only as fragmentary curves. All of them, however, showed a rapid movement of about 1 cm. in dorsal direction at the time of atrial systole, for which reason the relationship with atrial activity is obvious. For this reason, these sequences were studied in some patients with mitral

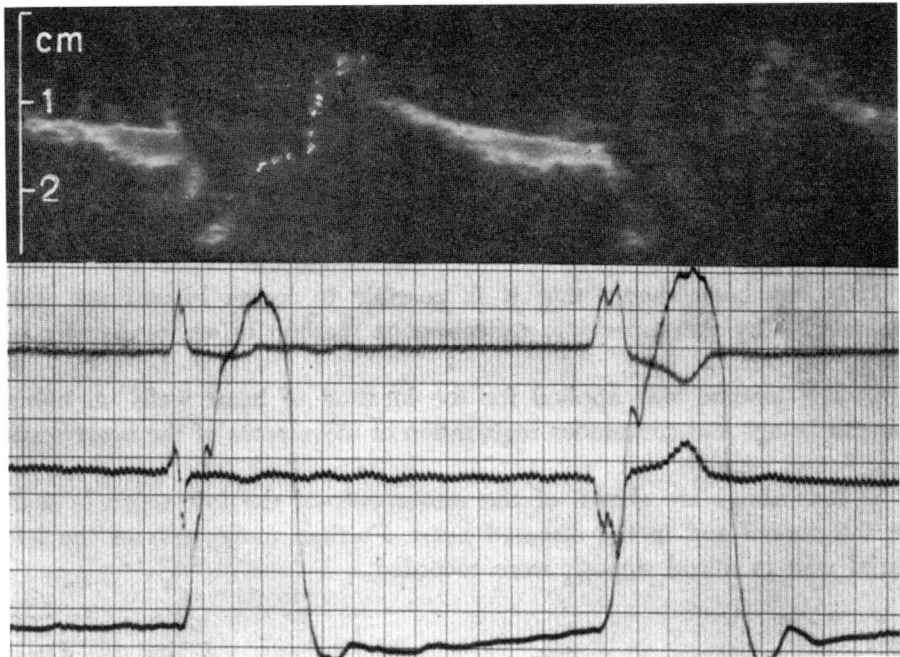

Fig. 11. UCG-curve showing the movements of left auricular wall in a case of mitral stenosis with auricular fibrillation. As in fig. 10, there is a gradual movement in dorsal direction after opening of the atrio-ventricular valves. A rapid movement is recorded at the time of the isometric contraction of the ventricle. At the time of the isometric relaxation of the ventricle, the reflecting surface returned in ventral direction.

valvular disease and enlarged left atrium. Better curves then were obtained from the left I: 3. Fig. 10 shows a curve for a patient with pure mitral stenosis. Valvulotomy had been done before and post-operatively there were no signs of mitral regurgitation. The curve lies at a depth corresponding to the position of the anterior wall of the left atrium, and shows at the time of the atrial systole a rapid movement in dorsal direction. In cases of mitral stenosis with auricular fibrillation, in which effective mechanical contraction of the atrium is absent, this movement is missing (Fig. 11). In both cases, the wall during the first part of ventricular diastole is gradually displaced in dorsal direction. Fig. 11 shows a retraction of the wall during ventricular systole, which corresponds to the systolic collapse seen in pressure curves from the left atrium and which is due to the pull exerted by ventricular contraction.

The echosignals obtained from left I: 3 over the region of the auricle correspond thus in position to the anterior wall of the left atrium. The movements of the echosignals correspond to the variation in the volume of the left atrium and to the contractions and displacements caused by the ventricular activity.

Summary.

1) It has been shown that it is possible to locate blood-heart wall boundaries by the supersonic reflectoscope method using frequencies of about 2.5 Mc.

2) The method was applied for the locating of heart walls on living human beings and continuous registration of movements of the heart walls was found possible.

3) Recordings are shown of the movements of the left ventricle wall in the normal and in the diseased heart. Further, movements of the left atrial wall in mitral stenosis were recorded.

The authors wish to express their sincere gratitude to Professor H. Malmros and Professor S. v. Friesen for invaluable support and interest in the study. Further thanks are due to Siemens Reiniger Werke, Germany, for placing the apparatus at our disposition.

References.

1. C. J. WIGGERS, Circulatory Dynamics, New York, Grune and Stratton, 1952. Pp. 53 ff.
2. R. F. RUSHMER et al. Continuous Measurements of Left Ventricular Dimensions in Intact, Unanesthetized Dogs. Circulation Research 2: 14 (1954).
3. W. D. KEIDEL, Über eine neue Methode zur Registrierung der Volumänderungen des Herzens am Menschen. Zeitschr. f. Kreislaufforschung 39, 257 (1949).
4. F. A. FIRESTONE, Supersonic reflectoscope, an instrument for inspecting the interior of solid parts by means of sound waves. J. Acoust. Soc. Am. 17, 287, (1945).
5. L. BERGMANN, Der Ultraschall, p. 530 (1949).
6. R. ESCHE, Untersuchung zur Ultraschallabsorption in tierischen Geweben und Kunststoffen. Akustische Beihefte 2, AB 71 (1952).
7. L. BERGMANN, Der Ultraschall p. 649 (1949).
8. T. HÜTER, Messung der Ultraschallabsorption in tierischen Geweben und ihre Abhängigkeit von der Frequenz Naturwiss. 35, 285 (1948).
9. E. L. CARSTENSEN, K. Li and H. P. Schwan. Determination of the acoustic properties of blood and its components. J. Acoust. Soc. Am. 25, 286 (1953).

10. G. D. Ludwig, The Velocity of Sound through Tissues and the Acoustic Impedance of Tissues. J. Acoust. Soc. Am., 22, 862 (1950).
11. A. H. Frucht, Die Geschwindigkeit des Ultraschalles in menschlichen und tierischen Geweben. Naturwiss. 39, 491 (1952).
12. J. J. Wild and J. M. Reid. The Effects of Biological Tissue on 15 Mc pulsed Ultrasound. J. Acoust. Soc. Am. 25, 270 (1953).
13. W. Güttner, G. Fiedler and J. Pätzold, Über Ultraschallabbildungen am menschlichen Schädel. Acustica 2, 148, (1952).

Tryckt den 30 april 1954.
Håkan Ohlssons boktryckeri, Lund.

Index

2-D ultrasound *see* two-dimensional (2-D) ultrasound
3-D ultrasound *see* three-dimensional (3-D) ultrasound
4-D ultrasound *see* four-dimensional (4-D) ultrasound

abdominal circumference (AC) 67
Abdulla, Usama 66
acoustic streaming 175
ACR/NEMA standard 185
Acta Paediatrica Scandinavica 17
Acuson 181, 182–4, 185, 186
Acuson128 system 68–9, 132, 182
Acuson128CDI system 184
Acuson128CV system 184
Adams, Judith 75
Adiels, M. 183
ADR 2130: 57, 68, 178–9
Advanced Diagnostic Research (ADR) 68, 178–9
Advanced Technology Laboratories (ATL) 179, 180, 181, 183, 184, 186
Aegis ultrasound miniPACS 185
Agilent HSG 184
aging 29
air–mucosa echo (AME) 173
Aixplorer 147
Alam, Mahbubul 15
Albert Lasker Clinical Medical Research Award vi, ix, 5, 12, 13
Allan, Lindsey 73
Aloka 184
Amedic AB 181, 182, 183, 184
American Journal of Surgery 87
American Society of Echocardiography 34
amniocentesis 73, 74
A-mode ultrasound 50, 63–4
  early pregnancy 68
  fetal biometry 67
  ophthalmology 161, 164, 165
  otorhinolaryngology 172, 173, 174
amyloidosis 28
Andersen, Frank 72
Andersson, Torbjörn 123, 185
Andolf, E. 59
anencephaly 55, 68
angiography 106, 113, 114
  carotid 98, 99
  paediatric 33
ankle–brachial pressure index (ABPI) 98
aortic aneurysms 115
aortic dissections 115
aortic valve examination 11
Areskog, H. 179

arterial disease, Doppler ultrasound in 97–8, 99–101
arterial dissections 115
arterial mapping of lower extremities, duplex ultrasound in 106–7
arteriography, ultrasonic 90
Arteriosonde 178
Aspelin, Peter 121
atherosclerosis 114, 115, 116–17
athlete's heart 29
atrial septal defects 37
Ausonics 180
automated functional imaging (AFI) 25
automatic border detection (ABD) 24
automatic segmental motion assessment (ASMA) 24
Aviso 162
Axberg, Monica 186
axial eye length measurements 161
Aztely, Mats 123

Baba, Kazunon 69, 76
back-wall echo (BWE) 173, 174
Baker, Don 83, 85–6, 87, 89, 178
Ballot, Buys 84
Bang, Jens 65, 67, 74, 76, 135
Barnes, R.W. 90
Barnett, Ellis 75
Baum, G. 161
Beach, Kirk W. 90, 92
  photo 93
Bell, John 81
Benacerraf, Beryl 73
Benoit, Bernard 69
Bergmann, Ludwig 2
Berning, Jens 136
B-flow imaging 141
biometric A-scans 161
biopsy devices 124, 125, 132–3, 180, 181, 182
biparietal diameter (BPD) 66, 67
Birnholz, Jason 179
bi-stable displays 121
blood–brain barrier 112
Blood Flow Classes (BFC) 57
B-mode ultrasound
  carotid arterial disease 98
  carotid intima–media thickness 116–17
  early pregnancy 68
  elastography 147
  fetal biometry 67
  industrial development 179–80
  ophthalmology 161, 162, 163, 164–5
  otorhinolaryngology 172, 173–4
  state of the art in radiology 139–41
  venous disease 101
Bohr, Niels 2

Bom, N. 14
Boman, Kurt 15–16
Bond, J.P. 13
Bourne, Tom 75
brain examination, origins of 5–6
    see also echo-encephalography
Brodin, Lars-Åke 15
Bronson, N. 162
Brown, Tom G. vi, 50, 63, 64
Brüel and Kjaer 130–1
Burns, Peter 159

Cacciatore, Bruno 75
Campbell, Stuart 67, 68, 71, 74, 75, 76
capacitative micromachined transducers
    (cMUTs) 139, 142–3
cardiac catheterization 33, 36
cardiac cycle, filling phase 24
cardiac output, measurement of 24
cardiac resynchronization 25
cardiology see echocardiography
cardiopulmonary bypass 37
cardiovascular magnetic resonance (CMR)
    imaging 27
carotid angiography 98, 99
carotid arterial disease 98–9, 100, 113
carotid interventions 108
carotid intima–media thickness (CIMT) 102, 106,
    116–17
Carrera, J.M. 73
cataract surgery 161
Cederlund, Jan 1
cephalometry 67
cervical length and preterm delivery 72
CFM700 CDI 184
CGR 181
Chaoui, Rabih 73, 77
chemotherapy 28
children see paediatric entries
chorionic villus sampling (CVS) 73, 74
choroidal haemangioma 167
Christensson, Bo 10
Circulation 17
Clarke, Sir Cyril A. 95
Clarke, Lisa 175
cleft lip 55
coarctatio aortae 98
colour Doppler ultrasound
    cross-licensing 138
    development 90
    echocardiography 19, 35
    industrial development 180, 184
    obstetrics and gynaecology 69, 71–2, 73, 75
    paediatric cardiology 19, 35
    venous disease 101
colour kinesis 24
Combison 330: 184
compounding 139, 140
compression elastography 146–7
computed tomography (CT) 6
    and contrast-enhanced ultrasound, comparison
        between 157, 158

Denmark 133
    and echo-encephalography 47–8
    ophthalmology 168, 169
    rhinosinusitis 172
    and ultrasound in radiology 126, 137
continuous wave (CW) Doppler
    carotid arterial disease 98
    development 87–8
    obstetrics 71
    physics 84–5
contrast-enhanced ultrasound (CEUS) 153–9
    echocardiography 24
    state of the art in radiology 143–6, 150
    transthoracic Doppler echocardiography 15
    vascular disease 106, 109–13, 115
cordocentesis 74
coronary artery disease (CAD) 26–8, 116
Cosgrove, David 122, 179, 180
Cossman, David 122
Cournand, Andre vi
Crang-Svalenius, Elizabeth 55
Cranley, Jack 82
crown–rump length (CRL), fetal 68
Curie, Pierre 63
Cushing, Harvey 43
Cypress 185

Daffos, Fernand 74
Danish Ultrasound Society 133–4
dating pregnancies 67
Dawes, Geoffrey 70
deep venous thrombosis (DVT) 101–2, 109–10
Denmark, early development of diagnostic
    ultrasound in 129–36
Deprest, Jan 75
DeVore, Greg 73, 77
Dewbury, Keith 122, 179
diabetes 29, 98
diagnostic ultrasound, early development in
    Denmark 129–36
Diamove 56
diaphragmatic hernia, fetal 75
Diasonics/Diasonics-Sonotron 183, 184
Diasonograph 50–1, 64–5, 66, 67, 122
diastolic function, assessment of 23–5
    paediatric 35
DICOM 3.0 Standard 185
disciform macula degeneration 167–8
dobutamine stress echocardiography (DSE) 27
Donald, Ian vi, 6, 50, 54, 63, 64, 65, 66, 70, 75
    photos 53, 65
Doppler, Christian Johann 63, 84
Doppler effect 63, 84, 96
Doppler rescue 111
Doppler ultrasound
    contrast agents 154–5
    duplex scanning see duplex ultrasound
    echocardiography 12, 19, 22–3, 24–5, 26, 27
    industrial development 179
    left ventricular function, assessment
        of 22–3, 24–5
    myocardial ischaemia 27

obstetrics 57–8, 71–2
otorhinolaryngology 172, 175, 176
paediatric cardiology 19
state of the art in radiology 141–2
valvular heart disease 26
vascular disease 81–93, 97–8
Doptone 87, 89, 95–6, 178
double-action rongeur 43
Down syndrome 55, 73
Drumm, John 71
ductus venosus pulsatility 72
duplex ultrasound (DU) 106
    in arterial disease in the lower extremity 99–101, 106–7
    in carotid arterial disease 98–9
    in clinical studies 102–3
    contrast-enhanced 109–13
    development 90–1
    diagnostic applications 108–9
    intraoperative and postoperative 107–8
    quality control 103
    Strandness 81, 87
    in venous disease 101–2
Dussik, Friedrich 44
Dussik, Karl 9, 44
Dymling, S.O. 175

early pregnancy assessment 67–8, 75
Ebstein's malformation of the tricuspid valve 17–18
echocardiography 21, 29
    contrast agents 155–7
    coronary artery disease 26–8
    development in Denmark 135–6
    development in Sweden 8–19, 64
    heart failure 21
    left ventricular function, assessment of 14, 15, 21–5, 40
    origins v, ix, 1–5
    subclinical disease 28–9
    'The Use of Ultrasonic Reflectoscope' paper (Edler & Hertz) 189–207
    valvular heart disease 25–6
echo-encephalography
    development in Sweden 43–9
    origins v, ix, 5–6
Ecton 185
ectopic pregnancy 75
Edler, Inge v, ix, 1, 8–9
    acclaim and international distinctions vi, ix, 4, 5, 12, 13
    contrast enhanced ultrasound 153
    Copenhagen National Hospital, cooperation with 135
    Doppler echocardiography 12, 15
    echocardiography 1, 3, 4, 10–11, 21, 33, 44, 64
    industrial development of ultrasound 178
    Lasker Award vi, ix, 5, 12, 13
    Lund 1–3, 8–9, 10–11, 12, 44, 64
    paediatric cardiology 16, 33
    personality 2
    personal recollections vi
    photos 3, 4, 9

retirement 14
'The Use of Ultrasonic Reflectoscope' paper (with Hertz) 189–207
World Congress on Ultrasound in Medicine (Vienna, 1969) 16
Edler, Karin 10
Effert, Sven 13
Egeblad, Hernrik 135, 136
Eik-Nes, Sturla 54, 57, 71, 72
ejection fraction (EF) 22–3, 40
Ekoline20 179
elastography 114, 146–9
Elbit 184
Elegra 184
Ellis, Richard 83, 86, 87
Elmqvist, Rune x
Elvin, Anders 126
endocarditis 36
endocrine orbitopathy 169
endometrial cancer 58
endophthalmitis 162
endovascular aneurysm repair (EVAR) 107–8, 114
Engsner, Gunnar 46
epicardial imaging 37
EQUALIS (External Quality Assurance in Laboratory Medicine in Sweden) 103
ergonomic improvements 138
European Association of Echocardiography (EAE) 35
European Committee for Medical Ultrasound Society (ECMUS) 59
European Congress of Cardiology (Rome, 1960) 11
European Federation of Societies for Ultrasound in Medicine and Biology 133, 135
eye tumours 165–8

Fabry's disease 28–9
Feichtinger, Wilfred 76
Feigenbaum, Harvey 13–14, 15, 179
Fenning, Nick Raine 77
Fernström, Ingmar 121
fetal abnormalities 55, 68, 72–3
fetal activity 70–1
fetal aortic pulsations 57
fetal biometry 66–7, 70
fetal biophysical profile test 71
fetal breathing movements 55–6, 70–1
fetal chromosome abnormalities 73
fetal echocardiography 38–9, 73, 76–7
fetal heartbeat 67, 68
Fetal Medicine Foundation (FMF) 78
fetal parameters 54
fetal physiological functions, studies of 55–8
fetal therapy 74–5
fetal weight prediction 67
Fetasonde 178
fetoscopy 74
Fibroscan 147
Filly, Roy 75
Fischer-Colbrie, W. 101
Fitzgerald, D.E. 71
Fledelius, Hans C. 135

flow-mediated dilatation (FMD) of the brachial artery 115–16
foot ergometer 95
Forsberg, Lillemor 121, 123
Forssmann, Werner vi
Foster, F.S. 162
four-dimensional (4-D) ultrasound
 industrial development 185
 obstetrics and gynaecology 69, 77
 state of the art 142–3
Franck, James 2
Franklin, Dean 85, 86, 87
freehand (compression) elastography 146–7
Fujifilm 187, 188
Fujitsu 184
functional echocardiography 40–1
fusion imaging 144–5

Gallagher, Bob 183
gamma knife 43
Gammelgaard, P.A. 129
Garrett, William 68
Gellinek, Wolfgang 2
Gembruch, Ulrich 73
General Electric (GE) 183, 184, 185, 186, 187
Gennser, Gerhard 55
Gentofte Group 130, 133–4
Gentofte scanner 130, 131, 132
Giles, Warwick 71
Gill, Robert 71
Gjöres, Jan Erik 96
glaucoma 161
Goldberg, B. 130, 179
Gosling, R.G. 95
Gottesfeld, Ken 65, 66
Gramiak, Raymond 109, 153
Granit, Ragnar 43
Gratacos, Eduard 75
Grennert, Lars 54, 67
Griffin, David 71
Griffith, James 14
Grumman 181
Gudmundsson, Saemundur 58
Gustafson, Arne 3, 9–10, 11, 16
Gustafson, Torsten 2
gynaecology, ultrasound in
 development in Sweden 50–4, 58–60, 126
 and development of ultrasound in radiology 121
 history 6–7, 63–6, 75–6, 77–8

Hackelör, Jochen 54, 75
haemodynamics, non-invasive 25–6
 paediatric cardiology 35
Hagen(-Ansert), Sandra 179, 180
Hahnemann, Niels 74
Hanafy, Amin 182
Hancke, Søren 134
hand carried ultrasound (HCU) systems 185–6
handedness, and fetal ultrasound 59
Hanse, Jens Falbe 135
Hansmann, Manfred 54, 66, 67, 74
Harkins, Henry 81
harmonic imaging 155–6

cross-licensing 138
obstetrics and gynaecology 69
second 24
state of the art in radiology 138, 139–40
vascular disease 111
harmonic power Doppler 156
Harrison, M.R. 74–5
Hasch, Ernst 133, 135
Hatle, Liv 15, 26
Haubet, Axel 133
heart examination 1–5
 see also echocardiography
heart failure 21
Hegedüs, Lazlo 134
Helmer, Rudolf 82
Henningsen, Per 135
Henry, Walter 14
hepatic transit time 145
Hertz, Birgit 2
Hertz, Gustav 2
Hertz, Heinrich 2
Hertz, Hellmuth v, ix, x, 2
 Copenhagen National Hospital, cooperation with 136
 echocardiography 1–3, 4–5, 8, 9, 10, 11–12, 14, 33, 44, 64
 and Holm 129
 Lasker Award vi, ix, 5, 12, 13
 Lund 1–3, 4–5, 7, 8, 9, 10, 44, 64
 obstetrics and gynaecology 54
 paediatric cardiology 33
 personality 2
 personal recollections vi
 photos 3, 9
 'The Use of Ultrasonic Reflectoscope' (with Edler) 189–207
 World Congress on Ultrasound in Medicine (Vienna, 1969) 16
Hewlett-Packard (HP) 181, 184
high-frequency B-scans 161, 162, 163
high-intensity focused ultrasound (HIFU) 149–50
Hildell, Jan 121
Hitachi 184
Hobbins, John 68, 74
Höglund, Christer 15
Hokanson, Eugene 86, 90
Hollander, Hans Jurgen 66
Holm, Hans Henrik 65, 67, 122, 123, 129, 133, 134, 135, 179
 photo 130
Holmer, Nils Gunnar 48, 173
Howry, Douglass 64, 65, 66
HP 77020 Echocardiography system 181
HP Colour Flow Option 184
Hughes, W.F. 161
hydrocephalus 45, 47, 48, 49
hydrophones 63
hyperphonography 44
hypertrophic cardiomyopathy 25
hypoplastic left heart syndrome (HLHS) 39

Iams, Jay 72
industrial development of ultrasound 178–88

infiltrative diseases 28–9
infrainguinal bypass surveillance 100–1
ink-jet writer 5
International Pediatric and Congenital Cardiac Code 35
International Society of Ultrasound in Obstetrics and Gynecology (ISUOG) 78
Interspec 184
interstitial ablative therapy 143–4
intracardiac ultrasound, paediatric 38
intracranial bleeding 6
intracranial pressure (ICP) 46, 48
intraoperative ultrasound, vascular disease 107–8
intrauterine growth-restricted (IGUS) fetus 57, 67, 71, 72
intravascular ultrasound (IVUS) 106, 113–14, 115
in vitro fertilization (IVF), oocyte collection for 58, 69, 76
Irving, Henry 122
Itoh, A. 147

Jacobs, Ian 76
Jannert, M. 173
Jansson, F. 161
Jeppsson, Stig 6, 45–7
Jesseph, J.E. 81
Jogestrand, Tomas 102
Johnson & Johnson (J&J) 180, 183
Jönsson, Marianne 184, 186
Jörgensen, Connie 55, 59
Jouppila, Pentti 179
Joyner, Claude R. 13, 153
Jurkovic, Davor 77

Kadar, Nick 75
Kaneko, Ziro 85
Karacagil, S. 101
Karlefors, Tord 10
Karner, Göran 122, 123, 179
Karp, Wilhelm 121
Karstrup, Steen 132–3
Kato, K. 85
Keidel, W.D. 173
Kemeter, Pieter 76
Kiedel, W.D. 9
Kieler, H. 59
Kimmelmann, B.A. 130
KinetDx 185
kinetic echography 169
King, D.H. 95
Kiserud, Torvid 72
Kleinman, Charles 73
Kockum's shipyard, Malmö 2, 8
Kolmården Ultrasound Course 122, 123, 126
Kone Corporation/Kone AB 180, 181, 182
Kontron AB 178
Kossoff, George 66, 71, 179, 180
Kranzbühler 179, 180, 181
Kratochwil, Alfred 58, 65, 67, 123
Kremkau, Frederick 153
Kretztechnik and Kretztechnik/Medison 184–5
Kristensen, Jørgen Kvist 129, 134
Kristiansson, Karl-Axel 48

Kuhnt–Junius macula degeneration 167–8
Kullander, Stig 54
kwashiorkor 46

Lagergren, Curt 123
Lagergren, J. 179
Landelius, John 15, 181
Langevin, Paul 63
Larsén, Åke 178, 179, 182, 184, 186
Larsson, Börje 43
Larsson, John 181, 183, 184
laser ablation 74
Lasker Award vi, ix, 5, 12, 13
Laurin, J. 54
Lee, Fred 122
Lees, William 122
left atrium (LA) size 23, 24
left ventricular (LV) dysfunction, chronic 27–8
left ventricular (LV) function, assessment of 14, 15, 21–5
  paediatric cardiology 40
left ventricular (LV) volumes, measurement of 39–40
Lehtinen, A. 161
Leksell, Lars v, vi, ix, 43
  Lund 1, 5–6, 43–5, 47, 50
Lenz, Susan 76
Le Quesne, Gary W. 122
Levi, Salvator 73
LIC 178
Lilley, William 74
Lindell, Sven-Eric 178
Lindgren, P.G. 123–4, 125, 180, 181, 182, 185, 187
Lindström, Kjell ix
  contrast-enhanced ultrasound 153
  Doppler echocardiography 12, 15, 16
  echo-encephalography 48
  fetal breathing movements 55
  personal recollections vi
  two-dimensional echocardiography 14
  WHO Working Group on Radiation and Ultrasound Safety 59
Lindvall, Kaj 14
Linton, Robert 82
Lithander, Brita 46
London Ultrasound Course 122
Loren Parks 178
lower extremities
  arterial disease in the 99–101
  arterial mapping of the 106–7
low-frequency B-scans 161, 162
Ludwig, George 63–4
Lund 1, 7
  brain examination 5–6
  and Copenhagen National Hospital, cooperation between 135–6
  echocardiography 1–5, 8–12, 14, 15, 16, 19, 33, 64
  echo-encephalography 5–6, 43–8
  historical context v, vi, ix
  industrial development of ultrasound 178
  obstetrics and gynaecology 6–7, 50–5, 57–8
  paediatric cardiology 16, 19, 33
  radiology 121

Lundbäck, Stig 15
Lundström, Nils-Rune 4, 16–19

McCleod, Fran 89
McKissock, Wylie 44
McLaughlin, Glen 186
McVicar, John vi, 63
magnetic resonance imaging (MRI)
   and contrast-enhanced ultrasound, comparison
      between 157
   and echo-encephalography 47–8
   elastography 146
   ophthalmology 168, 169
   and ultrasound in radiology 126, 137
Mahoney, Maurice 74
Makowsky, Ed 67
malignant melanoma 165–7
'Malmö model' of obstetric ultrasound screening 54
Mann, W. 173
Manning, Frank 71
Mantoni, Margit 135
marasmus 46
MarkV 179
Maršál, Karel 55, 57, 59, 70, 71, 187
Maslak, Sam 68, 181–2
Massachusetts Institute of Technology (MIT) 44, 63
mechanical sector scanner, 2-D
   echocardiography 14
Medata AB/Medata Nordic AB 181, 183, 184
Medison 185
Meire, Hylton 122, 179
melanoma, malignant 165–7
Merritt, C. 184
Merz, Eberhard 76
metastatic carcinoma 167
microbubble contrast agents 143–6, 149–50, 153–9
   vascular disease 106, 109–13
microcirculation 111
MicroMaxx 186
Miles, Richard 90
Mingograph ink-jet recorder x
mitral insufficiency 1, 3
mitral stenosis 1, 3, 16
mitral valve (MV) disease 26
mitral valve (MV) examination 3, 11, 13, 15
mitral valve (MV) inflow 23–4
M-mode ultrasound
   echocardiography 10, 14, 17, 18, 22, 33, 64
   elastography 147
   industrial development 179
   left ventricular function, assessment of 22
   origins and development 10, 14, 64
   paediatric cardiology 17, 18, 33
Mohr, Jan 74
molecular imaging with ultrasound 111–12, 145
Morley, Patricia 75
Mozersky, D.J. 90
Mundt, G.H. 161
Museum of Medical History, Lund 11
myocardial contrast echocardiography
   (MCE) 27, 28
myocardial function, direct measurement of 24
myocardial infarction 112, 117

myocardial ischaemia, diagnosing 27, 28
myocardial perfusion 156, 157
myocardial viability, diagnosing 27, 28
myopia 161

NanoMaxx 187
needle-guide units 124, 125
neurology *see* echo-encephalography
nevus, benign (elevated) 167
New England Journal of Medicine 87
Nicolaides, Kypros 71, 72, 73, 74, 75
Nightingale, K.R. 175
Nilsson, Anders 126
Nippa, Jurgen 89
Nobel Prizes
   Physics 2
   Physiology and Medicine vi, ix, 5, 43
Nolsö, Christian 122
Northevd, Allan 130, 135
Nyberg, David 75

Öberg, Lars 123
obesity 29
obstetrics, ultrasound in
   development in Denmark 133, 135
   development in Sweden 50–60, 126
   and development of ultrasound in radiology 121
   history 63–75, 76–8
   origins 6–7
   safety 51, 59
   see also fetal echocardiography
occlusive arterial disease 97–8
Octoson 66, 71, 180
Oksala, A. 161
Olivecrona, Herbert 43
Olli Elektromedicin 180
oocyte collection for *in vitro* fertilization 58, 69, 76
ophthalmology 161
   biometric A-scans 161
   high-frequency B-scans 162, 163
   low-frequency B-scans 162
   standardized echography 162–70
orbital myositis 169
Organon Teknika 185
Ossoinig, K. 162
otitis media with effusion 176
otorhinolaryngology 172
   Doppler ultrasound 174–5
   future 176
   paranasal sinuses 173–4
   safety issues 175–6
   sinus infection staging 174–5
ovarian cancer 59, 75, 76
ovarian cysts 59
ovarian tumours 52, 53, 75

paediatric echocardiography 4, 33–4
   development in Sweden 16–19, 33
   fetal 38–9
   functional 40–1
   three-dimensional 39–40
   transoesophageal 36–8
   transthoracic 34–6

paediatric echo-encephalography 6, 45, 46, 49
pancreatic carcinoma 149
paranasal sinuses 172, 173–4, 176
Pardi, Giorgio 74
Parks Medical Electronics 178, 181, 183
Parsons, John 76
Pasteur, Louis 7
patent foramen ovale 37
Patrick, John 70
Pavlin, C.J. 162
Pax Vobiscum project 185
Pedersen, Jan Fog 132, 135
Pedersen, Sören Torp 122
pelvic masses 52, 53, 75–6
pericardial effusion 11, 14
peripheral blood flow 95–6, 97
Persson, Per-Håkan 54, 67
Persson, Stig ix
phased array systems 14, 63, 181
Philips 181, 183, 184
Physionics 65
Picker machine 65, 183
picture archiving and communications system (PACS) workstations 137, 138, 185
piezo electric effect 63
placenta growth factor (PlGF) 72
placenta praevia 66
placentography 66
plaques 113–14, 115
Platt, Larry 71
plethysmography 81–2, 95
pneumo-encephalography 45, 47
polycystic kidneys 68
polycystic ovaries 75
polyhydramnios 68
positron emission tomography (PET) 27
postoperative ultrasound, vascular disease 107
post-systolic thickening 27
power pulse inversion 156–7
Prechtl, Heinz 70
pre-eclampsia 57, 71, 72
pregnancy-associated plasma protein-A (PAPP-A) 72
preterm delivery 72
Pretorius, Dolores 76
Proceedings of the Royal Physiographical Society in Lund 3, 11
pseudo-gliomas 168
pulmonary artery stenosis 37
pulmonary venous flow 23
pulsatility index (PI) 72
pulsed Doppler 89–90, 98
pulse inversion imaging 156–7
punctures, ultrasound-guided 123–4, 132–3
PW-Doppler 500A 179

quantitative echography 169
Quantum 180, 184

radar 63
radiofrequency (RF) ablation 149–50
radiology, ultrasound in development in Sweden 121–7
state of the art 137–50
radiosurgery 43
Radke, Hub 81
Rasmussen, Knud 134–5
Rasmussen, Steen Nørby 134
Read, John 64
real-time scanners 68–77
Reid, J.M. 13, 90, 196
resonance frequency 154
retinoblastomas 168
revascularization, chronic left ventricular dysfunction 27
Revonta, M. 173
rhesus disease in the fetus 74
rhinosinusitis 172, 174–5, 176
Richards, Dickinson vi
right ventricular (RV) function, assessment of 41
right ventricular (RV) volume, measurement of 39, 40
Roberts, Alistair 70
Robinson, Hugh 67–8
Roche Bio-Electronics 178
Rodeck, C.H. 74
roentgenograms 45
Roijer, Anders 15
Romero, Roberto 75
rongeur, double-action 43
Rosfors, R. 101
'Rudy Box' 82, 83
Rushmer, Robert F. 83, 85–6, 178

Sabbagha, Rudi 67
safety of ultrasound 59, 78, 175–6
Salford, Leif G. 47–8
Saraste, M. 184
Sassone, A.M. 75
Satomura, Shigeo 85
scan converter 66
Schedin, Monica 184
Schultz, Dick 86
scintigraphy 27
second harmonic imaging 24
Sectra-Imtec AB 185
Selbing, Anders 54–5
Sequoia 185, 186
Shah, Pravin M. 153
shear wave elastography 147–9
Siemens P10 187
Siemens/Siemens-Reiniger-Werke 2, 3, 8, 10, 178, 184, 185, 186, 187, 191
Sigma-motor pump 96
Sillesen, Henrik 134
Simeone, F.A. 82
single-photon emission computed tomography (SPECT) 27
sinusitis 172
sinus secretions 172, 174–5
Siösten, Anna-Karin 126
Sivertsson, R. 179
Sjögren, Iréne 46–7
Sjövall, Alf vi, 6, 50
Smidt-Jensen, Steen 74
Smith Kline Instruments (SKI) 178, 179

smoothing algorithms 140–1
Societas Internationalis de Diagnostica Ultrasonica in Ophthalmologia 161
Soldner, Richard 65
Sonazoid 157
sonohistology 141
sonoporation 145
Sonosite 186, 187
sonothrombolysis 112
Sonovue 157
Spacelabs 180
speckle-tracking algorithms 141
spectral broadening 89
spectral Doppler 89, 142
Spencer, Merrill 90
spina bifida 68
Squibb/Squibb Medical Systems (SMS) 180, 181, 183
SSD-880CW 184
SSH-65A 184
standardized echography 161, 162–70
static (compression) elastography 146–7
static scanners, obstetrics and gynaecology 64–8
Steptoe, Patrick 76
stereotactic surgery 43
stimulated acoustic emission 155
strain and strain rate 25, 27, 41
Strandness, Donald Eugene Jr (Gene) 81, 82, 86–9, 90–1, 99, 179
  photos 82, 91
stress echocardiography
  chronic left ventricular dysfunction 27
  contrast ultrasound 24
  dobutamine (DSE) 27
  myocardial ischaemia 27
  three-dimensional ultrasound 115
stroke 98–9, 112, 117, 146
subclavian steal syndrome 108
subclinical diseases 25, 28–9
Sumner, David S. 82, 86, 90, 91–2
  photo 93
Sundén, Bertil vi, ix, 1, 6, 7, 16, 50–2, 59–60, 68
  photo 53
supraventricular tachycardia 39
Sweden, development of ultrasound in
  echocardiography 8–19
  echo-encephalography 43–9
  industrial development 178–88
  obstetrics and gynaecology 50–60
  radiology 121–7
  vascular disease 95–103
  see also Lund
Swedish Board of Accreditation and Conformity Assessment (SWEDAC) 103
Swedish Board of Technical Development 4–5, 12, 14
Swedish Cardiological Society 13
Swedish Council on Technology Assessment in Health Care 102
Swedish Medical Research Council 6
Swedish National Board of Health and Welfare 54, 99, 102
Swedish Quality Board for Carotid Surgery 99
Swedish Society for Clinical Physiology 103
Swedish Society of Radiology 122, 123, 126
systolic function, assessment of 22–3
  paediatric 35

Tabor, A. 135
Tailor, Anil 75–6
Takeuchi, Hsiao 65
Taussig, Helen B. 33
Technicare 180, 183
Thompson, Horace 65, 67
thoracic circumference (TC) 67
three-dimensional (3-D) ultrasound
  echocardiography 19, 26, 38, 39–40
  industrial development 184
  obstetrics and gynaecology 63, 69, 70, 76–7
  paediatric cardiology 19, 38, 39–40
  state of the art 142–3
  valvular heart disease 26
  vascular disease 106, 115
thrombocytopenia, alloimmune 74
thrombolysis 112, 145–6
thrombus neovascularization 109
Thorelius, Lars 127
Thulesius, Olav 95, 96, 97
Thurstone, F.L. 14
time–distance recording 56
time gain compensation (TGC) 141
time-intensity curves 145
Timmerman, Dirk 76
Timor-Tritsch, Ilan 75
tissue Doppler
  echocardiography 15, 22–3, 41
  left ventricular function, assessment of 22–3
  paediatric cardiology 41
  state of the art in radiology 141–2
tissue perfusion, quantification of 159
tissue sensitivity in standardized echography 164, 165
topographic echography 169
Törngren, Anders 121, 123
Torp-Pedersen, Søren 129
Toshiba 183, 184
transducers 16, 139
transient ischaemic attacks (TIAs) 98–9
translabial ultrasound 58
transoesophageal echocardiography (TOE)
  development 15
  failed attempt 11
  paediatric cardiology 19, 36–8
  valvular heart disease 26
transposition of the great arteries 39
transthoracic echocardiography (TTE) 34–6
transvaginal sonography (TVS) 58, 65, 67, 69, 75–6
trauma 158
Travenol Tru-Cut needle 124, 125
Trudinger, Brian 71
twin pregnancies 6–7, 52, 54, 67
twin-to-twin transfusion syndrome 74

two-dimensional (2-D) ultrasound
  echocardiography 11–12, 14–15, 18–19, 22, 33, 34–5
  obstetrics and gynaecology 63, 64, 76, 77
  paediatric cardiology 18–19, 33, 34–5
  vascular disease 115

Ueno scale 147
Ultraschall-Impulsgerät 191
ultrasonic biomicroscopy (UBM) 162, 163, 164
Ultrasound in Obstetrics and Gynecology 60
UM6 CDI system 184
UM8 system 184
UM9CDI system 184
United States Atomic Energy Commission 44
University of Washington (UW) 81, 83, 85–7
Uterine Artery Score 57

Václavinková, Vlasta 58
Vahlquist, Bo 46
Valentin, Lill 59, 60, 76
valve function, assessment of 35
valvular heart disease 25–6
Van Nagell, John 76
Varian 181
vascular disease, ultrasound in
  development in Sweden 95–103
  Doppler ultrasound 81, 83–93
  early vascular laboratories 81–3
  state of the art 106–17
vector flow imaging 141, 142
venous disease, duplex ultrasound in 101–2, 109–10
ventricular dilatation 48
ventricular size, index of 46, 47
ventriculography 47
Vidoson 56, 74, 178
Ville, Yves 74
Vingmed 184
virtual histology intravascular sonography 113–14
Vivid I 186
Voluson730 69, 76, 185
von Friesen, Sten 2
von Ramm, Olaf 14
von Siever, Karin 126
Vscan 187

Wabloprodukter 178, 179, 180
Waldenström, U. 55
Wallentin, Ingemar 14, 184
Wandt, Birger 15
Washington, University of (UW) 81, 83, 85–7
water delay scanning 64, 66
Watson-Watt, Sir Robert 63
Wei, K. 157
Wells, Peter N.T. x
West, Kurt 46–7
Westberg, Gunnar 121, 123
Westling, Håkan x
White, D.N. 46
Whitney, R.J. 82
Wikland, M. 58
Wikstrand, John 102
Wilcox, Marty 179
Wild, John Julian 64, 196
Willenheimer, Ronnie 15
Willocks, James 66
Winsor, Travis 82
Winter, Reidar 15
Wladimiroff, Yuri 71
World Congress on Ultrasound in Medicine
  (Vienna, 1969) 12, 16
World Congress on Ultrasound in Obstetrics
  (Stockholm, 2003) 60
World Federation for Ultrasound in
  Medicine and Biology (WFUMB) 59, 60, 133, 176
World Health Organization (WHO) 59, 176
Wranne, Bengt 14
Wylie, Jack 88

Yoo, S.-J. 73
Young, Thomas 63
Younge, Robert 181–2

Zbornikova, Vera 98
Zonare 186–7
z.one rev.2 system 186–7
Zone Sonography 187
z.one system 186
z-score method, paediatric cardiology 36